WIND TURBINE TECHNOLOGY

Principles and Design

WIND TURBINE TECHNOLOGY

Principles and Design

Edited by

Muyiwa Adaramola, PhD

Apple Academic Press

TORONTO NEW JERSEY

Apple Academic Press Inc. 3333 Mistwell Crescent Oakville, ON L6L 0A2 Canada	Apple Academic Press Inc. 9 Spinnaker Way Waretown, NJ 08758 USA

International Standard Book Number-13: 978-1-77188-015-2 (Hardcover)

Library of Congress Control Number: 2013958425

Library and Archives Canada Cataloguing in Publication

Wind turbine technology: principles and design/edited by Muyiwa Adaramola, PhD.

Includes bibliographical references and index.
ISBN 978-1-77188-015-2 (bound)
1. Wind turbines--Design and construction. 2. Wind turbines--Technological innovations.
I. Adaramola, Muyiwa, editor of compilation

TJ828.W45 2014   621.31'2136   C2014-900070-7

Apple Academic Press also publishes its books in a variety of electronic formats. Some content that appears in print may not be available in electronic format. For information about Apple Academic Press products, visit our website at **www.appleacademicpress.com** and the CRC Press website at **www.crcpress.com**

ABOUT THE EDITOR

MUYIWA ADARAMOLA, PhD

Dr. Muyiwa S. Adaramola earned his BSc and MSc in Mechanical Engineering from Obafemi Awolowo University, Nigeria and University of Ibadan, Nigeria, respectively. He received his PhD in Environmental Engineering at the University of Saskatchewan Saskatoon, Canada. He has worked as a researcher at the Norwegian University of Science and Technology, focusing on wind energy, wind turbine performance, and wind turbine wake. Currently, Dr. Adaramola is an Associate Professor in Renewable Energy at the Norwegian University of Life Sciences, Ås, Norway.

CONTENTS

Acknowledgment and How to Cite ix
List of Contributors xi
Introduction xv

Part I: Aerodynamics

1. **Wind Turbine Blade Design** **1**
Peter J. Schubel and Richard J. Crossley

2. **A Shrouded Wind Turbine Generating High Output Power with Wind-lens Technology** **35**
Yuji Ohya and Takashi Karasudani

3. **Ecomoulding of Composite Wind Turbine Blades Using Green Manufacturing RTM Process** **57**
Brahim Attaf

4. **Aerodynamic Shape Optimization of a Vertical-Axis Wind Turbine Using Differential Evolution** **79**
Travis J. Carrigan, Brian H. Dennis, Zhen X. Han, and Bo P. Wang

Part II: Generators and Gear Systems

5. **Performance Evaluation of an Induction Machine with Auxiliary Winding for Wind Turbine Power** **125**
Riadh W. Y. Habash, Qianjun Tang, Pierre Guillemette, and Nazish Irfan

6. **Time Domain Modeling and Analysis of Dynamic Gear Contact Force in a Wind Turbine Gearbox with Respect to Fatigue Assessment** **141**
Wenbin Dong, Yihan Xing, and Torgeir Moan

Part III: Tower and Foundation

7. **Wind Turbine Tower Vibration Modeling and Monitoring by the Nonlinear State Estimation Technique (NSET)** **173**
Peng Guo and David Infield

Part IV: Control Systems

8. Two LQRI Based Blade Pitch Controls for Wind Turbines 199

Sungsu Park and Yoonsu Nam

9. Power Control Design for Variable-Speed Wind Turbines 227

Yolanda Vidal, Leonardo Acho, Ningsu Luo, Mauricio Zapateiro, and Francesc Pozo

10. H_∞ Based Control for Load Mitigation in Wind Turbines 251

Asier Diaz de Corcuera, Aron Pujana-Arrese, Jose M. Ezquerra, Edurne Segurola, and Joseba Landaluze

Part V: Environmental Issues

11. Electromagnetic Interference on Large Wind Turbines 293

Florian Krug and Bastian Lewke

12. Noise Pollution Prevention in Wind Turbines: Status and Recent Advances 311

Ofelia Jianu, Marc A. Rosen, and Greg Naterer

Author Notes 330

Index 334

ACKNOWLEDGMENT AND HOW TO CITE

The editor and publisher thank each of the authors who contributed to this book, whether by granting their permission individually or by releasing their research as Open Source articles. The chapters in this book were previously published in various places in various formats. To cite the work contained in this book and to view the individual permissions, please refer to the "How to Cite" box at the beginning of each chapter. Each chapter was read individually and carefully selected by the editors. The result is a book that provides a nuanced study of the recent advances wind turbine technology.

LIST OF CONTRIBUTORS

Leonardo Acho
Control Dynamics and Applications Research Group (CoDAlab), Barcelona College of Industrial Engineering, Polytechnic University of Catalonia, Comte d'Urgell, 187, Barcelona 08036, Spain

Brahim Attaf
Team Europe, European Commission, 39 Boulevard Charles Moretti A6, 13014 Marseille, France

Travis J. Carrigan
Department of Mechanical and Aerospace Engineering, The University of Texas at Arlington, P.O. Box 19023, Arlington, TX 76019-0023, USA

Richard J. Crossley
Faculty of Engineering, Division of Materials, Mechanics and Structures, University of Nottingham, University Park, Nottingham NG7 2RD, UK

Brian H. Dennis
Department of Mechanical and Aerospace Engineering, The University of Texas at Arlington, P.O. Box 19023, Arlington, TX 76019-0023, USA

Asier Diaz de Corcuera
IKERLAN-IK4, Arizmendiarreta, 2, E-20500 Arrasate-Mondragon, The Basque Country, Spain

Wenbin Dong
Centre for Ships and Ocean Structures (CeSOS), Norwegian University of Science and Technology (NTNU), Otto Nielsens V.10, N-7491, Trondheim, Norway

Jose M. Ezquerra
IKERLAN-IK4, Arizmendiarreta, 2, E-20500 Arrasate-Mondragon, The Basque Country, Spain

Pierre Guillemette
Trias Innovations Group, Ottawa, ON, K1L 8K4, Canada

Peng Guo
School of Control and Computer Engineering, North China Electric Power University, Beijing 102206, China

Riadh W. Y. Habash
School of Electrical Engineering and Computer Science, University of Ottawa, Ottawa, ON, K1N 6N5, Canada

Zhen X. Han
Department of Mechanical and Aerospace Engineering, The University of Texas at Arlington, P.O. Box 19023, Arlington, TX 76019-0023, USA

David Infield
Institute for Energy and Environment, Department of Electronic and Electrical Engineering, University of Strathclyde, Glasgow G1 1XQ, UK

Nazish Irfan
School of Electrical Engineering and Computer Science, University of Ottawa, Ottawa, ON, K1N 6N5, Canada

Ofelia Jianu
Faculty of Engineering and Applied Science, University of Ontario Institute of Technology, Oshawa, Ontario, L1H 7K4, Canada

Takashi Karasudani
Research Institute for Applied Mechanics, Kyushu University/ Kasuga 816-8580, Japan

Florian Krug
Siemens AG, Wittelsbacherplatz 2, 80333 Munich, Germany

Joseba Landaluze
IKERLAN-IK4, Arizmendiarreta, 2, E-20500 Arrasate-Mondragon, The Basque Country, Spain

Bastian Lewke
Siemens Wind Power A/S, 7330 Brande, Denmark

Ningsu Luo
Modal Intervals and Control Engineering Research Group, Department of Electrical Engineering, Electronics and Automatic Control, Institute of Informatics and Applications, University of Girona, Campus Montilivi, P-IV, Girona 17071, Spain

Torgeir Moan
Centre for Ships and Ocean Structures (CeSOS), Norwegian University of Science and Technology (NTNU), Otto Nielsens V.10, N-7491, Trondheim, Norway and Department of Marine Technology, Norwegian University of Science and Technology (NTNU), Otto Nielsens V.10, N-7491, Trondheim, Norway

Yoonsu Nam
Department of Mechanical and Mechatronics Engineering, Kangwon National University, Kangwon 200-701, Korea

Greg Naterer
Faculty of Engineering and Applied Science, University of Ontario Institute of Technology, Oshawa, Ontario, L1H 7K4, Canada

Yuji Ohya
Research Institute for Applied Mechanics, Kyushu University/ Kasuga 816-8580, Japan

Sungsu Park
Department of Aerospace Engineering, Sejong University, Seoul 143-737, Korea

Francesc Pozo
Control Dynamics and Applications Research Group (CoDAlab), Barcelona College of Industrial Engineering, Polytechnic University of Catalonia, Comte d'Urgell, 187, Barcelona 08036, Spain

Aron Pujana-Arrese
IKERLAN-IK4, Arizmendiarreta, 2, E-20500 Arrasate-Mondragon, The Basque Country, Spain

Marc A. Rosen
Faculty of Engineering and Applied Science, University of Ontario Institute of Technology, Oshawa, Ontario, L1H 7K4, Canada

Peter J. Schubel
Faculty of Engineering, Division of Materials, Mechanics and Structures, University of Nottingham, University Park, Nottingham NG7 2RD, UK

Edurne Segurola
IKERLAN-IK4, Arizmendiarreta, 2, E-20500 Arrasate-Mondragon, The Basque Country, Spain

Qianjun Tang
School of Electrical Engineering and Computer Science, University of Ottawa, Ottawa, ON, K1N 6N5, Canada and Trias Innovations Group, Ottawa, ON, K1L 8K4, Canada

Yolanda Vidal
Control Dynamics and Applications Research Group (CoDAlab), Barcelona College of Industrial Engineering, Polytechnic University of Catalonia, Comte d'Urgell, 187, Barcelona 08036, Spain

Bo P. Wang
Department of Mechanical and Aerospace Engineering, The University of Texas at Arlington, P.O. Box 19023, Arlington, TX 76019-0023, USA

Yihan Xing
Centre for Ships and Ocean Structures (CeSOS), Norwegian University of Science and Technology (NTNU), Otto Nielsens V.10, N-7491, Trondheim, Norway

Mauricio Zapateiro
Control Dynamics and Applications Research Group (CoDAlab), Barcelona College of Industrial Engineering, Polytechnic University of Catalonia, Comte d'Urgell, 187, Barcelona 08036, Spain

INTRODUCTION

This book seeks to introduce some of the basic principle of wind turbine design. The different chapters discuss ways to analyze wind turbine performance, approaches for wind turbine improvement, fault detection in wind turbines, and how to mediate the adverse effects of wind turbine use. The book is broken into five sections: the first focuses on wind turbine blade design, the second goes into detail on generators and gear systems, the third focuses on wind turbine towers and foundations, the fourth is on control systems, and the final section discusses some of the environmental issues.

In Chapter 1, a detailed review of the current state of art for wind turbine blade design is presented, including theoretical maximum efficiency, propulsion, practical efficiency, HAWT blade design, and blade loads. Schubel and Crossley provide a complete picture of wind turbine blade design and shows the dominance of modern turbines' almost exclusive use of horizontal axis rotors. The aerodynamic design principles for a modern wind turbine blade are detailed, including blade plan shape/quantity, aerofoil selection, and optimal attack angles. A detailed review of design loads on wind turbine blades is offered, describing aerodynamic, gravitational, centrifugal, gyroscopic and operational conditions.

Ohya and Karasudani have developed a new wind turbine system that consists of a diffuser shroud with a broad-ring brim at the exit periphery and a wind turbine inside it in Chapter 2. The shrouded wind turbine with a brimmed diffuser has demonstrated power augmentation by a factor of about 2–5 compared with a bare wind turbine, for a given turbine diameter and wind speed. This is because a low-pressure region, due to a strong vortex formation behind the broad brim, draws more mass flow to the wind turbine inside the diffuser shroud.

According to ecodesign considerations and green manufacturing requirements, the choice of moulding process for the production of composite wind turbine blades must provide the existence of a common area of intersection engendered by a simultaneous interaction between quality, health, and environment aspects (i.e. Q, H, and E for abbreviations, resp.). This common area can be maximized via ecoalternatives in order to minimize negative adverse environmental and/or human health impacts. With this objective in mind, Chapter 3, by Attaf, focuses on the closed-mould manufacturing RTM (resin transfer moulding) process. The reason for this choice is that RTM process participates in the reduction of VOC (volatile organic compound) emissions such as styrene vapours and presents an industrial solution to wind turbine blades production coupled with high quality finishing, good mechanical properties, lower cost, and a total absence of bonding operation of half shells. In addition to these advantages, sustainable development issues and ecodesign requirements are still, however, the main objectives to be fulfilled in this analysis with an acceptable degree of tolerance to the new regulations and ecostandards leading the way for green design of composite wind turbine blades.

Chapter 4, by Carrigan and colleagues, aims to introduce and demonstrate a fully automated process for optimizing the airfoil cross-section of a vertical-axis wind turbine (VAWT). The objective is to maximize the torque while enforcing typical wind turbine design constraints such as tip speed ratio, solidity, and blade profile. By fixing the tip speed ratio of the wind turbine, there exists an airfoil cross-section and solidity for which the torque can be maximized, requiring the development of an iterative design system. The design system required to maximize torque incorporates rapid geometry generation and automated hybrid mesh generation tools with viscous, unsteady computational fluid dynamics (CFD) simulation software. The flexibility and automation of the modular design and simulation system allows for it to easily be coupled with a parallel differential evolution algorithm used to obtain an optimized blade design that maximizes the efficiency of the wind turbine.

In Chapter 5, Habash and colleagues reinforce with theoretical and experimental evaluation of the effectiveness of employing an induction generator to enhance the performance of a small wind energy converter (SWEC). With this generator, the SWEC works more efficiently and therefore can produce more energy in a unit turbine area. To verify the SWEC performance, a model has been proposed, simulated, built, and experimentally tested over a range of operating conditions. The results demonstrate a significant increase in output power with an induction generator that employs an auxiliary winding, which is only magnetically coupled to the stator main winding. It is also shown that the operating performance of the induction machine with the novel proposed technique is significantly enhanced in terms of suppressed signal distortion and harmonics, severity of resistive losses and overheating, power factor, and preventing high inrush current at starting.

The gearbox is one of the most expensive components of the wind turbine system. In order to refine the design and hence increase the long-term reliability, there has been increasing interest in utilizing time domain simulations in the prediction of gearbox design loads. In Chapter 6, by Dong and colleagues, three problems in time domain based gear contact fatigue analysis under dynamic conditions are discussed: (1) the torque reversal problem under low wind speed conditions, (2) statistical uncertainty effects due to time domain simulations and (3) simplified long term contact fatigue analysis of the gear tooth under dynamic conditions. Several recommendations to deal with these issues are proposed based on analyses of the National Renewable Energy Laboratory's 750 kW land-based Gearbox Reliability Collaborative wind turbine.

With appropriate vibration modeling and analysis the incipient failure of key components such as the tower, drive train and rotor of a large wind turbine can be detected. In Chapter 7, the Nonlinear State Estimation Technique (NSET) has been applied by Guo and Infield to model turbine tower vibration to good effect, providing an understanding of the tower vibration dynamic characteristics and the main factors influencing these. The developed tower vibration model comprises two different parts: a sub-model used for below rated wind speed; and another for above rated wind speed. Supervisory control and data acquisition system (SCADA) data from a single wind turbine collected from March to April 2006 is used in the modeling. Model validation has been subsequently undertaken and is presented. This research has demonstrated the effectiveness of the NSET approach to tower vibration; in particular its conceptual simplicity, clear physical interpretation and high accuracy. The developed and validated tower vibration model was then used to successfully detect blade angle asymmetry that is a common fault that should be remedied promptly to improve turbine performance and limit fatigue damage. The work also shows that condition monitoring is improved significantly if the information from the vibration signals is complemented by analysis of other relevant SCADA data such as power performance, wind speed, and rotor loads.

As the wind turbine size has been increasing and their mechanical components are built lighter, the reduction of the structural loads becomes a very important task of wind turbine control in addition to maximum wind power capture. In Chapter 8, Park and Nam present a separate set of collective and individual pitch control algorithms. Both pitch control algorithms use the LQR control technique with integral action (LQRI) and utilize Kalman filters to estimate system states and wind speed. Compared to previous works in this area, the authors' pitch control algorithms can control rotor speed and blade bending moments at the same time to improve the trade-off between rotor speed regulation and load reduction, while both collective and individual pitch controls can be designed separately. Simulation results show that the proposed collective and individual pitch controllers achieve very good rotor speed regulation and significant reduction of blade bending moments.

Chapter 9, by Vidal and colleagues, considers power generation control in variable-speed variable-pitch horizontal-axis wind turbines operating at high wind speeds. A dynamic chattering torque control and a proportional integral (PI) pitch control strategy are proposed and validated using the National Renewable Energy Laboratory wind turbine simulator FAST (Fatigue, Aerodynamics, Structures, and Turbulence) code. Validation results show that the proposed controllers are effective for power regulation and demonstrate high-performances for all other state variables (turbine and generator rotational speeds; and smooth and adequate evolution of the control variables) for turbulent wind conditions. To highlight the improvements of the provided method, the proposed controllers are compared to relevant previously published studies.

Chapter 10, by Diaz de Corcuera and colleagues, demonstrates a strategy to design multivariable and multi-objective controllers based on the $H\infty$ norm reduction applied to a wind turbine. The wind turbine model has been developed in the GH Bladed software and it is based on a 5 MW wind turbine defined in the Upwind European project. The designed control strategy works in the above rated power production zone and performs generator speed control and load reduction on the drive train and tower. In order to do this, two robust H∞ MISO (Multi-Input Single-Output) controllers have been developed. These controllers generate collective pitch angle and generator torque set-point values to achieve the imposed control objectives. Linear models obtained in GH Bladed 4.0 are used, but the control design methodology can be used with linear models obtained from any other modelling package. Controllers are designed by setting out a mixed sensitivity problem, where some notch filters are also included in the controller dynamics. The obtained H∞ controllers have been validated in GH Bladed and an exhaustive analysis has been carried out to calculate fatigue load reduction on wind turbine components, as well as to analyze load mitigation in some extreme cases. The analysis compares the proposed control strategy based on H∞ controllers to a baseline control strategy designed using the classical control methods implemented on the present wind turbines.

Electromagnetic interference (EMI) can both affect and be transmitted by mega-watt wind turbines. In Chapter 11, Krug and Lewke provide a general overview on EMI with respect to mega-watt wind turbines. Possibilities of measuring all types of electromagnetic interference are shown. Electromagnetic fields resulting from a GSM transmitter mounted on a mega-watt wind turbine will be analyzed in detail. This cellular system operates as a real-time communication link. The method-of-moments is used to analytically describe the electro-magnetic fields. The electromagnetic interference will be analyzed under the given boundary condition with a commercial simulation tool. Different transmitter positions are judged on the basis of their radiation patterns. The principal EMI mechanisms are described and taken into consideration.

The global push towards sustainability has led to increased interest in alternative power sources other than coal and fossil fuels. One of these sustainable sources is to harness energy from the wind through wind turbines. However, a significant hindrance preventing the widespread use of wind turbines is the noise they produce. Chapter 12, by Jianu and colleague, reviews recent advances in the area of noise pollution from wind turbines. To date, there have been many different noise control studies. While there are many different sources of noise, the main one is aerodynamic noise. The largest contributor to aerodynamic noise comes from the trailing edge of wind turbine blades. The aim of this paper is to critically analyze and compare the different methods currently being implemented and investigated to reduce noise production from wind turbines, with a focus on the noise generated from the trailing edge.

PART I

AERODYNAMICS

CHAPTER 1

WIND TURBINE BLADE DESIGN

PETER J. SCHUBEL AND RICHARD J. CROSSLEY

1.1 INTRODUCTION

Power has been extracted from the wind over hundreds of years with historic designs, known as windmills, constructed from wood, cloth and stone for the purpose of pumping water or grinding corn. Historic designs, typically large, heavy and inefficient, were replaced in the 19th century by fossil fuel engines and the implementation of a nationally distributed power network. A greater understanding of aerodynamics and advances in materials, particularly polymers, has led to the return of wind energy extraction in the latter half of the 20th century. Wind power devices are now used to produce electricity, and commonly termed wind turbines.

The orientation of the shaft and rotational axis determines the first classification of the wind turbine. A turbine with a shaft mounted horizontally parallel to the ground is known as a horizontal axis wind turbine or (HAWT). A vertical axis wind turbine (VAWT) has its shaft normal to the ground (Figure 1).

The two configurations have instantly distinguishable rotor designs, each with its own favourable characteristics [1]. The discontinued mainstream development of the VAWT can be attributed to a low tip speed

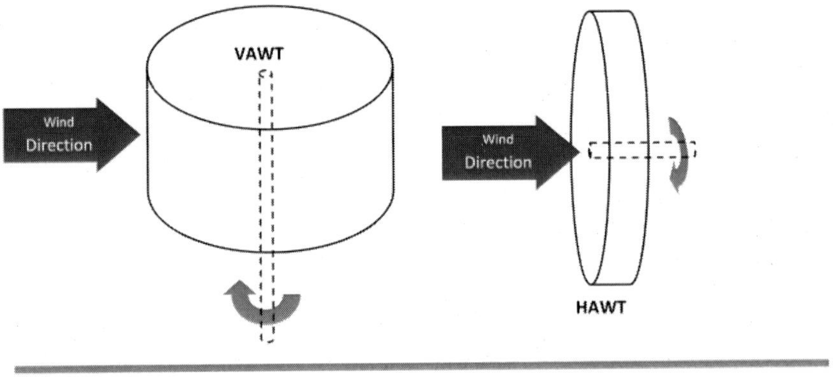

FIGURE 1: Alternative configurations for shaft and rotor orientation.

ratio and difficulty in controlling rotor speed. Difficulties in the starting of vertical turbines have also hampered development, believed until recently to be incapable of self-starting [2]. However, the VAWT requires no additional mechanism to face the wind and heavy generator equipment can be mounted on the ground, thus reducing tower loads. Therefore, the VAWT is not completely disregarded for future development. A novel V-shaped VAWT rotor design is currently under investigation which exploits these favourable attributes [3]. This design is currently unproven on a megawatt scale, requiring several years of development before it can be considered competitive. In addition to the problems associated with alternative designs, the popularity of the HAWT can be attributed to increased rotor control through pitch and yaw control. The HAWT has therefore emerged as the dominant design configuration, capitalised by all of today's leading large scale turbine manufacturers.

1.2 THEORETICAL MAXIMUM EFFICIENCY

High rotor efficiency is desirable for increased wind energy extraction and should be maximised within the limits of affordable production. Energy (P) carried by moving air is expressed as a sum of its kinetic energy [Equation (1)]:

$$P = \frac{1}{2}\rho A V^3 \qquad \begin{aligned} \rho &= \text{Air Density} \\ A &= \text{Swept area} \\ V &= \text{Air Velocity} \end{aligned} \tag{1}$$

A physical limit exists to the quantity of energy that can be extracted, which is independent of design. The energy extraction is maintained in a flow process through the reduction of kinetic energy and subsequent velocity of the wind. The magnitude of energy harnessed is a function of the reduction in air speed over the turbine. 100% extraction would imply zero final velocity and therefore zero flow. The zero flow scenario cannot be achieved hence all the winds kinetic energy may not be utilised. This principle is widely accepted [4,5] and indicates that wind turbine efficiency cannot exceed 59.3%. This parameter is commonly known as the power coefficient Cp, where max Cp = 0.593 referred to as the Betz limit [6]. The Betz theory assumes constant linear velocity. Therefore, any rotational forces such as wake rotation, turbulence caused by drag or vortex shedding (tip losses) will further reduce the maximum efficiency. Efficiency losses are generally reduced by:

- Avoiding low tip speed ratios which increase wake rotation
- Selecting aerofoils which have a high lift to drag ratio
- Specialised tip geometries

In depth explanation and analysis can be found in the literature [4,6].

1.3 PROPULSION

The method of propulsion critically affects the maximum achievable efficiency of the rotor. Historically, the most commonly utilised method was drag, by utilising a sail faced normal to the wind, relying on the drag factor (Cd) to produce a force in the direction of the prevailing wind. This method proved inefficient as the force and rotation of the sail correspond to the wind direction; therefore, the relative velocity of the wind is reduced as rotor speed increases (Table 1).

TABLE 1: The two mechanisms of propulsion compared.

Propulsion	Drag	Lift
Diagram	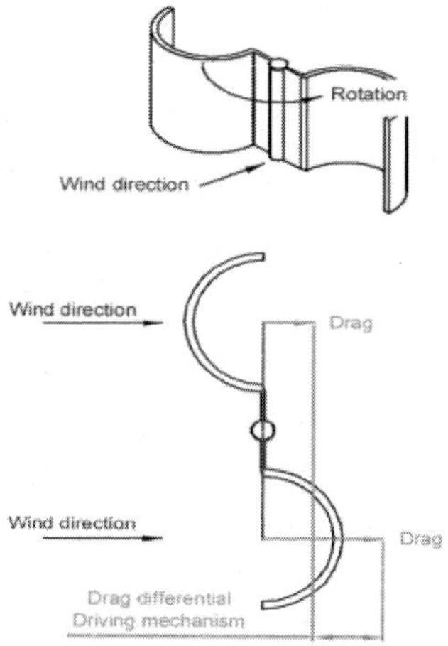	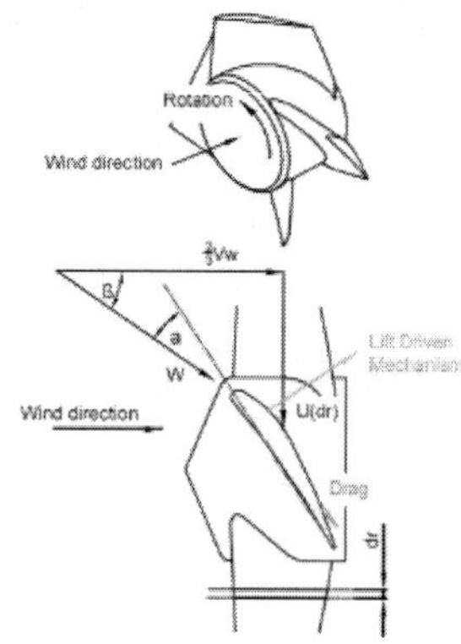
Relative Wind Velocity	= wind velocity – blade velocity	$= \sqrt{\frac{2}{3} wind\ velocity^2 - blade\ velocity(dr)?}$
Maximum Theoretical Efficiency	16% [4]	50% [6]

Reducing efficiency further is the drag of the returning sail into the wind, which was often shielded from the oncoming wind. Unshielded designs rely on curved blade shapes which have a lower drag coefficient when returning into the wind and are advantageous as they work in any wind direction. These differential drag rotors can be seen in use today on cup anemometers and ventilation cowls. However, they are inefficient power producers as their tip speed ratio cannot exceed one [4].

An alternative method of propulsion is the use of aerodynamic lift (Table 1), which was utilised without precise theoretical explanation for over 700 years in windmills then later in vintage aircraft. Today, due to its difficult mathematical analysis, aerodynamics has become a subject of its own.

Multiple theories have emerged of increasing complexity explaining how lift force is generated and predicted. Aerodynamic force is the integrated effect of the pressure and skin friction caused by the flow of air over the aerofoil surface [7]. Attributed to the resultant force caused by the redirection of air over the aerofoil known as downwash [8]. Most importantly for wind turbine rotors, aerodynamic lift can be generated at a narrow corridor of varying angles normal to the wind direction. This indicates no decrease in relative wind velocity at any rotor speed (Table 1).

For a lift driven rotor (Table 1) the relative velocity at which air strikes the blade (W) is a function of the blade velocity at the radius under consideration and approximately two thirds of the wind velocity (Betz theory Section 2) [4]. The relative airflow arrives at the blade with an angle of incidence (β) dependant on these velocities. The angle between the blade and the incidence angle is known as the angle of attack (α).

1.4 PRACTICAL EFFICIENCY

In practice rotor designs suffer from the accumulation of minor losses resulting from:

- Tip losses
- Wake effects
- Drive train efficiency losses
- Blade shape simplification losses

Therefore, the maximum theoretical efficiency has yet to be achieved [9]. Over the centuries many types of design have emerged, and some of the more distinguishable are listed in Table 2. The earliest designs, Persian windmills, utilised drag by means of sails made from wood and cloth. These Persian windmills were principally similar to their modern counterpart the Savonius rotor (No. 1) which can be seen in use today in ventilation cowls and rotating advertising signs. Similar in principle is the cup type differential drag rotor (No. 2), utilised today by anemometers for calculating airspeed due to their ease of calibration and multidirectional operation. The American farm windmill (No. 3) is an early example of a high torque lift driven rotor with a high degree of solidity, still in use today for water pumping applications. The Dutch windmill (No. 4) is another example of an early lift type device utilised for grinding corn which has now disappeared from mainstream use, yet a small number still survive as tourist attractions. The Darrieus VAWT (No. 5) is a modern aerodynamic aerofoil blade design which despite extensive research and development has so far been unable to compete with the modern HAWT design, although recent developments [2,3] could see a resurgence of this rotor type. Due to its efficiency and ease of control, the aerofoil three bladed HAWT (No. 6) has become the wind turbine industry benchmark, with a fully established international supply chain securing its dominance for the foreseeable future.

1.5 HAWT BLADE DESIGN

A focus is now being made on the HAWT due to its dominance in the wind turbine industry. HAWT are very sensitive to changes in blade profile and design. This section briefly discusses the major parameters that influence the performance of HAWT blades.

1.5.1 TIP SPEED RATIO

The tip speed ratio defined as the relationship between rotor blade velocity and relative wind velocity [Equation (2)] is the foremost design parameter around which all other optimum rotor dimensions are calculated:

$$\lambda = \frac{\Omega r}{V_w} \tag{2}$$

Where λ = Tip speed ratio, Ω = rotational velocity (rad/s), r= radius, and V_w = windspeed.

Aspects such as efficiency, torque, mechanical stress, aerodynamics and noise should be considered in selecting the appropriate tip speed (Table 3). The efficiency of a turbine can be increased with higher tip speeds [4], although the increase is not significant when considering some penalties such as increased noise, aerodynamic and centrifugal stress (Table 3).

TABLE 2: Modern and historical rotor designs.

Ref No.	Design	Orientation	Use	Propulsion	* Peak Efficiency	Diagram
1	Savonius rotor	VAWT	Historic Persian windmill to modern day ventilation	Drag	16%	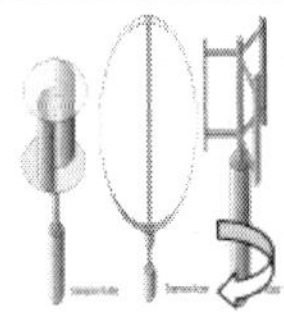
2	Cup	VAWT	Modern day cup anemometer	Drag	8%	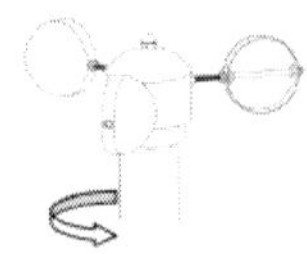
3	American farm windmill	HAWT	18th century to present day, farm use for Pumping water, grinding wheat, generating electricity	Lift	31%	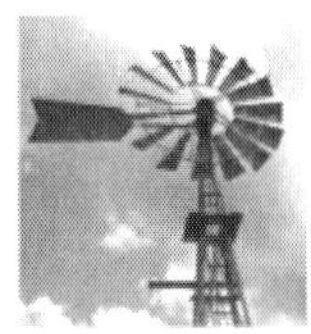
4	Dutch Windmill	HAWT	16th Century, used for grinding wheat.	Lift	27%	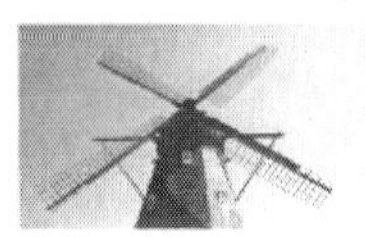
5	Darrieus Rotor (egg beater)	VAWT	20th century, electricity generation	Lift	40%	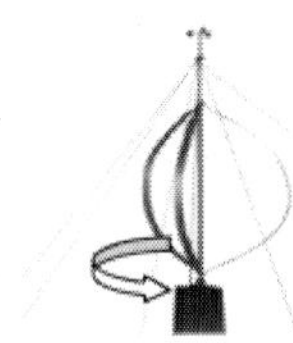
6	Modern Wind Turbine	HAWT	20th century, electricity generation	Lift	Blade qty / efficiency 1 / 43% 2 / 47% 3 / 50%	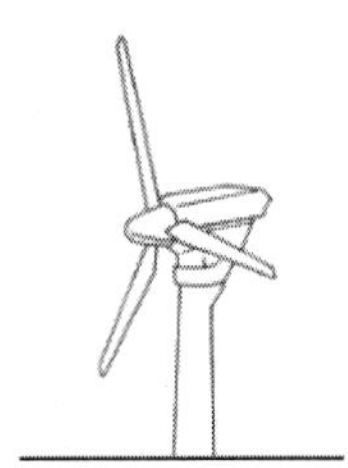

** Peak efficiency is dependent upon design, values quoted are maximum efficiencies of designs in operation to date [1].*

TABLE 3: Tip speed ratio design considerations.

Tip Speed Ratio	Low	High
Value	Tip speeds of one to two are considered low	Tip Speeds higher than 10 are considered high
Utilisation	traditional wind mills and water pumps	Mainly single or two bladed prototypes
Torque	Increases	Decreases
Efficiency	Decreases significantly below five due to rotational wake created by high torque [4]	Insignificant increases after eight
Centrifugal Stress	Decreases	Increases as a square of rotational velocity [4]
Aerodynamic Stress	Decreases	Increases proportionally with rotational velocity [4]
Area of Solidity	Increases, multiple 20+ blades required	Decreases significantly
Blade Profile	Large	Significantly Narrow
Aerodynamics	Simple	Critical
Noise	Increases to the 6th power approximately [4]	

A higher tip speed demands reduced chord widths leading to narrow blade profiles. This can lead to reduced material usage and lower production costs. Although an increase in centrifugal and aerodynamic forces is associated with higher tip speeds. The increased forces signify that difficulties exist with maintaining structural integrity and preventing blade failure. As the tip speed increases the aerodynamics of the blade design become increasingly critical. A blade which is designed for high relative wind speeds develops minimal torque at lower speeds. This results in a higher cut in speed [10] and difficulty self-starting. A noise increase is also associated with increasing tip speeds as noise increases approximately proportionately to the sixth power [4,11]. Modern HAWT generally utilise a tip speed ratio of nine to ten for two bladed rotors and six to nine for three blades [1]. This has been found to produce efficient conversion of the winds kinetic energy into electrical power [1,6].

1.5.2 BLADE PLAN SHAPE AND QUANTITY

The ideal plan form of a HAWT rotor blade is defined using the BEM method by calculating the chord length according to Betz limit, local air velocities and aerofoil lift. Several theories exist for calculating the optimum chord length which range in complexity [1,4,10,12], with the simplest theory based on the Betz optimisation [Equation (3)] [1]. For blades with tip speed ratios of six to nine utilising aerofoil sections with negligible drag and tip losses, Betz's momentum theory gives a good approximation [1]. In instances of low tip speeds, high drag aerofoil sections and blade sections around the hub, this method could be considered inaccurate. In such cases, wake and drag losses should be accounted for [4,12]. The Betz method gives the basic shape of the modern wind turbine blade (Figure 2). However, in practice more advanced methods of optimization are often used [12–14].

$$C_{opt} = \frac{2\pi r}{n}\frac{8}{9C_L}\frac{U_{wd}}{\lambda V_r} \quad \text{where} \quad V_r = \sqrt{V_w^2 + U^2} \tag{3}$$

Where r= radius (m), n = blade quantity, C_L = Lift coefficient, λ = local tip speed ratio, V_r = local resultant air velocity (m/s), U = wind speed (m/s), U_{wd} = design windspeed (m/s), and C_{opt} = optimum chord length.

Assuming that a reasonable lift coefficient is maintained, utilising a blade optimisation method produces blade plans principally dependant on design tip speed ratio and number of blades (Figure 3). Low tip speed ra-

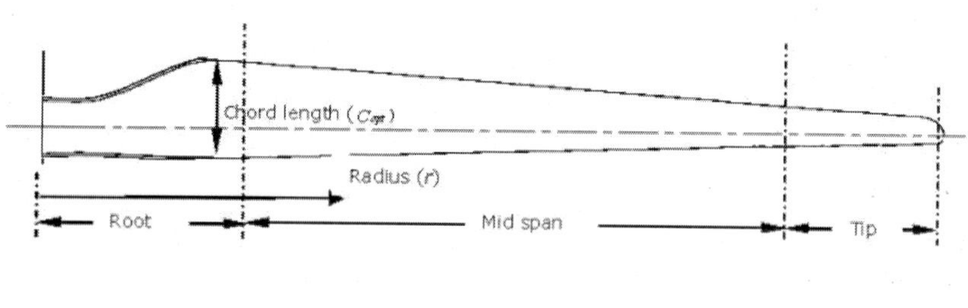

FIGURE 2: A typical blade plan and region classification.

tios produce a rotor with a high ratio of solidity, which is the ratio of blade area to the area of the swept rotor. It is useful to reduce the area of solidity as it leads to a decrease in material usage and therefore production costs. However, problems are associated with high tip speeds (Section 5.1).

Generally, in practice the chord length is simplified to facilitate manufacture and which involves some linearization of the increasing chord length (Figure 4). The associated losses signify that simplification can be justified by a significant production cost saving.

For optimum chord dimensioning (Equation 3) the quantity of blades is considered negligible in terms of efficiency. However, in practice when blade losses are considered a 3% loss is incurred for two bladed designs [1] and a 7%–13% loss for one bladed design [6] when compared to three blades. A four bladed design offers marginal efficiency increases which do not justify the manufacturing cost of an extra blade. Tower loading

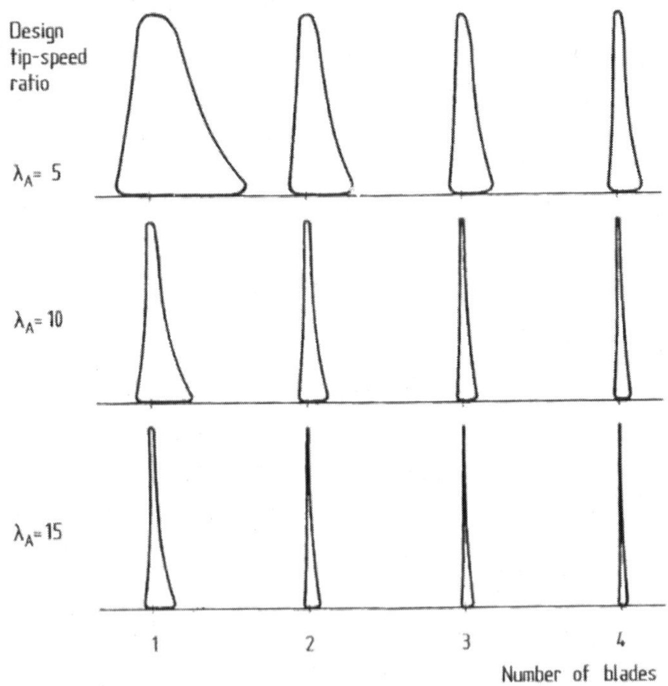

FIGURE 3: Optimal blade plan shape for alternate design tip speed ratios and number of blades [1].

must also be considered when choosing the appropriate blade quantity [6]. Four, three, two and one bladed designs lead to increased dynamic loads, respectively [16].

The imposing size and location of wind turbines signify that the visual impact must be considered. Three bladed designs are said to appear smoother in rotation therefore more aesthetically pleasing. Faster one and two bladed designs have an apparent jerky motion [1]. Three bladed rotors are also thought to appear more orderly when in the stationary position [17].

1.5.3 CONFIGURATION

A favourable reduction in rotor nacelle weight and manufacturing costs occur with the use of fewer blades [16]. However, dynamic structural and balancing difficulties of the polar asymmetrical rotor are apparent [16]. Increased wear, inferior aesthetic qualities and bird conservation problems are also associated with one and two bladed rotors [17,18]. The three blade turbine (Figure 5) has been widely adopted (Table 4) as the most efficient

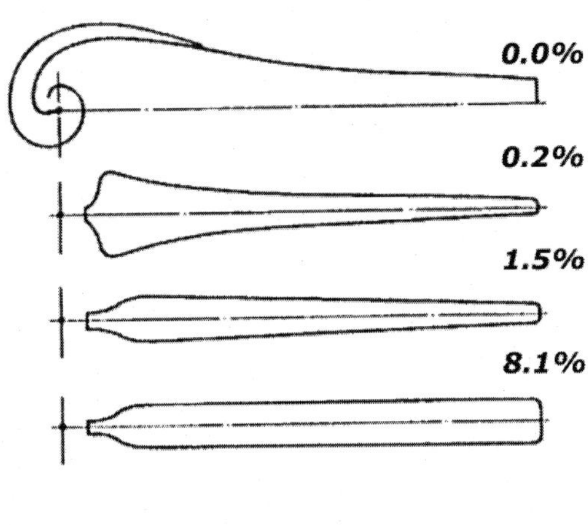

FIGURE 4: Efficiency losses as a result of simplification to ideal chord length [15].

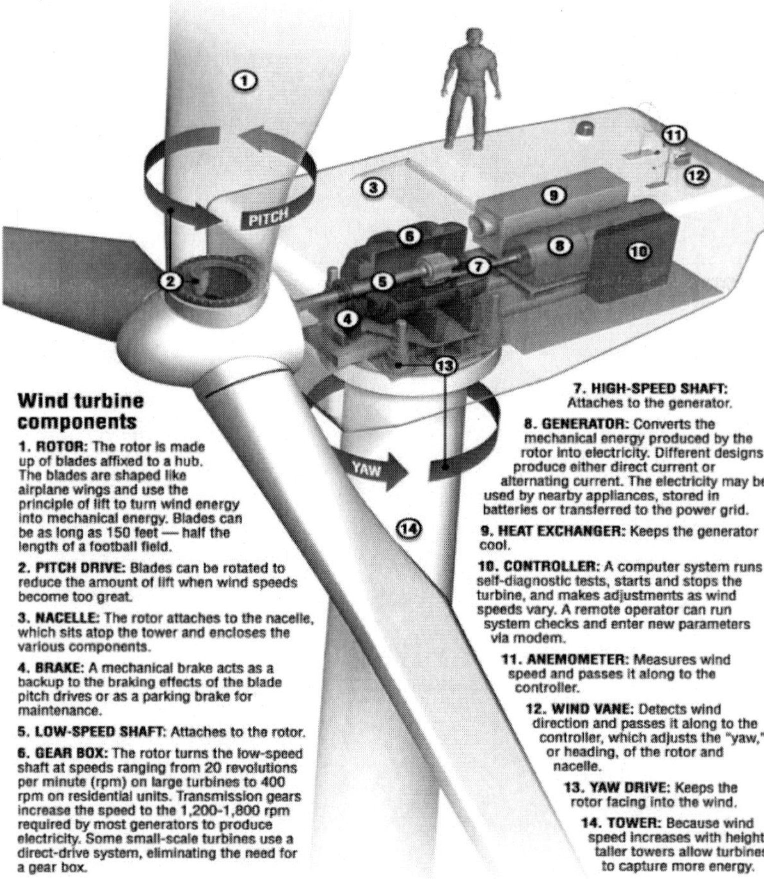

FIGURE 5: Typical configuration of a modern large scale wind turbine (www.desmoinesregister.com).

design to meet environmental, commercial and economic constraints and therefore dominates today's large scale wind turbine industry. Modern commercially available wind turbines include complex control and safety systems, remote monitoring and maintenance with provision for the survival of lightning strike (Table 5).

TABLE 4: A selection of turbine size and weight configurations.

Turbine Name	Pitch or Stall	Rotor Dia (m)	No. of Blades	Nacelle and Rotor Weight (kg)	Weight per Swept Area (kg/m²)
Mitsubishi MWT-1000 (1 MW)	P	57	3	Unspecified	
Nordex N90 (2.3 MW)	P	90	3	84,500	13.3
Nordex N80 (2.5 MW)	P	80	3	80,500	16
Repower 5M (5 MW)	P	126	3	Unspecified	
Siemens SWT-3.6-107 (3.6 MW)	P	107	3	220,000	24.5
Siemens SWT-2.3-93 (2.3 MW)	P	93	3	142,000	20.9
Gamesa G90-2MW (2 MW)	P	90	3	106,000	16.7
Gamesa G58-850 (850 kW)	P	58	3	35,000	13.3
Enercon E82 (2 MW)	P	82	3	Unspecified	
GE wind 3.6sl (3.6 MW)	P	111	3	Unspecified	
Vestas V164 (7.0 MW)	P	164	3	Unspecified	
Vestas V90 (2 MW)	P	90	3	106,000	16.7
Vestas V82 (1.65 MW)	P	82	3	95,000	18

TABLE 5: A Typical modern 2MW wind turbine specification.

Rotor	
Diameter	90 m
Swept Area	6362 m²
Rotational Speed	9–19 rpm
Direction of Rotation	Clockwise from front
Weight (including hub)	36 T
Top Head Weight	106 T

TABLE 5: *Cont.*

Blades		
Quantity	3	
Length	44 m	
Aerofoils	Delft University and FFA-W3	
Material	Pre impregnated epoxy glass fibre + carbon fibre	
Mass	5800 kg	
Tower		
Tubular modular design	Height	Weight
3 Section	67 m	153 T
4 Section	78 m	203 T
5 Section	100 m	255 T
Gearbox		
Type	1 planetary stage, 2 helical stages	
Ratio	1:100	
Cooling	Oil pump with oil cooler	
Oil heater	2.2 kW	
2.0 MW Generator		
Type	Doubly fed machine	
Voltage	690 V ac	
Frequency	50 Hz	
Rotational speed	900–1900	
Stator current	1500A @ 690v	
Mechanical Design		
Drive train with main shaft supported by two spherical bearings that transmit the side loads directly onto the frame by means of the bearing housing. This prevents the gearbox from receiving additional loads. Reducing and facilitating its service.		
Brake		
Full feathering aerodynamic braking with a secondary hydraulic disc brake for emergency use.		
Lightening Protection		
In accordance with IEC 61024-1. Conductors direct lightening from both sides of the blade tip down to the root joint and from there across the nacelle and tower structure to the grounding system located in the foundations. As a result, the blade and sensitive electrical components are protected.		
Control System		
The generator is a doubly fed machine (DFM), whose speed and power is controlled through IGBT converters and pulse width modulation (PWM) electronic control. Real time operation and remote control of turbines, meteorological mast and substation is facilitated via satellite-terrestrial network. TCP/IP architecture with a web interface. A predictive maintenance system is in place for the early detection of potential deterioration or malfunctions in the wind turbines main components.		

1.5.4 AERODYNAMICS

Aerodynamic performance is fundamental for efficient rotor design [19]. Aerodynamic lift is the force responsible for the power yield generated by the turbine and it is therefore essential to maximise this force using appropriate design. A resistant drag force which opposes the motion of the blade is also generated by friction which must be minimised. It is then apparent that an aerofoil section with a high lift to drag ratio [Equation (4)], typically greater than 30 [20], be chosen for rotor blade design [19]:

$$\text{Lift to Drag ratio} = \frac{\text{Coefficient of lift}}{\text{Cofficient of drag}} = \frac{C_L}{C_D} \tag{4}$$

The co-efficient for the lift and drag of aerofoils is difficult to predic-mathematically, although freely available software, such as XFOIL [21] model results accurately with the exception of post stall, excessive angles of attack and aerofoil thickness conditions [22,23]. Traditionally aerofoils are tested experimentally with tables correlating lift and drag at given angles of attack and Reynolds numbers [24]. Historically wind turbine aerofoil designs have been borrowed from aircraft technologies with similar Reynolds numbers and section thicknesses suitable for conditions at the blade tip. However, special considerations should be made for the design of wind turbine specific aerofoil profiles due to the differences in operating conditions and mechanical loads.

The effects of soiling have not been considered by aircraft aerofoils as they generally fly at altitudes where insects and other particulates are negligible. Turbines operate for long periods at ground level where insect and dust particulate build up is problematic. This build up known as fouling can have detrimental effects on the lift generated. Provision is therefore made for the reduced sensitivity to fouling of wind turbine specific aerofoil designs [25].

The structural requirements of turbine blades signify that aerofoils with a high thickness to chord ratio be used in the root region. Such aerofoils are rarely used in the aerospace industry. Thick aerofoil sections generally have a lower lift to drag ratio. Special consideration is therefore made for increasing the lift of thick aerofoil sections for use in wind turbine blade designs [25,26].

National Advisory Committee for Aeronautics (NACA) four and five digit designs have been used for early modern wind turbines [1]. The classification shows the geometric profile of a NACA aerofoil where the 1st digit refers to maximum chamber to chord ratio, 2nd digit is the camber position in tenths of the chord and the 3rd & 4th digits are the maximum thickness to chord ratio in percent [24]. The emergence of wind turbine specific aerofoils such as the Delft University [23], LS, SERI-NREL and FFA [6] and RISO [26] now provide alternatives specifically tailored to the needs of the wind turbine industry.

The angle of attack is the angle of the oncoming flow relative to the chord line, and all figures for C_L and C_D are quoted relative to this angle. The use of a single aerofoil for the entire blade length would result in inefficient design [19]. Each section of the blade has a differing relative air velocity and structural requirement and therefore should have its aerofoil section tailored accordingly. At the root, the blade sections have large minimum thickness which is essential for the intensive loads carried resulting in thick profiles. Approaching the tip blades blend into thinner sections with reduced load, higher linear velocity and increasingly critical aerodynamic performance. The differing aerofoil requirements relative to the blade region are apparent when considering airflow velocities and structural loads (Table 6).

TABLE 6: The aerofoil requirements for blade regions [26].

Parameter	Blade Position (Figure 2)		
	Root	Mid Span	Tip
Thickness to chord ratio (%) ([d/c] Figure 2)	>27	27–21	21–15
Structural load bearing requirement	High	Med	Low
Geometrical compatibility	Med	Med	Med
Maximum lift insensitive to leading edge roughness		High	
Design lift close to maximum lift off-design		Low	Med
Maximum CL and post stall behaviour		Low	High
Low Aerofoil Noise			High

An aerodynamic phenomenon known as stall should be considered carefully in turbine blade design. Stall typically occurs at large angles of attack depending on the aerofoil design. The boundary layer separates at the tip rather than further down the aerofoil causing a wake to flow over the upper surface drastically reducing lift and increasing drag forces [6]. This condition is considered dangerous in aviation and is generally avoided. However, for wind turbines, it can be utilised to limit the maximum power output to prevent generator overload and excessive forces in the blades during extreme wind speeds and could also occur unintentionally during gusts. It is therefore preferable that the onset of the stall condition is not instantaneous for wind turbine aerofoils as this would create excessive dynamic forces and vibrations [1].

The sensitivity of blades to soiling, off design conditions including stall and thick cross sections for structural purposes are the main driving forces for the development of wind turbine specific aerofoil profiles [1,26]. The use of modern materials with superior mechanical properties may allow for thinner structural sections with increased lift to drag ratios at root sections. Thinner sections also offer a chance to increase efficiency through reducing drag. Higher lift coefficients of thinner aerofoil sections will in turn lead to reduced chord lengths reducing material usage [Equation (3)].

1.5.5 ANGLE OF TWIST

The lift generated by an aerofoil section is a function of the angle of attack to the inflowing air stream (Section 5.4). The inflow angle of the air stream is dependent on the rotational speed and wind speed velocity at a specified radius. The angle of twist required is dependent upon tip speed ratio and desired aerofoil angle of attack. Generally the aerofoil section at the hub is angled into the wind due to the high ratio of wind speed to blade radial velocity. In contrast the blade tip is likely to be almost normal to the wind.

The total angle of twist in a blade maybe reduced simplifying the blade shape to cut manufacturing costs. However, this may force aerofoils to operate at less than optimum angles of attack where lift to drag ratio is reduced.

Such simplifications must be well justified considering the overall loss in turbine performance.

1.5.6 OFF-DESIGN CONDITIONS AND POWER REGULATION

Early wind turbine generator and gearbox technology required that blades rotate at a fixed rotational velocity therefore running at non design tip speed ratios incurring efficiency penalties in all but the rated wind conditions [1]. For larger modern turbines this is no longer applicable and it is suggested that the gearbox maybe obsolete in future turbines [27]. Today the use of fixed speed turbines is limited to smaller designs therefore the associated off-design difficulties are omitted.

The design wind speed is used for optimum dimensioning of the wind turbine blade which is dependent upon site wind measurements. However, the wind conditions are variable for any site and the turbine must operate at off-design conditions, which include wind velocities higher than rated. Hence a method of limiting the rotational speed must be implemented to prevent excessive loading of the blade, hub, gearbox and generator. The turbine is also required to maintain a reasonably high efficiency at below rated wind speeds.

As the oncoming wind velocity directly affects the angle of incidence of the resultant airflow onto the blade, the blade pitch angle must be altered accordingly. This is known as pitching, which maintains the lift force of the aerofoil section. Generally the full length of the blade is twisted mechanically through the hub to alter the blade angle. This method is effective at increasing lift in lower than rated conditions and is also used to prevent over speed of the rotor which may lead to generator overload or catastrophic failure of the blade under excessive load [1].

Two methods of blade pitching are used to reduce the lift force and therefore the rotational velocity of the rotor during excessive wind speeds. Firstly decreasing the pitch angle reduces the angle of attack which therefore reduces the lift generated. This method is known as feathering. The alternative method is to increase the pitch angle which increases the angle of attack to a critical limit inducing the stall condition and reducing lift. The feathering requires the maximum amount of mechanical movement in pitching the blade. However, it is still favoured as stalling can result in excessive dynamic loads. These loads are a result of the unpredictable transition from attached to detached airflow around the blade which may lead to undesirable fluttering [1].

Utilising the stall condition a limiting speed can be designed into the rotor blade known as passive stall control [1]. Increased wind velocity and rotor speed produce an angle at which stall is initiated therefore automatically limiting the rotor speed. In practice accurately ensuring stall occurs is difficult and usually leads to a safety margin. The use of a safety margin indicates that normal operation occurs at below optimum performance, consequently this method is utilised only by smaller turbines [28]. Full blade feathered pitching at the hub is used by the majority of today's wind turbine market leaders (Table 4). Feathered pitching offers increased performance, flexibility and the capability of fully pitching the blades to a parked configuration. Manufacturers are reported as using collective pitch [29], in that all the blades are pitched at identical angles. However, further load reductions can be found by pitching blades individually [30]. This requires no extra mechanism in most designs and it is expected to be widely adopted [29,30].

1.5.7 SMART BLADE DESIGN

The current research trend in blade design is the so called "Smart Blades", which alter their shape depending on the wind conditions. Within this category of blade design are numerous approaches which are either aerodynamic control surfaces or smart actuator materials. An extensive review of this subject is given by Barlas [31]. The driver behind this research is to limit ultimate (extreme) loads and fatigue loads or to increase dynamic energy capture. Research is mainly initiated based on similar concepts from helicopter control and is being investigated by various wind energy research institutes. The work package "Smart rotor blades and rotor control" in the Upwind EU framework programme, the project "Smart dynamic control of large offshore wind turbines" and the Danish project "ADAPWING" all deal with the subject of Smart rotor control. In the framework of the International Energy Agency, two expert meetings were

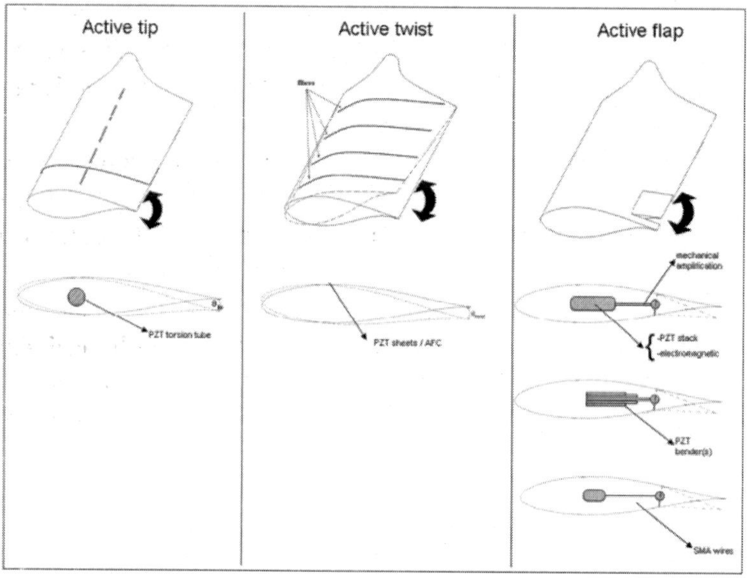

FIGURE 6: Schematics of smart structure concepts.

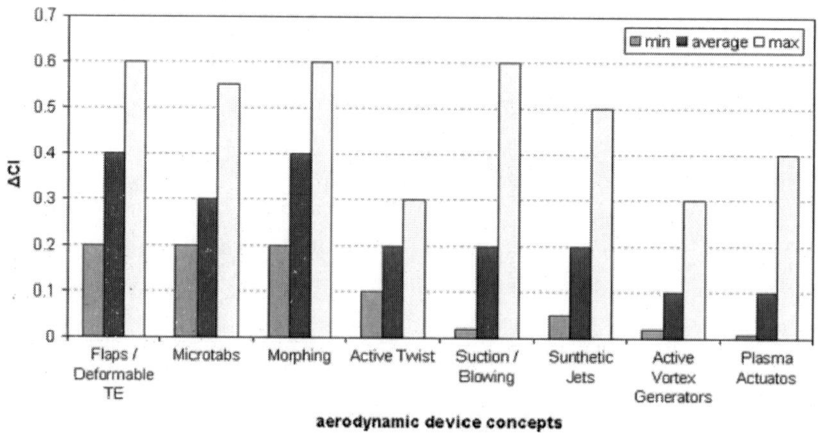

FIGURE 7: Comparison of aerodynamic device concepts in terms of lift control capability [31].

held on "The application of smart structures for large wind turbine rotors", by Delft University and Sandia National Labs, respectively. The proceedings show a variety of topics, methods and solutions, which reflects the on-going research [32,33].

The use of aerodynamic control surfaces includes aileron style flaps, camber control, active twist and boundary layer control. Figures 6 and 7 show a comparison graph of aerodynamic performance (lift control capability) of a variety of aerodynamic control surface based concepts.

Smart actuator materials include conventional actuators, smart material actuators, piezoelectric and shape memory alloys. Traditional actuators probably do not meet minimum requirements for such concepts. Furthermore, proposed concepts of aerodynamic control surfaces (distributed along the blade span) require fast actuation without complex mechanical systems and large energy to weight ratios. Promising solution for this purpose is the use of smart material actuator systems. By definition, smart materials are materials which possess the capability to sense and actuate in a controlled way in response to variable ambient stimuli. Generally known types of smart materials are ferroelectric materials (piezoelectric, electrostrictive, magnetostrictive), variable rheology materials (electrorheological, magnetorheological) and shape memory alloys. Piezoelectric materials and shape memory alloys are generally the most famous smart materials used in actuators in various applications. The development of their technology has reached a quite high level and commercial solutions are available and widely used [31].

1.5.8 BLADE SHAPE SUMMARY

An efficient rotor blade consists of several aerofoil profiles blended at an angle of twist terminating at a circular flange (Figure 8) [4,34]. It may also include tip geometries for reducing losses. To facilitate production, several simplifications maybe made:

- Reducing the angle of twist.
- Linearization of the chord width.
- Reducing the number of differing aerofoil profiles.

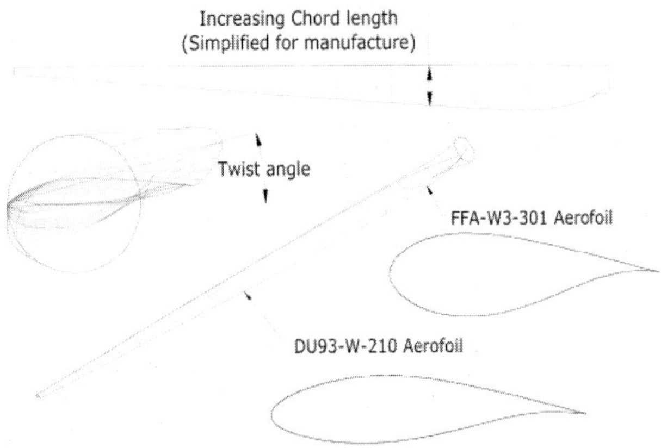

FIGURE 8: A typical modern HAWT blade with multiple aerofoil profiles, twist and linear chord length increase.

All manufacturing simplifications are detrimental to rotor efficiency and should be well justified. The introduction of new moulding techniques and materials has allowed the manufacture of increasingly complex blade shapes. However, the economics of production coupled with difficulty of design analysis still dictate final geometry. Leading wind turbine suppliers now include most optimisation features such as angle of twist, variable chord length and multiple aerofoil geometries.

1.6 BLADE LOADS

Multiple aerofoil sections and chord lengths, 22 specified stochastic load cases and an angle of twist with numerous blade pitching angles results in a complex engineering scenario. Therefore, the use of computer analysis software such as fluid dynamics (CFD) and finite element (FEA) is now commonplace within the wind turbine industry [35]. Dedicated commercially available software such as LOADS, YawDyn, MOSTAB, GH Bladed, SEACC and AERODYN are utilised to perform calculations based upon blade geometry, tip speed and site conditions [15].

To simplify calculations, it has been suggested that a worst case loading condition be identified for consideration, on which all other loads may be tolerated [4]. The worst case loading scenario is dependent on blade size and method of control. For small turbines without blade pitching, a 50 year storm condition would be considered the limiting case. For larger turbines (D > 70 m), loads resulting from the mass of the blade become critical and should be considered [4]. In practice several load cases are considered with published methods detailing mathematical analysis for each of the IEC load cases [6].

For modern large scale turbine blades the analysis of a single governing load case is not sufficient for certification. Therefore multiple load cases are analysed. The most important load cases are dependent on individual designs. Typically priority is given to the following loading conditions:

- emergency stop scenario [36]
- extreme loading during operation [6]
- parked 50 year storm conditions [34]

Under these operational scenarios the main sources of blade loading are listed below [6]:

1. Aerodynamic
2. Gravitational
3. Centrifugal
4. Gyroscopic
5. Operational

The load magnitude will depend on the operational scenario under analysis. If the optimum rotor shape is maintained, then aerodynamic loads are unavoidable and vital to the function of the turbine, considered in greater detail (Section 6.1). As turbines increase in size, the mass of the blade is said to increase proportionately at a cubic rate. The gravitational and centrifugal forces become critical due to blade mass and are also elaborated (Section 6.2). Gyroscopic loads result from yawing during operation. They are system dependant and generally less intensive than gravitational loads. Operational loads are also system dependant, resulting from pitching, yawing, breaking and generator connection and can be intensive during emergency stop or grid loss scenarios. Gyroscopic and operational loads can be reduced by adjusting system parameters. Blades which can withstand aerodynamic, gravitational and centrifugal loads are generally capable of withstanding these reduced loads. Therefore, gyroscopic and operational loads are not considered within this work.

1.6.1 AERODYNAMIC LOAD

Aerodynamic load is generated by lift and drag of the blades aerofoil section (Figure 9), which is dependent on wind velocity (VW), blade velocity (U), surface finish, angle of attack (α) and yaw. The angle of attack is dependent on blade twist and pitch. The aerodynamic lift and drag produced (Figure 9) are resolved into useful thrust (T) in the direction of rotation absorbed by the generator and reaction forces (R). It can be seen that the reaction forces are substantial acting in the flatwise bending plane, and must be tolerated by the blade with limited deformation.

For calculation of the blade aerodynamic forces the widely publicised blade element momentum (BEM) theory is applied [4,6,37]. Working along the blade radius taking small elements (δr), the sum of the aerodynamic forces can be calculated to give the overall blade reaction and thrust loads (Figure 9).

1.6.2 GRAVITATIONAL AND CENTRIFUGAL LOADS

Gravitational centrifugal forces are mass dependant which is generally thought to increase cubically with increasing turbine diameter [38]. Therefore, turbines under ten meters diameter have negligible inertial loads, which are marginal for 20 meters upward, and critical for 70 meter rotors and above [4]. The gravitational force is defined simply as mass multiplied by the gravitational constant, although its direction remains constant acting towards the centre of the earth which causes an alternating cyclic load case.

The centrifugal force is a product of rotational velocity squared and mass and always acts radial outward, hence the increased load demands of higher tip speeds. Centrifugal and gravitational loads are superimposed to give a positively displaced alternating condition with a wavelength equal to one blade revolution.

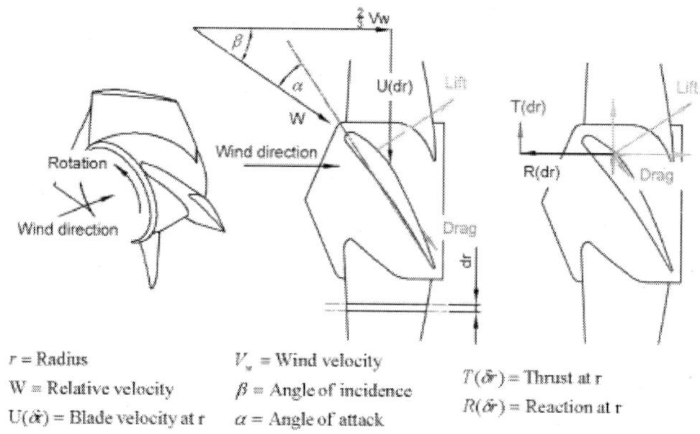

FIGURE 9: Aerodynamic forces generated at a blade element.

1.6.3 STRUCTURAL LOAD ANALYSIS

Modern load analysis of a wind turbine blade would typically consist of a three dimensional CAD model analysed using the Finite Element Method [39]. Certification bodies support this method and conclude that there is a range of commercial software available with accurate results [40]. These standards also allow the blade stress condition to be modelled conservatively using classical stress analysis methods.

Traditionally the blade would be modelled as a simple cantilever beam with equivalent point or uniformly distributed loads used to calculate the flap wise and edgewise bending moment. The direct stresses for root sections and bolt inserts would also be calculated. The following simple analysis (Sections 6.4–6.6) offers basic insight into the global structural loading of a wind turbine blade. In practice a more detailed computational analysis would be completed including local analysis of individual features, bonds and material laminates.

1.6.4 FLAPWISE BENDING

The flap wise bending moment is a result of the aerodynamic loads (Figure 9), which can be calculated using BEM theory (Section 6.1). Aerodynamic loads are suggested as a critical design load during 50 year storm and extreme operational conditions [6]. Once calculated, it is apparent that load case can be modelled as a cantilever beam with a uniformly distributed load (Figure 10) [4]. This analysis shows how bending occurs about the chord axis creating compressive and tensile stresses in the blade cross section (Figure 11). To calculate these stresses the second moment of area of the load bearing material must be calculated [Equation (6)]. Using classical beam bending analysis bending moments can be calculated at any section along the blade [41]. Local deflections and material stresses can then be calculated at any point along the beam using the fundamental beam bending equation [Equation (7)].

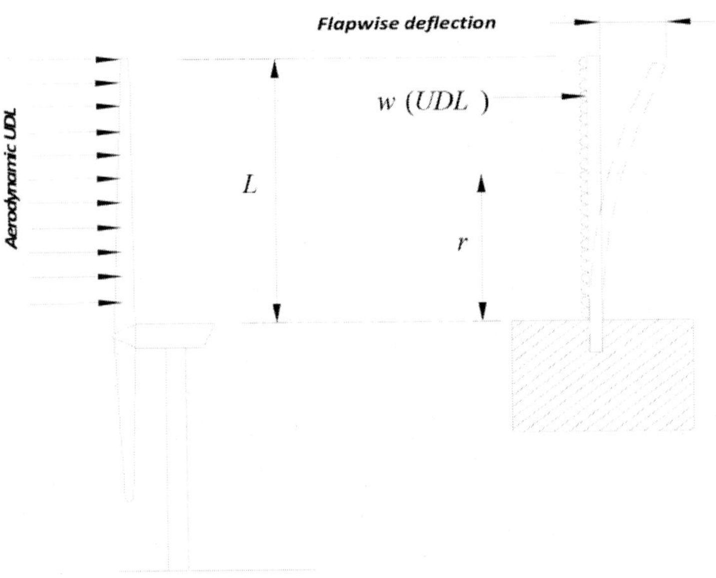

FIGURE 10: The blade modelled as a cantilever beam with uniformly distributed aerodynamic load.

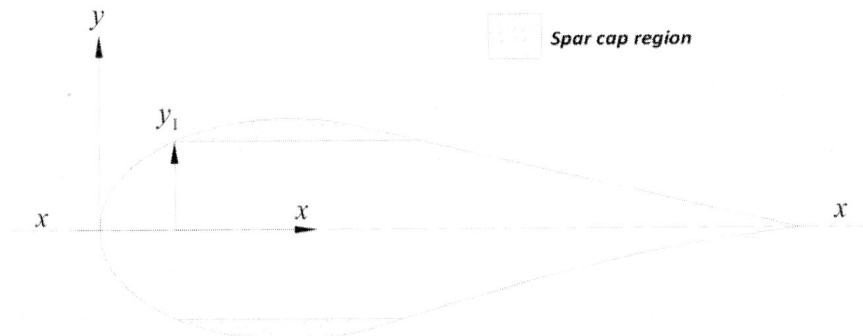

FIGURE 11: Flapwise bending about the axis xx.

$$I_{xx} = \iint (y - y_1)^2 \, dx \, dy \quad (5)$$

$$M = -\frac{1}{2}w(L - r)^2 \quad (6)$$

$$\frac{\sigma}{y} = \frac{M}{I} = \frac{E}{R} \quad (7)$$

Where L = total blade length, M = bending moment, w = UDL, r = radial distance from the hub, σ = stress, y = distance from the neutral axis, I = second moment of area, E = modulus of elasticity, and R = radius of curvature

When calculating the second moment of area [Equation (5)] it is apparent that increasing the distance from the central axis of bending gives a cubic increase. When substituted into the beam bending equation [Equation (7)], it can be seen that a squared decrease in material stress can be obtained by simply moving load bearing material away from the central plane of bending. It is therefore efficient to place load bearing material in the spar cap region of the blade at extreme positions from the central plane of bending (x) (Figure 11). This signifies why thick section aerofoils are structurally preferred, despite their aerodynamic deficiencies. This increase in structural efficiency can be used to minimise the use of structural materials and allow significant weight reductions [42]. The conflict between slender aerofoils for aerodynamic efficiency and thicker aerofoils for structural integrity is therefore apparent. Bending moments [Equation (6)] and therefore stress [Equation (7)] can be seen to increase towards the rotor hub. This signifies why aerofoil sections tend to increase in thickness towards the hub to maintain structural integrity.

1.6.5 EDGEWISE BENDING

The edgewise bending moment is a result of blade mass and gravity. Therefore this loading condition can be considered negligible for smaller

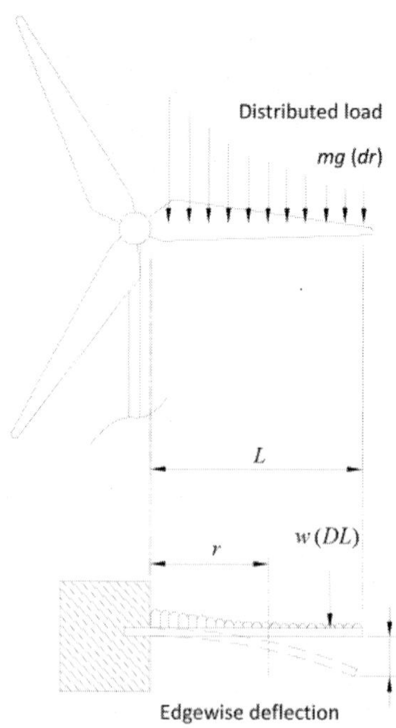

FIGURE 12: Gravitational load modelled as a cantilever beam.

blades with negligible blade mass [4]. Simple scaling laws dictate a cubic rise in blade mass with increasing turbine size. Therefore for increasing turbine sizes in excess of 70 m diameter, this loading case is said to be increasingly critical [4].

The bending moment is at its maximum when the blade reaches the horizontal position. In this case the blade may once again be modelled as a cantilever beam (Figures 12 and 13). The beam now has a distributed load which increases in intensity towards the hub as the blade and material thicknesses increase. The actual values for second moment of area, bending moments, material stress and deflections can be calculated in a similar procedure to flapwise bending (Section 6.4). It should be noted that in the edgewise loading condition, the plane of central bending is now normal to the chord line. For flapwise bending it is beneficial to concentrate load bearing material centrally in the spar cap region at extreme positions on the aerofoil profile, away from flapwise plane of bending (xx). This positioning is inefficient for edgewise bending as the centre of the spar cap is

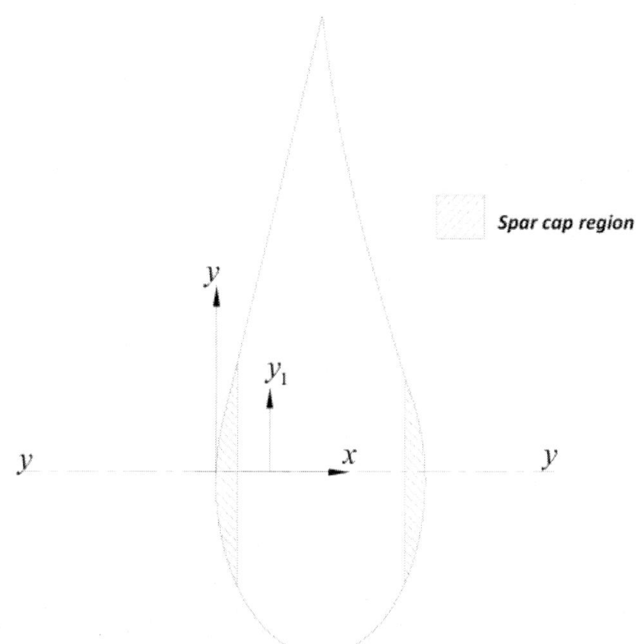

FIGURE 13: Edgewise bending about yy.

increasingly close to the central plane of bending (yy). Careful consideration is therefore giving to position structural material efficiently for both the flapwise and edgewise bending conditions [42].

1.6.6 FATIGUE LOADS

The major loading conditions applied to the blade are not static. Fatigue loading can occur when a material is subjected to a repeated non continuous load which causes the fatigue limit of the material to be exceeded. It is possible to produce a wind turbine blade capable of operating within the fatigue limit of its materials. However, such a design would require excessive amounts of structural material resulting in a heavy, large, expensive and inefficient blade. Fatigue loading conditions are therefore unavoidable in efficient rotor blade design.

Fatigue loading is a result of gravitational cyclic loads (Section 6.5) which are equal to the number of rotations throughout the lifetime of the turbine, typically 20 years. In addition smaller stochastic loads are created by the gusting wind contributing up to 1×10^9 cyclic loadings during the turbine lifetime [43]. Therefore the design of many wind turbine components maybe governed by fatigue rather than ultimate load [6]. Fatigue analysis and testing is required for both IEC [44] and DNV [40] certification [45].

1.6.7 STRUCTURAL BLADE REGIONS

The modern blade can be divided into three main areas classified by aerodynamic and structural function (Figure 14):

- The blade root. The transition between the circular mount and the first aerofoil profile—this section carries the highest loads. Its low relative wind velocity is due to the relatively small rotor radius. The low wind velocity leads to reduced aerodynamic lift leading to large chord lengths. Therefore the blade profile becomes excessively large at the rotor hub. The problem of low lift is compounded by the need to use excessively thick aerofoil sections to improve structural integrity at this load intensive region. Therefore the root region of the blade will typically consist of thick aerofoil profiles with low aerodynamic efficiency.

- The mid span. Aerodynamically significant—the lift to drag ratio will be maximised. Therefore utilising the thinnest possible aerofoil section that structural considerations will allow.
- The tip. Aerodynamically critical—the lift to drag ratio will be maximised. Therefore using slender aerofoils and specially designed tip geometries to reduce noise and losses. Such tip geometries are as yet unproven in the field [1], in any case they are still used by some manufacturers.

1.7 CONCLUSIONS

For reasons of efficiency, control, noise and aesthetics the modern wind turbine market is dominated by the horizontally mounted three blade design, with the use of yaw and pitch, for its ability to survive and operate under varying wind conditions. An international supply chain has evolved around this design, which is now the industry leader and will remain so for the immediate foreseeable future. During the evolution of this design many alternatives have been explored and have eventually declined in popularity. Manufacturers seeking greater cost efficiency have exploited the ability to scale the design, with the latest models reaching 164 m in diameter. The scale of investment in creating alternative designs of comparative size now ensures that new challengers to the current configuration are unlikely.

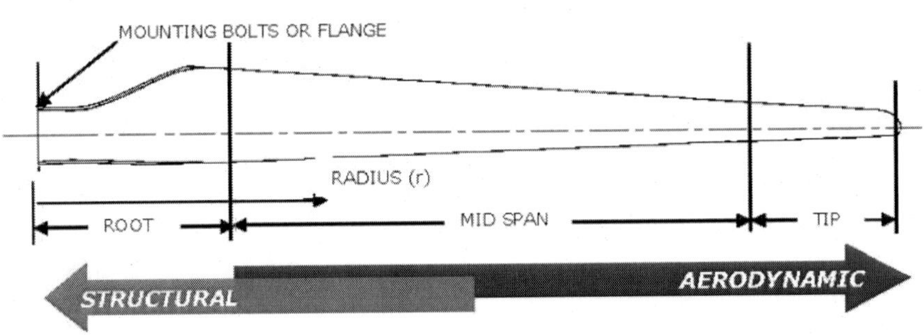

FIGURE 14: The three blade regions.

A comprehensive look at blade design has shown that an efficient blade shape is defined by aerodynamic calculations based on chosen parameters and the performance of the selected aerofoils. Aesthetics plays only a minor role. The optimum efficient shape is complex consisting of aerofoil sections of increasing width, thickness and twist angle towards the hub. This general shape is constrained by physical laws and is unlikely to change. However, aerofoil lift and drag performance will determine exact angles of twist and chord lengths for optimum aerodynamic performance.

A basic load analysis reveals that the blade can be modelled as a simple beam with a built in support at the hub end. A uniformly distributed load can be used to represent aerodynamic lift during operation. The increasing bending moment towards the support indicate that structural requirements will also determine blade shape especially in areas around the hub which require increased thickness.

Currently manufacturers are seeking greater cost effectiveness through increased turbine size rather than minor increases through improved blade efficiency. This is likely to change as larger models become problematic through construction, transport and assembly issues. Therefore, it is likely that the general shape will remain fixed and will increase in size until a plateau is reached. Minor changes to blade shape may then occur as manufacturers incorporate new aerofoils, tip designs and structural materials. A conflict of increased aerodynamic performance in slender aerofoils versus structural performance of thicker aerofoils is also evident.

REFERENCES

1. Hau, E. Wind Turbines, Fundamentals, Technologies, Application, Economics, 2nd ed.; Springer: Berlin, Germany, 2006.
2. Dominy, R.; Lunt, P.; Bickerdyke, A.; Dominy, J. Self-starting capability of a darrieus turbine. Proc. Inst. Mech. Eng. Part A J. Power Energy 2007, 221, 111–120.
3. Holdsworth, B. Green Light for Unique NOVA Offshore Wind Turbine, 2009. Available online: http://www.reinforcedplastics.com (accessed on 8 May 2012).
4. Gasch, R.; Twele, J. Wind Power Plants; Solarpraxis: Berlin, Germany, 2002.
5. Gorban, A.N.; Gorlov, A.M.; Silantyev, V.M. Limits of the turbine efficiency for free fluid flow. J. Energy Resour. Technol. Trans. ASME 2001, 123, 311–317.
6. Burton, T. Wind Energy Handbook; John Wiley & Sons Ltd.: Chichester, UK, 2011.
7. Hull, D.G. Fundamentals of Airplane Flight Mechanics; Springer: Berlin, Germany, 2007.

8. Anderson, D.; Eberhardt, S. Understanding Flight; McGraw-Hill: New York, NY, USA, 2001.
9. Yurdusev, M.A.; Ata, R.; Cetin, N.S. Assessment of optimum tip speed ratio in wind turbines using artificial neural networks. Energy 2006, 31, 2153–2161.
10. Duquette, M.M.; Visser, K.D. Numerical implications of solidity and blade number on rotor performance of horizontal-axis wind turbines. J. Sol. Energy Eng.-Trans. ASME 2003, 125, 425–432.
11. Oerlemans, S.; Sijtsma, P.; Lopez, B.M. Location and quantification of noise sources on a wind turbine. J. Sound Vib. 2006, 299, 869–883.
12. Chattot, J.J. Optimization of wind turbines using helicoidal vortex model. J. Sol. Energy Eng. Trans. ASME 2003, 125, 418–424.
13. Fuglsang, P.; Madsen, H.A. Optimization method for wind turbine rotors. J. Wind Eng. Ind. Aerodyn. 1999, 80, 191–206.
14. Jureczko, M.; Pawlak, M.; Mezyk, A. Optimisation of wind turbine blades. J. Mater. Proc. Technol. 2005, 167, 463–471.
15. Habali, S.M.; Saleh, I.A. Local design, testing and manufacturing of small mixed airfoil wind turbine blades of glass fiber reinforced plastics Part I: Design of the blade and root. Energy Convers. Manag. 2000, 41, 249–280.
16. Thresher, R.W.; Dodge, D.M. Trends in the evolution of wind turbine generator configurations and systems. Wind Energy 1998, 1, 70–86.
17. Gipe, P. The Wind Industrys Experience with Aesthetic Criticism. Leonardo 1993. 26, 243–248.
18. Chamberlain, D.E. The effect of avoidance rates on bird mortality predictions made by wind turbine collision risk models. Ibis 2006, 148, 198–202.
19. Maalawi, K.Y.; Badr, M.A. A practical approach for selecting optimum wind rotors. Renew. Energy 2003, 28, 803–822.
20. Griffiths, R.T. The effect of aerofoil charachteristics on windmill performance. Aeronaut. J. 1977, 81, 322–326.
21. Drela, M. XFoil; Massachusetts Institute of Technology: Cambridge, MA, USA, 2000.
22. Drela, M. Xfoil User Primer; Massachusetts Institute of Technology: Cambridge, MA, USA, 2001.
23. Timmer, W.A.; van Rooij, R.P.J.O.M. Summary of the Delft University wind turbine dedicated airfoils. J. Sol. Energy Eng. Trans. ASME 2003, 125, 488–496.
24. Abbott, I.H.; Doenhoff, A.V. Theory of Wind Sections; McGraw-Hill: London, UK, 1949.
25. Rooij, R.P.J.O.M.; Timmer, W. Roughness sensitivity considerations for thick rotor blade airfoils. J. Solar Energy Eng. Trans. ASME 2003, 125, 468–478.
26. Fuglsang, P.; Bak, C. Development of the Riso wind turbine airfoils. Wind Energy 2004, 7, 145–162.
27. Polinder, H. Comparison of direct-drive and geared generator concepts for wind turbines. IEEE Trans. Energy Convers. 2006, 21, 725–733.
28. Gupta, S.; Leishman, J.G. Dynamic stall modelling of the S809 aerofoil and comparison with experiments. Wind Energy 2006, 9, 521–547.
29. Stol, K.A.; Zhao, W.X.; Wright, A.D. Individual blade pitch control for the controls advanced research turbine (CART). J. Sol. Energy Eng. Trans. ASME 2006, 128, 498–505.

30. Bossanyi, E.A. Individual blade pitch control for load reduction. Wind Energy 2003, 6, 119–128.
31. Barlas T.K.; van Kuik, G.A.M. Review of state of the art in smart rotor control research for wind turbines. Prog. Aerosp. Sci. 2010, 46, 1–27.
32. Barlas, T.; Lackner, M. The Application of Smart Structures for Large Wind Turbine Rotor Blades. In Proceedings of the Iea Topical Expert Meeting; Delft University of Technology: Delft, The Netherlands, 2006.
33. Thor, S. The Application of Smart Structures for Large Wind Turbine Rotor Blades. In Proceedings of the IEA Topical Expert Meeting; Sandia National Labs: Alberquerque, NM, USA, 2008.
34. Kong, C.; Bang, J.; Sugiyama, Y. Structural investigation of composite wind turbine blade considering various load cases and fatigue life. Energy 2005, 30, 2101–2114.
35. Quarton, D.C. The Evolution of Wind Turbine Design Analysis—A Twenty Year Progress Review; Garrad Hassan and Partners Ltd.: Bristol, UK, 1998; pp. 5–24.
36. Ahlstrom, A. Emergency stop simulation using a finite element model developed for large blade deflections. Wind Energy 2006, 9, 193–210.
37. Kishinami, K. Theoretical and experimental study on the aerodynamic characteristics of a horizontal axis wind turbine. Energy 2005, 30, 2089–2100.
38. Brondsted, P.; Lilholt, H.; Lystrup, A. Composite materials for wind power turbine blades. Ann. Rev. Mater. Res. 2005, 35, 505–538.
39. Jensen, F.M. Structural testing and numerical simulation of a 34 m composite wind turbine blade. Compos. Struct. 2006, 76, 52–61.
40. Veritas, D.N. Design and Manufacture of Wind Turbine Blades, Offshore and Onshore Turbines; Standard DNV-DS-J102; Det Norske Veritas: Copenhagen, Denmark, 2010.
41. Case, J.; Chilver, A.H. Strength Of Materials; Edward Arnold Ltd.: London, UK, 1959.
42. Griffin, D.A.; Zuteck, M.D. Scaling of composite wind turbine blades for rotors of 80 to 120 meter diameter. J. Sol. Energy Eng. Trans. ASME 2001, 123, 310–318.
43. Shokrieh, M.M.; Rafiee, R. Simulation of fatigue failure in a full composite wind turbine blade. Compos. Struct. 2006, 74, 332–342.
44. Wind Turbines. Part 1: Design Requirements; BS EN 61400-1:2005; BSi British Standards: London, UK, January 2006.
45. Kensche, C.W. Fatigue of composites for wind turbines. Int. J. Fatigue 2006, 28, 1363–1374.

CHAPTER 2

A SHROUDED WIND TURBINE GENERATING HIGH OUTPUT POWER WITH WIND-LENS TECHNOLOGY

YUJI OHYA AND TAKASHI KARASUDANI

2.1 INTRODUCTION

For the application of an effective energy resource in the future, the limitation of fossil fuels is clear and the security of alternative energy sources is an important subject. Furthermore, due to concerns for environmental issues, i.e., global warming, etc., the development and application of renewable and clean new energy are strongly expected. Among others, wind energy technologies have developed rapidly and are about to play a big role in a new energy field. However, in comparison with the overall demand for energy, the scale of wind power usage is still small; especially, the level of development in Japan is extremely small. As for the reasons, various causes are conceivable. For example, the limited local area suitable for wind power plants, the complex terrain compared to that in European or North American countries and the turbulent nature of the local wind are pointed out. Therefore, the introduction of a new wind power system that

Originally printed under the terms of the Creative Commons Attribution License. Ohya Y and Karasudani T. A Shrouded Wind Turbine Generating High Output Power with Wind-lens Technology. Energies **2010**,3 (2010). pp. 634–649; doi:10.3390/en3040634.

produces higher power output even in areas where lower wind speeds and complex wind patterns are expected is strongly desired.

Wind power generation is proportional to the wind speed cubed. Therefore, a large increase in output is brought about if it is possible to create even a slight increase in the velocity of the approaching wind to a wind turbine. If we can increase the wind speed by utilizing the fluid dynamic nature around a structure or topography, namely if we can concentrate the wind energy locally, the power output of a wind turbine can be increased substantially. Although there have been several studies of collecting wind energy for wind turbines reported so far [1–7], it has not been an attractive research subject conventionally. Unique research that was carried out intensively in the past is the examination of a diffuser-augmented wind turbine (DAWT) by Gilbert et al. [2], Gilbert and Foreman [3], Igra [4] and others around 1980. In these studies, there was a focus on concentrating wind energy in a diffuser with a large open angle, a boundary layer controlled with several flow slots was employed to realize a flow that goes along the inside surface of the diffuser. Thus, the method of boundary layer control prevents pressure loss by flow separation and increases the mass flow inside the diffuser. Based on this idea, a group in New Zealand [5,6] developed the Vortec 7 diffuser augmented wind turbine. They used a multi-slotted diffuser to prevent separation within the diffuser. Bet and Grassmann [7] developed a shrouded wind turbine with a wing-profiled ring structure. It was reported that their DAWT showed an increase in power output by the wing system by a factor of 2.0, compared to the bare wind turbine. Although several other ideas have been reported so far, most of them do not appear to be reaching commercialization.

The present study, regarding the development of a wind power system with high output, aims at determining how to collect the wind energy efficiently and what kind of wind turbine can generate energy effectively from the wind. There appears hope for utilizing the wind power in a more efficient way. In the present study, this concept of accelerating the wind was named the "wind-lens" technology. For this purpose, we have developed a diffuser-type structure that is capable of collecting and accelerating the approaching wind. Namely, we have devised a diffuser shroud with a large brim that is able to increase the wind speed from approaching wind substantially by utilizing various flow characteristics, e.g., the generation of low pressure region by vortex formation, flow entrainment by vortices and so on, of the inner or peripheral flows of a diffuser shroud equipped with a brim. Although it adopts a diffuser-shaped structure surrounding a wind turbine like the others [1–7], the feature that distinguishes it from the others is a large brim attached at the exit of diffuser shroud. Furthermore, we placed a wind turbine inside the diffuser shroud equipped with a brim and evaluated the power output generated. As a result, the shrouded wind turbine equipped with a brimmed diffuser demonstrated power augmentation for a given turbine diameter and wind speed by a factor of about 4–5 compared to a standard micro wind turbine.

Furthermore, for the practical application to a small- and mid-size wind turbine, we have been developing a compact-type brimmed diffuser. The combination of a diffuser shroud and a brim is largely modified from the one with a long diffuser with a large brim. The compact "wind-lens turbines" showed power augmentation of 2–3 times as compared to a bare wind turbine. The application examples for a few projects are introduced.

2.2 DEVELOPMENT OF A COLLECTION-ACCELERATION DEVICE FOR WIND (DIFFUSER SHROUD EQUIPPED WITH A BRIM, CALLED "WIND-LENS")

2.2.1 SELECTION OF A DIFFUSER-TYPE STRUCTURE AS THE BASIC FORM

A large boundary-layer wind tunnel of the Research Institute for Applied Mechanics, Kyushu University, was used. It has a measurement section of 15 m long × 3.6 m wide × 2 m high with a maximum wind velocity of 30 m/s. Two types of hollow-structure models, a nozzle and a diffuser type, were tested (Figure 1). The distributions of wind velocity U and static pressure p along the central axis of the hollow-structure model were measured with an I-type hot-wire and a static-pressure tube. In the case of using a big hollow-structure model, paying attention to the blockage effect in the wind tunnel, we removed the ceiling and both side walls ranging

6 m in the center portion of the measurement section. Namely, we used our wind tunnel with an open-type test section to avoid the blockage effect. The smoke-wire technique was employed for the flow visualization experiment.

The experiments revealed that a diffuser-shaped structure can accelerate the wind at the entrance of the body, as shown in Figure 2 [8–10]. The reason is clarified through the flow visualization, as shown in Figure 3. Figure 3a,b shows the flows inside and outside the nozzle- and diffuser-type models. The flow is from left to right. As seen in the Figure 3(a), the wind tends to avoid the nozzle-type model, while the wind flows into the diffuser-type model as it is inhaled, as seen in Figure 3(b).

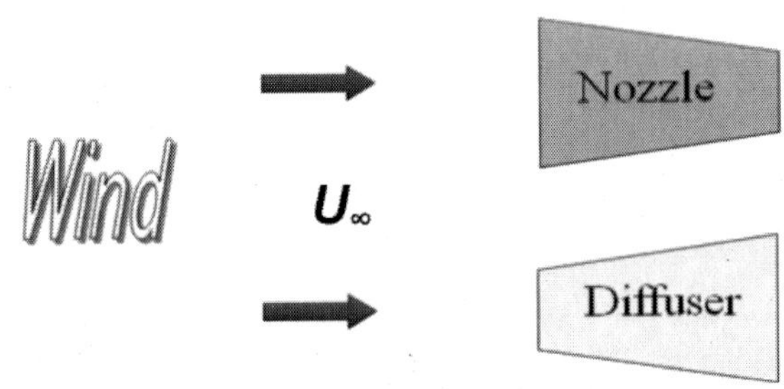

FIGURE 1: Two types of hollow structures.

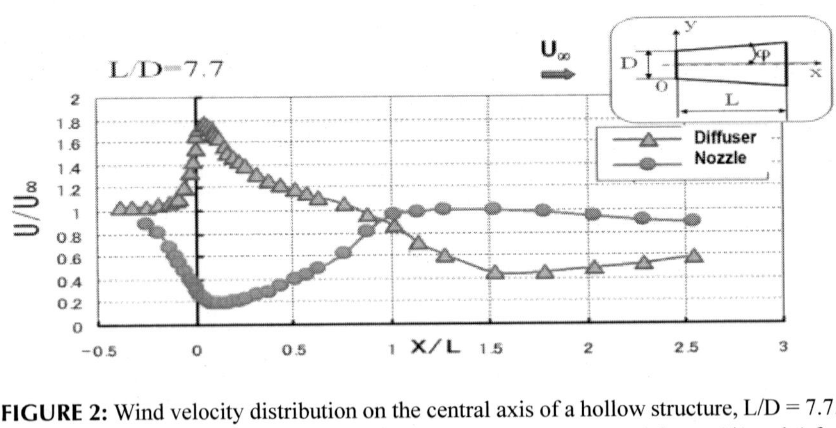

FIGURE 2: Wind velocity distribution on the central axis of a hollow structure, L/D = 7.7. The area ratios μ (outlet area/inlet area) of the hollow-structure models are 1/4 and 4 for the nozzle- and diffuser-type models, respectively.

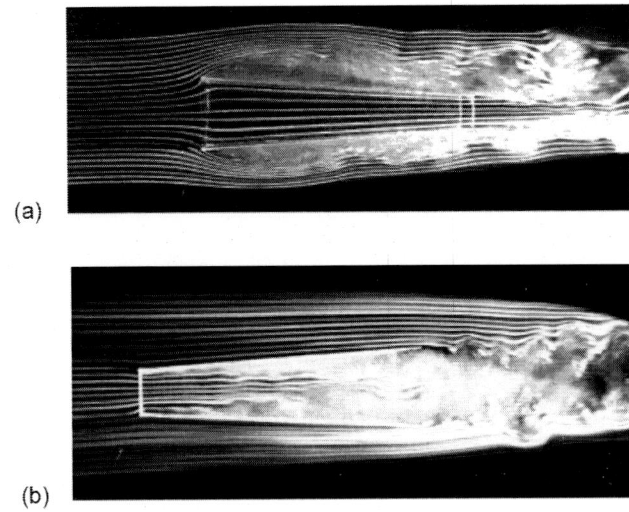

FIGURE 3: Flows around nozzle- and diffuser-type models. L/D = 7.7. The smoke flows from left to right. (a) Nozzle-type model, (b) Diffuser-type model.

2.2.2 IDEA OF A RING-TYPE PLATE WHICH FORMS VORTICES (IT IS CALLED "BRIM")

If we use a long type diffuser, the wind speed is accelerated further near the entrance of the diffuser. However, a long heavy structure is not preferable in the practical sense. Then we added a ring-type plate, called "brim", to the exit periphery of a short diffuser. The plate forms vortices behind it and generates a low-pressure region behind the diffuser, as shown in Figure 4. Accordingly, the wind flows into a low-pressure region, the wind velocity is accelerated further near the entrance of the diffuser. Figure 5 illustrates the flow mechanism. A shrouded wind turbine equipped with a brimmed diffuser came into existence in this way. We call it the "wind-lens turbine". Next we add an appropriate structure for entrance, called an inlet shroud, to the entrance of the diffuser with a brim. The inlet shroud makes wind easy to flow into the diffuser. Viewed as a whole, the collection-acceleration device consists of a venturi-shaped structure with a brim [8–10].

As for other parameters, we have examined the diffuser opening angle, the hub ratio, and the center-body length [10-12]. Then the optimal shape of a brimmed diffuser was found [10]. In addition, we are now examining the turbine blade shape in order to acquire higher output power. As illustrated in Figure 6, when a brimmed diffuser is applied (see also Figure 7), a remarkable increase in the output power coefficient (C_w=P/0.5ρAU^3, P: output power, A: swept area of turbine blades) of approximately 4–5 times that of a conventional wind turbine is achieved in field experiment. A simple theory for the present wind-lens turbine was given by Inoue et al [13]. The output performance is decided by the two factors of the pressure discovery coefficient of the diffuser shroud and the base pressure behind it.

2.2.3 CHARACTERISTICS OF A WIND TURBINE WITH BRIMMED DIFFUSER SHROUD

Figure 7 shows the first prototype of a wind turbine equipped with a brimmed diffuser shroud (rated power 500 W, rotor diameter of 0.7 m). The diffuser length of this model is 1.47 times as long as the diameter of the diffuser throat D (Lt = 1.47 D, for Lt, see Figure 8). The width of the brim is h = 0.5D. For the field experiment, some data are apparently

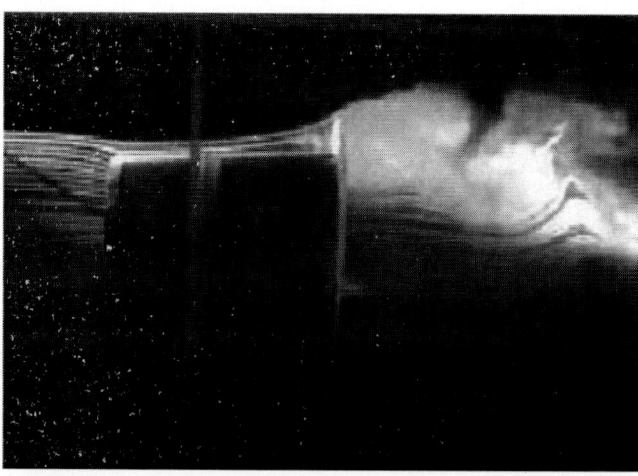

FIGURE 4: Flow around a circular-diffuser model with a brim. The smoke flows from left to right. L/D = 1.5. The area ratio μ (outlet area/inlet area) of the circular-diffuser model is 1.44. Karman vortices are formed behind brim.

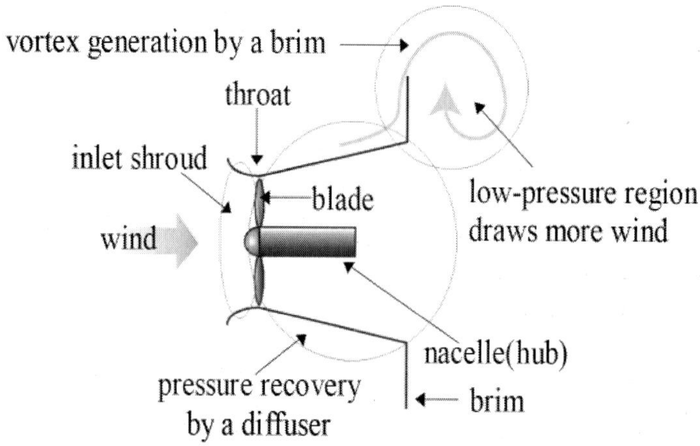

FIGURE 5: Flow around a wind turbine with brimmed diffuser (wind-lens).

significantly larger than the "wind tunnel-curve"; this is because the fluctuation in wind speed (variance component) in the field gives a higher value than the wind tunnel value at a constant wind speed. The important features of this wind turbine equipped with a brimmed diffuser shroud are as follows.

1. Four-fivefold increase in output power compared to conventional wind turbines due to concentration of the wind energy ("wind-lens" technology).
2. Brim-based yaw control: The brim at the exit of the diffuser makes wind turbines equipped with a brimmed diffuser rotate following the change in the wind direction, like a weathercock. As a result, the wind turbine automatically turns to face the wind.
3. Significant reduction in wind turbine noise: Basically, an airfoil section of the turbine blade, which gives the best performance in a low-tip speed ratio range, is chosen. Since the vortices generated from the blade tips are considerably suppressed through the interference with the boundary layer within the diffuser shroud, the aerodynamic noise is reduced substantially [14].

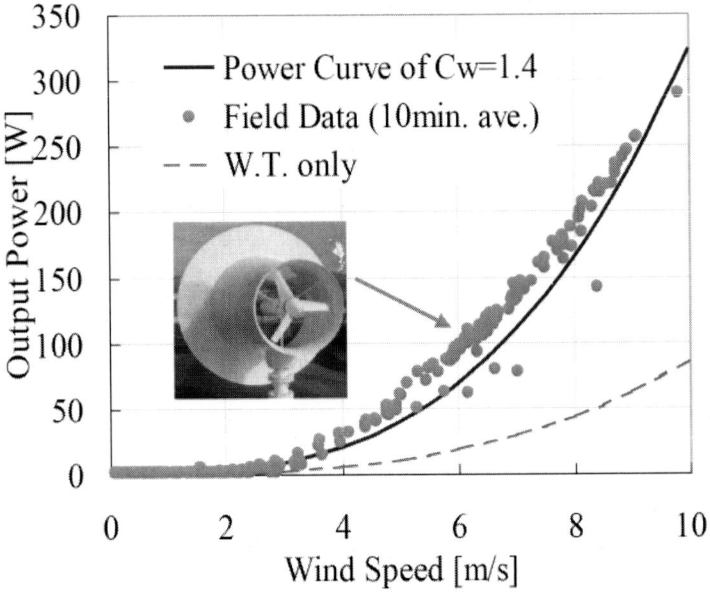

FIGURE 6: Field experiment of 500 W wind turbine with wind-lens. C_w is the power coefficient.

4. Improved safety: The wind turbine, rotating at a high speed, is shrouded by a structure and is also safe against damage from broken blades.
5. As for demerits, wind load to a wind turbine and structural weight are increased.

2.3 DEVELOPMENT OF A SHROUDED WIND TURBINE WITH COMPACT BRIMMED DIFFUSER

For the practical application to a small-size and mid-size wind turbine, we have been developing a compact-type brimmed diffuser. For the 500 W

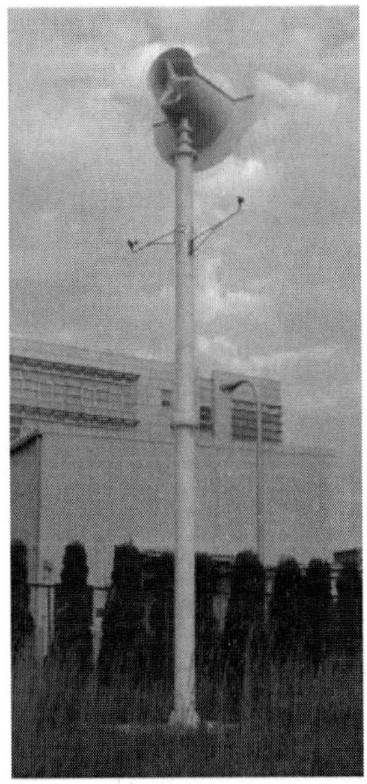

FIGURE 7: 500 W wind-lens turbine (rotor diameter 0.7 m).

wind-lens turbine, the length of brimmed diffuser L_t is 1.47D and still relatively long as a collection-acceleration structure for wind (for L_t, see Figure 8). If we apply this brimmed diffuser to a larger wind turbine in size, the wind load to this structure and the weight of this structure becomes severe problems. Therefore, to overcome the above-mentioned problems, we propose a very compact collection-acceleration structure (compact brimmed diffuser), the length L_t of which is quite short compared to D, i.e., $L_t < 0.4D$. We made a couple of compact brimmed diffusers in a range of a relatively short one to a very short one of $L_t = 0.1D - 0.4D$. We conducted the output performance test of those wind-lens turbines with compact brimmed diffuser in a wind tunnel experiment and also carried out a field test using a prototype 5 kW type model.

2.3.1 EXPERIMENTAL METHOD IN OUTPUT PERFORMANCE TEST OF COMPACT WIND-LENS TURBINES

For the size of the brimmed diffuser in the present experiment, the throat diameter D is 1020 mm and the rotor diameter is 1000 mm. Figure 8 shows a schematic of a compact wind-lens turbine. We made four types of diffusers called A-, B-, C- and S-type with different sectional shapes, as shown in Figure 9. Table 1 shows the length ratios L_t /D and the area ratios μ of (exit area)/(throat area) for each diffuser model. All diffuser types show almost the same L_t /D, but show different area ratio μ. For the S-type diffuser, it has a straight sectional shape such as the 500 W prototype. For the other three types, A to C, curved sectional shapes are adopted, as shown in Figure 9. For C-type, we adopted a cycloid curve for the sectional shape. Here, the hub ratio D_h/D is 13% and the tip clearance s is 10 mm.

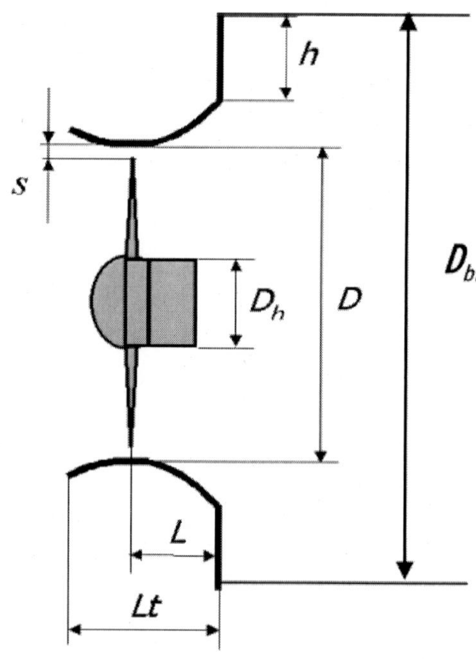

FIGURE 8: Schematic of wind-lens turbine.

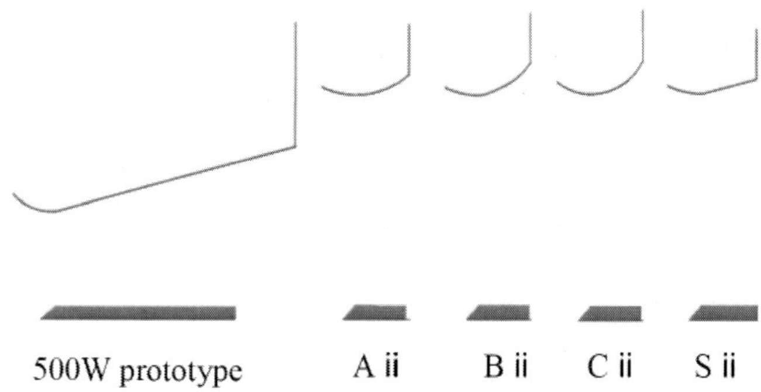

FIGURE 9: Sectional shapes of wind-lens.

TABLE 1: Parameters of wind-lens shapes

Diffuser	Prototype	Aii	Bii	Cii	Sii
Lt/D	1.470	0.225	0.221	0.221	0.225
μ	2.345	1.173	1.288	1.294	1.119

As for the experimental method, connecting a torque transducer (the rating 10 N·m) to the wind turbine and in the rear of it, an AC torque motor brake, was set for the loading. We measured the torque Q(N·m) and the rotational speed n (Hz) of the wind turbine in the condition that the turbine loading was gradually applied from zero. The calculated power output $P(W) = Q \times 2\pi n$ is shown as a performance curve. The shrouded wind turbine model with a compact brimmed diffuser was supported by a long straight bar from the measurement bed which was placed in the downstream and consists of a torque transducer, a revolution sensor and an AC torque motor brake, as shown in Figure 10. The approaching wind speed U_o was 8 m/s.

2.3.2 SELECTION OF COMPACT BRIMMED DIFFUSER SHAPE AS WIND-LENS

Figure 11 shows the experimental result of the shrouded wind turbines with compact brimmed diffuser of Aii, Bii, Cii and Sii type. The height of brim is 10%, i.e., h = 0.1D. The horizontal axis shows the blade tip speed ratio $\lambda = \omega r/Uo$, here ω is the angular frequency, $2\pi n$, and r is the radius of a wind turbine rotor (r = 0.58 m). The vertical axis shows the power coefficient C_w ($=P/(0.5\rho U_\infty^3 A)$, A is the rotor swept area, πr^2). The wind turbine blade with a specially designed wing-section contour was designed using a three-bladed wind turbine resulting in an optimum tip speed ratio of around 4.0. As shown in Figure 11, when a compact brimmed diffuser is applied, we have successfully achieved a remarkable increase in the output power coefficient approximately 1.9–2.4 times as large as a bare wind turbine. Namely, the C_w is 0.37 for a bare wind turbine, on the other hand, the C_w is 0.7–0.88 for a wind turbine with a compact brimmed diffuser. The experimental results shown in Figure 11 were obtained under the same wind speed and the swept area of a wind turbine.

First, we compare Aii type with Sii type in Figure 11. Both types have an almost same area ratio μ. The C_w of Aii is higher than Sii. It means that the curved sectional shape is preferable to the straight one. Furthermore, it is noted that the Bii and Cii types show higher C_w compared to Aii type. It means that if the boundary-layer flow along the inside wall of curved dif-

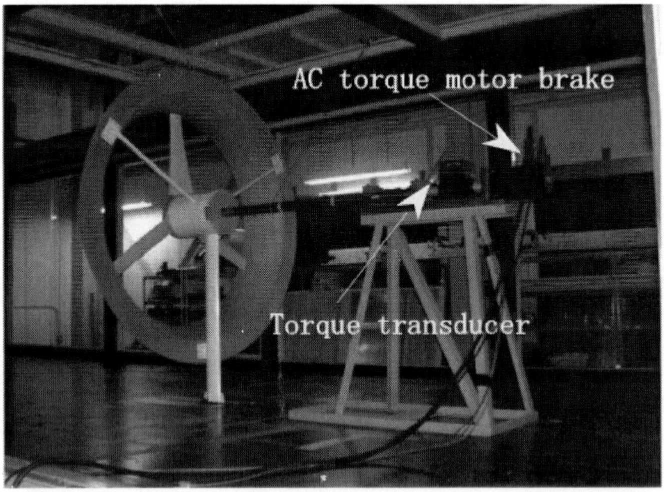

FIGURE 10: Output performance test of a wind-lens turbine in a wind tunnel.

fuser dose not show a large separation, Bii and Cii types, which have a larger area ratio μ compared to that of Aii, are suitable to a compact diffuser.

If we adopt the swept area A* instead of A (due to the rotor diameter), where A* is the circular area due to the brim diameter D_{brim} at diffuser exit, the output coefficient C_w* based on A* becomes 0.48–0.54 for those compact wind-lens turbines. It is still larger than the power coefficient C_w (around 0.4) of conventional wind turbines. It means that the compact wind-lens turbines clearly show higher efficiency compared to conventional wind turbines, even if the rotor diameter of a conventional wind turbine is extended to the brim diameter.

2.3.3 OUTPUT POWER OF WIND-LENS TURBINE WITH THE COMPACT DIFFUSER LENGTH

From the experimetal result shown in Figure 11, we discuss C-type diffuser as the compact collection-acceleration structure. For the next step, we investigated the length effect of the C-type diffuser on the output per-

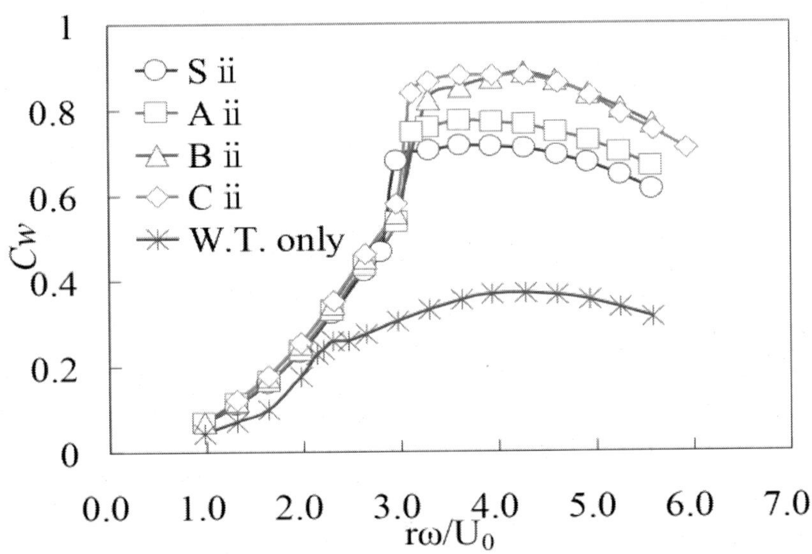

FIGURE 11: Power coefficients C_w of various wind-lens turbines vs. tip-speed ratio $\lambda = \omega r/U_o$. The brim height is 10%, i.e., h = 0.1D.

formance of wind-lens turbines. We prepared four kinds of C-type diffusers from C0 to Ciii, as described in Table 2. Figure 12 shows the result of output performance with the four C-type diffuser lengths. The brim height is 10%, i.e., h = 0.1D. Figure 13 also shows the variation of $C_{w,max}$ with the diffuser length Lt /D, here $C_{w,max}$ is the maximum value of C_w in the output performance curves as is shown in Figure 12. As expected, the $C_{w,max}$ value becomes smaller as the diffuser length Lt /D becomes smaller. However, when the brim height is larger than 10%, i.e., in case of h > 0.1D, the C_w of a wind-lens turbine with C0-type diffuser shows almost two-fold increase compared to a bare wind turbine and the one with Ciii-type diffuser shows 2.6-times increase. Thus, we can expect a 2–3-times increase in output performance, even if we use a very compact brimmed diffuser as the wind-lens structure.

TABLE 2: Parameters of C-type wind-lens. For C0–Ciii diffuser, see Figure 13.

Diffuser	C0	Ci	Cii	Ciii
Lt/D	0.1	0.137	0.221	0.371
μ	1.138	1.193	1.294	1.555

2.3.4 FIELD EXPERIMENT

As described above, one of the merits of wind-lens turbine is the brim-based yaw control. Namely, owing to the brim, the wind-lens turbine automatically turns to face the wind. However, for the comapct wind-lens structure, it is difficult to realize the wind-lens turbine as the upwind-type wind turbine. Therefore, we made a prototype compact wind-lens turbine as a downwind-type.

For the 5 kW downwind-type wind turbine, we selected the Cii-type diffuser (Lt /D = 0.22) as the wind-lens structure. The brim height is 10%, i.e., h = 0.1D. Here, D is 2560 mm and the rotor diameter is 2500 mm. Figure 14 shows the prototype 5 kW wind-lens turbine. We conducted a field experiment using this 5 kW wind turbine. Figure 15 shows the result of performance test on a windy day. The field data are plotted as 1 minute average data. The power curve is plotted along the C_w = 1.0 curve and

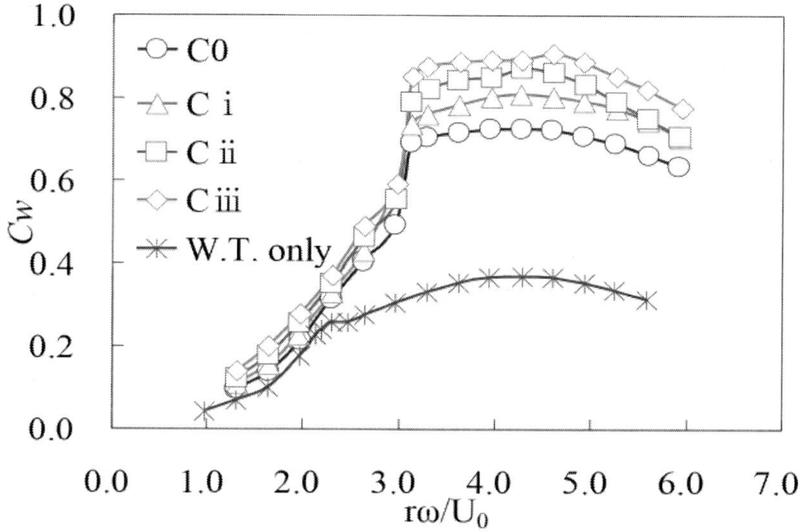

FIGURE 12: Power coefficients C_w of wind-lens turbines with C-type wind-lens (h = 0.1D). For C0–Ciii diffuser, see Figure 13.

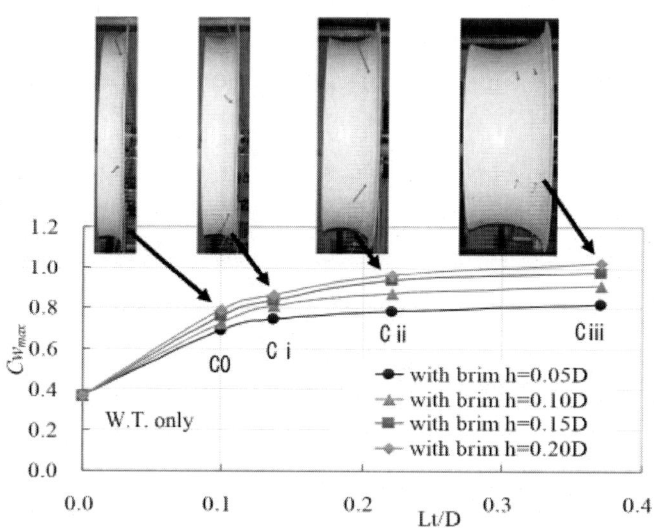

FIGURE 13: Maximum power coefficient $C_{w,max}$ versus C-type wind-lens length.

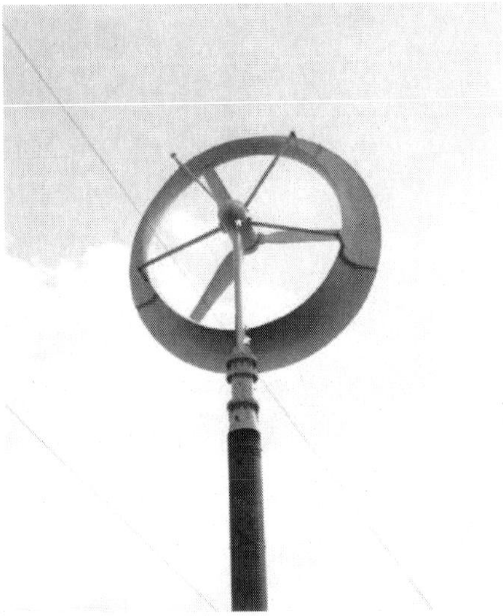

FIGURE 14: 5 kW wind-lens turbine (rotor diameter 2.5 m), downwind type

the high output performance of the present wind-lens turbine is demonstrated. We obtained 2.5-times increase in output power as compared to conventional (bare) wind turbines, due to concentration of the wind energy. Adopting the reference area A*, where A* is the circular area due to the brim diameter Dbrim at diffuser exit, the output coefficient C_w* based on A* reaches 0.54 for the present compact wind-lens turbines.

2.4 APPLICATION OF 5 KW WIND-LENS TURBINES FOR SUPPLYING STABLE ELECTRICITY TO AN IRRIGATION PLANT IN CHINA

Northwest China is an area facing deepening global environmental problems. To stop desertification and to turn the land into green land, irrigation and greenery projects began by capitalizing on the vast wind energy as a power source in the northwest, as shown in Figure 16. A small wind-lens turbine, which can be moved and installed easily, is the best means of power generation in this area without power grid infrastructure. The highly efficient wind-lens turbines offering the great small windmill per-

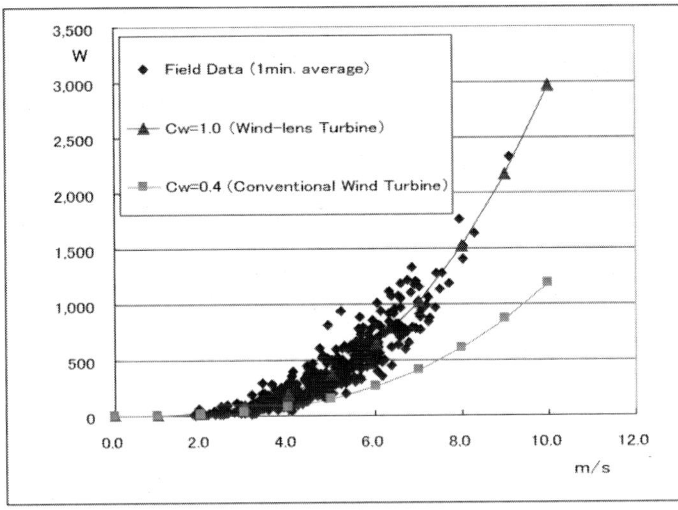

FIGURE 15: Field experiment of 5 kW wind-lens turbine. C_w is the power coefficient.

formance, developed by the authors' group, were improved, remodeled and enlarged through technological development for the application to a desert area. Six units of 5 kW wind-lens turbines were installed to build a wind farm for irrigation, and their effectiveness for the greenery project has been examined. Thus, a plant was constructed for pumping irrigation system by building a network of distributed power sources, ensuring that micro-grids will stably supply electric power by combining the network and power storage technology using batteries. This plant initiated to implement tree planting and greening the desert, and its effectiveness will be examined.

2.5 EFFICIENT UTILIZATION OF WIND ENERGY ON THE SEASHORE IN AN URBAN CITY

Three 5 kW wind-lens turbines have been recently installed in a seashore park in Fukuoka city, Japan. Fukuoka city faces the sea in the north, as shown in Figure 17. Since relatively strong winds are often observed in the winter season, Fukuoka city and our Kyushu University planned to make a collaborative research to install small wind-lens turbines, examining the effectiveness as a distributed power plant. Figure 17 shows the seaside park where the wind-lens turbines were installed. North is located in the upper side in this figure. In parallel with field measurements using wind poles, to implement the micro-siting for wind turbines, we carried out a numerical simulation of wind pattern over this complex area using RIAM-COMPACT [15], which is a calculation code based on a LES turbulence model. We assume the northern prevailing wind, say, a sea breeze. Figure 18 shows the calculation domain, extending 2800 m in the north-south direction (x-direction), 3500 m in the east-west direction (y-direction) and 900 m in the vertical direction (z-direction). The inflow condition is 1/7 power law in the vertical direction. The number of grid points is 161 × 201 × 51. The grid resolution is $\Delta x = \Delta y = 17.5$ m in horizontal directions and $\Delta z_{min} = 1$ m in the vertical direction, concentrating towards the ground. The Reynolds number based on the highest building h in the calculation domain is Re = 10,000. Figure 19 shows the result of the wind pattern at a height of 15 m, which is the hub height of small wind-lens turbines. We can see the accelerated areas around the entrance of a river and decelerated areas due to the high buildings near the shoreline. Judging from this result, we selected a suitable site, which is near the entrance of the large river in the left-hand side of Figure 17. Thus, three 5 kW wind-lens turbines were installed, as seen in Figure 20.

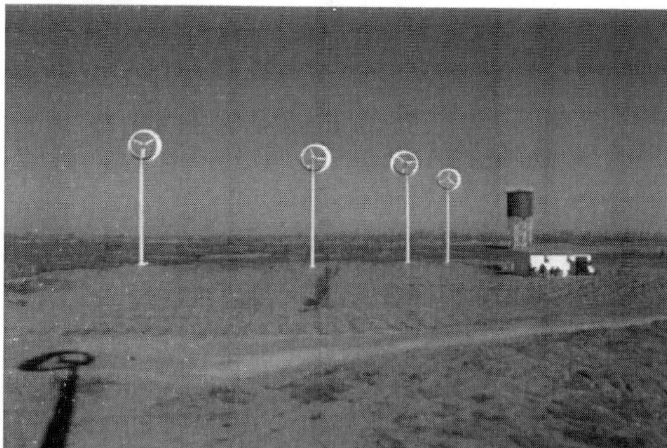

FIGURE 16: An irrigation-greenery plant using wind energy (5 kW wind-lens turbine farm) in a desert area in northwest China.

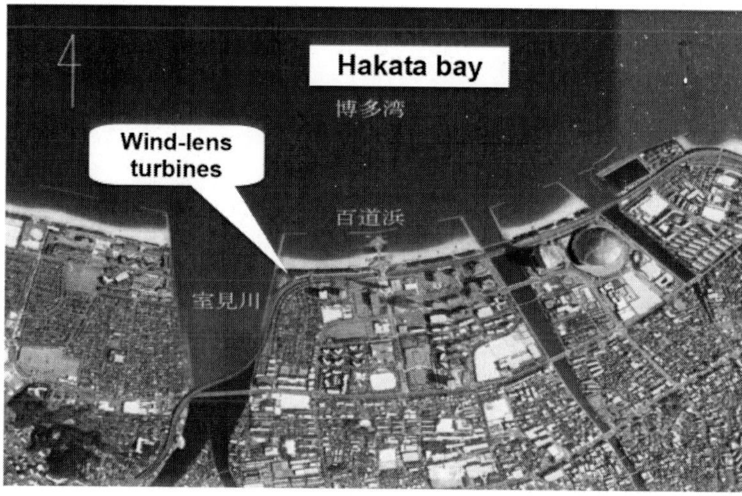

FIGURE 17: Seashore in Fukuoka city, where a few rivers are seen.

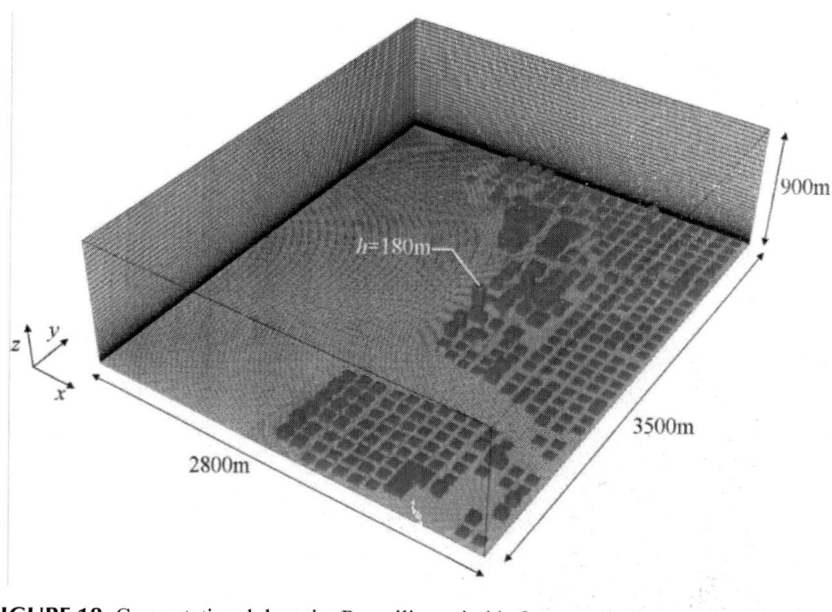

FIGURE 18: Computational domain. Prevailing wind is from north along x-direction. The inflow condition is 1/7 power law. The number of grid points is 161 × 201 × 51. The grid resolution is $\Delta x = \Delta y = 17.5$ m in horizontal directions and $\Delta z_{min} = 1$ m in the vertical direction. The Reynolds number based on the highest building h is Re = 10,000 in the calculation.

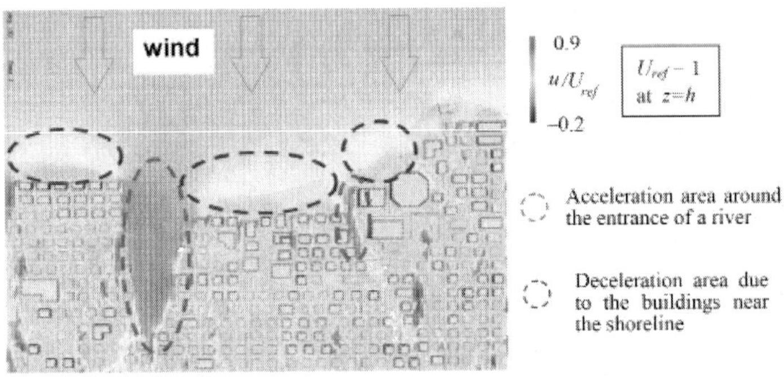

FIGURE 19: Result of numerical prediction of wind pattern at a height of 15 m for the seashore shown in Figures 17 and 18, using the RIAM-COMPACT.

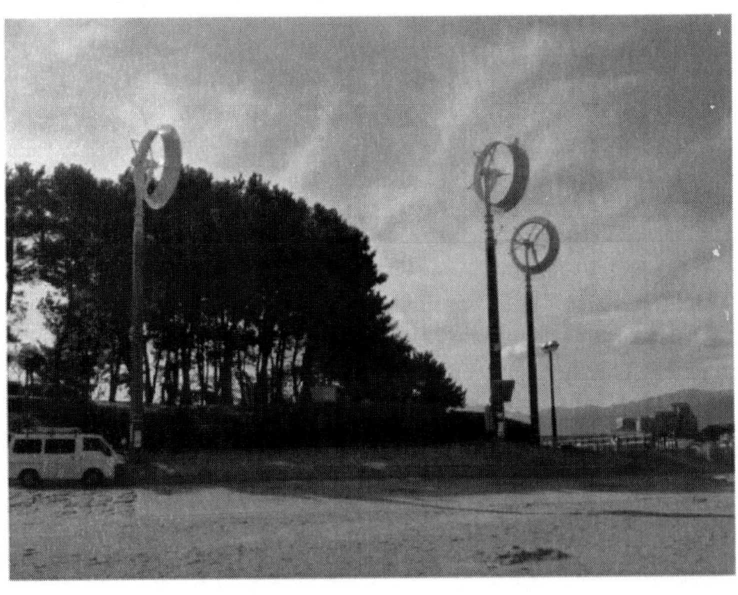

FIGURE 20: 5 kW Wind-lens turbines in a seashore park in Fukuoka city, Japan.

2.6 CONCLUSIONS

A collection-acceleration devise for wind, “the brimmed diffuser”, which shrouds a wind turbine, was developed. Significant increase in the output power of a micro-scale wind turbine was obtained. With a relatively long diffuser (L_t = 1.47D), a remarkable increase in the output power of approximately 4–5-times that of a conventional wind turbine is achieved. This is because a low-pressure region due to a strong vortex formation behind the broad brim draws more mass flow to the wind turbine inside the diffuser.

For the purpose of the practical application to a small- and mid-size wind turbine, we developed a very compact brimmed diffuser (wind-lens structure). Using this compact brimmed diffuser, we achieved two-three-fold increase in output power as compared to conventional (bare) wind turbines, due to concentration of the wind energy. We are now developing a wind-lens turbine of 100 kW at the rated wind speed of 12 m/s. The rotor diameter will be 12.8 m, which is much smaller than a conventinal wind turbine of the same rated power; two-thirds the size.

Incidentally, if we adopt the swept area A* instead of A (due to the rotor diameter), where A* is the circular area due to the brim diameter Dbrim at diffuser exit, the output coefficient C_w* based on A* becomes 0.48–0.54 for those compact wind-lens turbines. It is still larger than the power coefficient C_w (around 0.4) of conventional wind turbines. It means that the compact wind-lens turbines clearly show higher efficiency compared to conventional wind turbines, even if the rotor diameter of a conventional wind turbine is extended to the brim diameter.

For the examination of practical application, an international project and a local project using 5 kW wind-lens turbines were initiated. Six units of 5 kW wind-lens turbines were installed to build a wind farm for an irrigation plant in a desert area in northwest China, and their effectiveness for the greenery project has been examined. Three 5 kW wind-lens turbines have been recently installed in seashore in Fukuoka city, Japan, aiming at the efficient utilization of wind energy.

REFERENCES

1. Lilley, G.M.; Rainbird, W.J. A Preliminary Report on the Design and Performance of Ducted Windmills; Report No. 102; College of Aeronautics: Cranfield, UK, 1956.
2. Gilbert, B.L.; Oman, R.A.; Foreman, K.M. Fluid dynamics of diffuser-augmented wind turbines. J. Energy 1978, 2, 368–374.
3. Gilbert, B.L.; Foreman, K.M. Experiments with a diffuser-augmented model wind turbine. Trans. ASME, J. Energy Resour. Technol. 1983, 105, 46–53.
4. Igra, O. Research and development for shrouded wind turbines. Energ. Conv. Manage. 1981, 21, 13–48.
5. Phillips, D.G.; Richards, P.J.; Flay, R.G.J. CFD modelling and the development of the diffuser augmented wind turbine. In Proceedings of the Comp. Wind Engineer, Birmingham, UK, 2000, pp. 189–192.
6. Phillips, D.G.; Flay, R.G.J.; Nash, T.A. Aerodynamic analysis and monitoring of the Vortec 7 diffuser augmented wind turbine. IPENZ Trans. 1999, 26, 3–19.
7. Bet, F.; Grassmann, H. Upgrading conventional wind turbines. Renew. Energy 2003, 28, 71–78.
8. Ohya, Y.; Karasudani, T.; Sakurai, A. Development of high-performance wind turbine with a brimmed diffuser. J. Japan Soc. Aeronaut. Space Sci. 2002, 50, 477–482 (in Japanese).
9. Ohya, Y.; Karasudani, T.; Sakurai, A. Development of high-performance wind turbine with a brimmed diffuser, Part 2. J. Japan Soc. Aeronaut. Space Sci. 2004, 52, 210–213 (in Japanese).
10. Ohya, Y.; Karasudani, T.; Sakurai, A.; Abe, K.; Inoue, M. Development of a shrouded wind turbine with a flanged diffuser. J. Wind Eng. Ind. Aerodyn. 2008, 96, 524–539.
11. Abe, K.; Ohya, Y. An investigation of flow fields around flanged diffusers using CFD. J. Wind Eng. Ind. Aerodyn. 2004, 92, 315–330.
12. Abe, K.; Nishida, M.; Sakurai, A.; Ohya, Y.; Kihara, H.; Wada, E.; Sato, K. Experimental and numerical investigations of flow fields behind a small-type wind turbine with flanged diffuser. J. Wind Eng. Ind. Aerodyn. 2005, 93, 951–970.
13. Inoue, M; Sakurai, A.; Ohya, Y. A simple theory of wind turbine with brimmed diffuser. Turbomach. Int. 2002, 30, 46–51(in Japanese).
14. Abe, K.; Kihara, H.; Sakurai, A.; Nishida. M.; Ohya, Y.; Wada, E.; Sato, K. An experimental study of tip-vortex structures behind a small wind turbine with a flanged diffuser. Wind Struct. 2006, 9, 413–417.
15. Uchida, T.; Ohya, Y. Micro-siting technique for wind turbine generators by using large-eddy simulation. J. Wind Eng. Ind. Aerodyn. 2008, 96, 2121–2138.

CHAPTER 3

ECOMOULDING OF COMPOSITE WIND TURBINE BLADES USING GREEN MANUFACTURING RTM PROCESS

BRAHIM ATTAF

3.1 INTRODUCTION

In modern manufacturing industry of wind turbine blades [1], fibre-reinforced composite materials are chosen among other available engineering materials because of their significant and attractive advantages in terms of stiffness- and strength-to-weight ratio, thermal and chemical resistance properties, coupled with material cost effectiveness [2]. In addition to the economic advantage and technical-quality efficiency, further ecological aspects are still required in order to green up the moulding processes and this after an appropriate selection of matrix resin and fibre materials that are answering questions related to environmental and safety issues. These ecological aspects are based on balanced key criteria characterized mainly by a comprehensive consideration of environmental preservation and health protection besides quality assurance [3–5]; all of which must provide healthier, safe, clean, and sustainable process. Within this environmentally mindful context, the closed mould process provides an alter-

This chapter was originally published under the Creative Commons Attribution License. Attaf B. Ecomoulding of Composite Wind Turbine Blades Using Green Manufacturing RTM Process. ISRN Materials Science ***2012*** *(2012). http://dx.doi.org/10.5402/2012/734328.*

native solution to these requirements and satisfies the condition of green design method (i.e., ecodesign).

Further to that, the advantages achieved by the green moulding processes (e.g., closed mould process) with regard to other traditional moulding processes (e.g., open mould process) are performed at three levels of environmental consciousness, which of these focused on (i) the improvement of competitiveness and productivity via innovative engineering approaches, (ii) the minimization of energy consumption, and (iii) the reduction of emission levels via alternative solutions.

This new mode of composite manufacturing can greatly enhance the development of ecoefficient and reliable moulding processes and can therefore help boost potential development level for industrial wind energy field at short, medium, and long term. Among these closed-moulding processes, the most familiar one is the resin transfer moulding (RTM) process [6]. The present study will focus on techniques and formulation of resin flow in an anisotropic fibrous medium. Although some background analysis techniques of the state-of-the-art related to this subject can be found in the literature, [7] has addressed some very important research studies on the flow and rheology in polymer composites manufacturing.

By adopting the strategy in the context to go green can provide a sustainable moulding process which may reinforce the technological programme of Wind Energy Roadmap [1] and may help composite wind turbine blades manufacturers to achieve the following key ecodesign aims: (i) reduction of VOC emissions, (ii) use of nontoxic chemicals, (iii) use of no carcinogenic substances, (iv) generation of gelcoats with low emission of odours, and so forth.

With this objective as a key target, a further aim of this study is to send a strong message to nongreen composite companies to encourage them to join the green movement by setting up new strategies to reform the old manufacturing practices.

In one hand, this ecoaction will provide sustainable methods to develop new products with very cost-effective way for wind energy activities; while on the other hand, it will play a key role in stimulating innovation, creativity, and competitiveness in the worldwide industry of wind turbine blades.

3.2 METHODOLOGY OF ECOMOULDING

The current scientific research investigation is directed towards a methodology of analysis to provide an ecoefficient moulding process that minimizes environmental impact and ensures health protection whilst maintaining quality assurance criterion. This ecocompatible solution can help designers and analysts to assess and improve environmental and health aspects.

3.2.1 CONCEPT OF ECOMOULDING

The diagram shown in Figure 1 represents the ecomoulding model as an interaction between quality, health, and environment aspects. As it can be seen from Figure 1, this interaction yields a certain number of subsets. However, only subset $\overset{\therefore}{F}$ (hereafter denoted as $F_{\therefore}$) is fulfilling the required condition of ecomoulding. The three dots ($\therefore$) above the character "F" are only a brief description of the diagram illustrated in Figure 1, showing interaction between health, quality, and environment aspects. In other terms, the three dots represent the three pillars that characterize the basic elements of the sustainable development concept [8].

3.2.2 APPLICATION OF PROBABILITY APPROACH

To evaluate the number of chances providing the realization of the event $F_{\therefore}$ (subset of the event), it is necessary to use the notion of probability. Therefore, the event $F_{\therefore}$ and the associated probability, denoted , can be written respectively as [9]

$$\overset{\therefore}{F} = Q \cap H \cap E \tag{1}$$

$$P\left(\overset{\therefore}{F}\right) = P(Q \cap H \cap E) \tag{2}$$

According to the dependency of sets Q, H, and E and the rules of multiplication in the probability theory, (2) can be written as follows:

$$P\left(\frac{\therefore}{F}\right) = P(Q)\times P_Q(H)\times P_{Q\cap H}(E) \tag{3}$$

As the moulding process depends on the probability value expressed by (3), it is convenient to assign to each of Q, H, and E aspects a specific coefficient representing the probability of approval. In the searched case, it may therefore be considered that

1. $\alpha = P(Q)$ is an eco-coefficient representing the probability of approval in terms of quality assurance;
2. $\beta = P_Q(H)$ is an eco-coefficient representing the probability of approval with regard to health protection known that quality is achieved;
3. $\gamma = P_{Q\cap H}(E)$ is an eco-coefficient representing the probability of approval with regard to environmental preservation, known that health and quality are achieved.

The condition to green up the moulding process (subset $F_{\therefore}$ as shown in Figure 1) is performed by considering the mathematical product of the above-mentioned eco-coefficients. For notation simplicity, the quantity obtained by the rule of multiplication may be represented by a single variable called "ecofactor" and denoted by the Greek letter λ.

According to this approach, (3) can therefore be written as

$$\lambda = \alpha\times\beta\times\gamma \tag{4}$$

This ecofactor is considered to be as a key performance indicator (KPI). It is made for the purpose of discussion and analysis and will be used to provide better assessment of Q-H-E performance in relation to the moulding process. For instance, if the ecofactor λ approaches unity (100%), the process used for moulding is fully satisfying the green design requirements and ensuring its sustainability. However, if the ecofactor λ

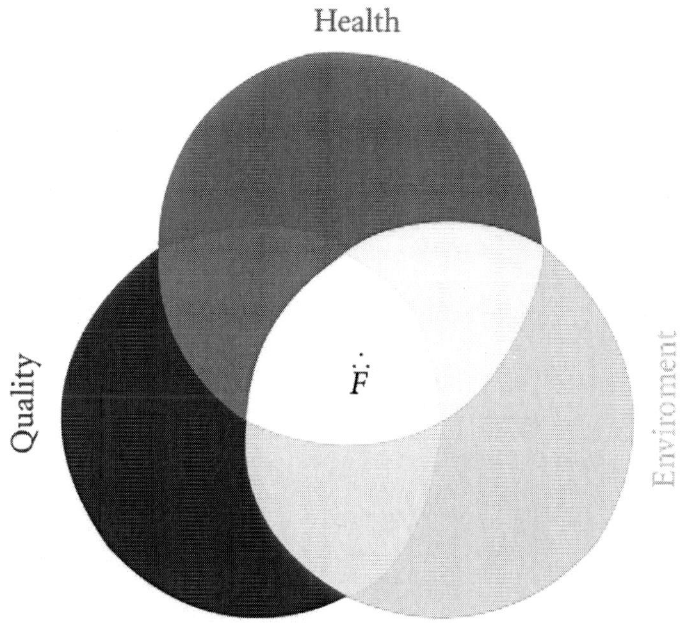

FIGURE 1: Model of ecomoulding process.

is not close to the target value required by sustainability standards, it is recommended to search for possible new alternatives that provide new eco-coefficients and then new derived ecofactor. Table 1 recapitulates the assessment operation for different intervals and shows a rating satisfaction measure in the form of colour gauges.

3.3 BLADE STRUCTURE, MATERIAL, AND MECHANICAL CHARACTERIZATION

3.3.1 SANDWICH STRUCTURE

The design and selection procedure of the airfoil section are discussed in [10] by considering the basic aerodynamic theory. In the current research study, the airfoil section of the typical blade is a sandwich structure separated by a thick lighter element called core (polystyrene). The upper and lower surfaces (skin of the blade) are manufactured from glass-fibre reinforced laminates. To further increase the longitudinal blade stiffness, two composite longitudinal stiffeners were incorporated into the internal structure of the sandwich, as shown in Figure 2. The stiffeners are located at 25% C and 55% C with regard to the blade leading edge, where the letter C characterizes the chord of the considered airfoil (see Figure 2). Stiffeners are made of the same material used for upper and lower laminated surfaces.

TABLE 1: Probability colour gauges for different eco-factor values of λ.

Interval	Assessment	Gauge
$\lambda_5 \leq \lambda \leq 1$	Excellent	
$\lambda_4 \leq \lambda < \lambda_5$	Very good	
$\lambda_3 \leq \lambda < \lambda_4$	Good	
$\lambda_2 \leq \lambda < \lambda_3$	Fair	
$\lambda_1 \leq \lambda < \lambda_2$	Poor	
$0 \leq \lambda < \lambda_1$	Very poor	

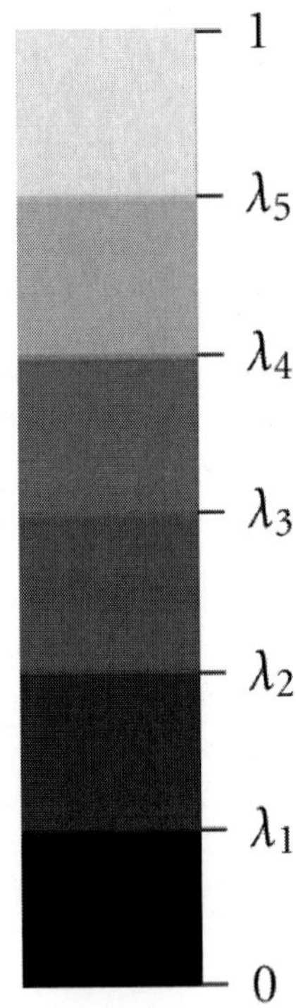

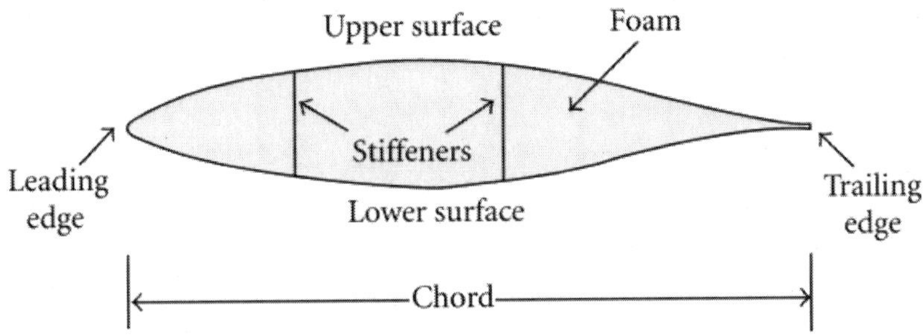

FIGURE 2: Airfoil-shaped cross section.

3.3.2 MECHANICAL CHARACTERISTICS

Blade structure requires high strength and high stiffness in the longitudinal directions and this dictates that the majority of fibres should be uniaxially (or nearly uniaxially) aligned but that some hoop strength should also be provided. The moduli of elasticity for layers parallel and perpendicular to the fibres are denoted by E_1 and E_2, respectively. The blade skin is manufactured by several stacking sequences of unidirectional E-glass fibre (UD 900 g/mm^2), orientated principally in the 0° direction (along the blade length) with some layers orientated at ±45°.

The properties of the composites were based on 60% fibre volume fraction. The material properties are listed in Table 2.

TABLE 2: Composite material properties.

Material	Material properties				
	E_1(MPa)	E_2(MPa)	G_{12}(MPa)	v_{12}	Density (kg·m^{-3})
UD99/Epoxy	25350	6265	2235	0.35	4.0

3.3.3 GEOMETRY AND DIMENSIONS

Figure 3 illustrates the principal lateral dimensions of a wind turbine blade. The blade structure was divided into four zones with different thicknesses;

thus four material zones were considered. Each material is affected to the corresponding zone. On the other hand and according to stress distributions along the blade length, a decrease in thickness from blade root to free end was considered for each zone. In addition, a fifth material zone was considered for the two internal stiffeners; each one has a thickness of 3 mm. Figure 3 illustrates how the different zones of materials and their positions relative to the blade structure were sectioned. These are defined as follows:

1. Zone A corresponds to the upper or lower surface area with a thickness of 12 mm.
2. Zone B corresponds to the upper or lower surface area with a thickness of 9 mm.
3. Zone C corresponds to the upper or lower surface area with a thickness of 6 mm.
4. Zone D corresponds to the upper or lower surface area with a thickness of 3 mm.

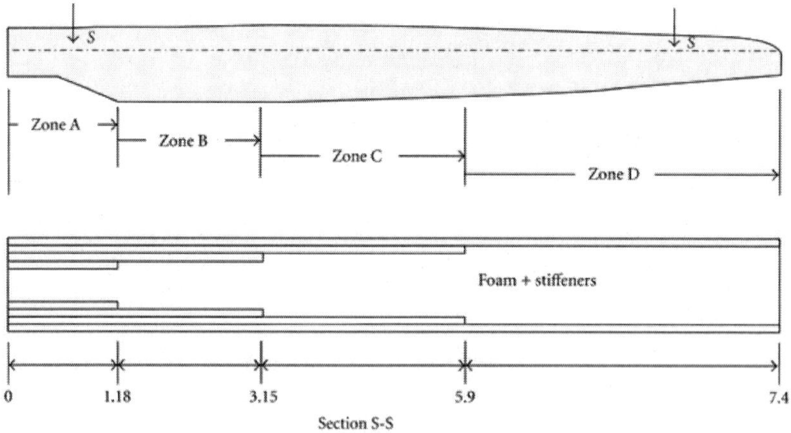

FIGURE 3: Different thicknesses assigned to different zones.

3.4 RTM MOULDING PROCESS

This technique of moulding involves injecting the resin in liquid state into a closed mould cavity, in which the dry fibre reinforcements (glass-fibres preform) that were previously placed rely primarily on pressure difference that occurs inside the closed cavity, allowing the resin to flow and therefore impregnate the preformed dry reinforcements [11, 12]. Figure 4 illustrates the sequence of the RTM process, which is summarized by the following stages:

- Stage 1: selection of fibre reinforcements (and matrix resin) recommended by the design office.
- Stage 2: preparation of fibrous preform (orientation of fibres and stacking sequence).
- Stage 3: placement of fibrous preform, closing the mould and venting operation.

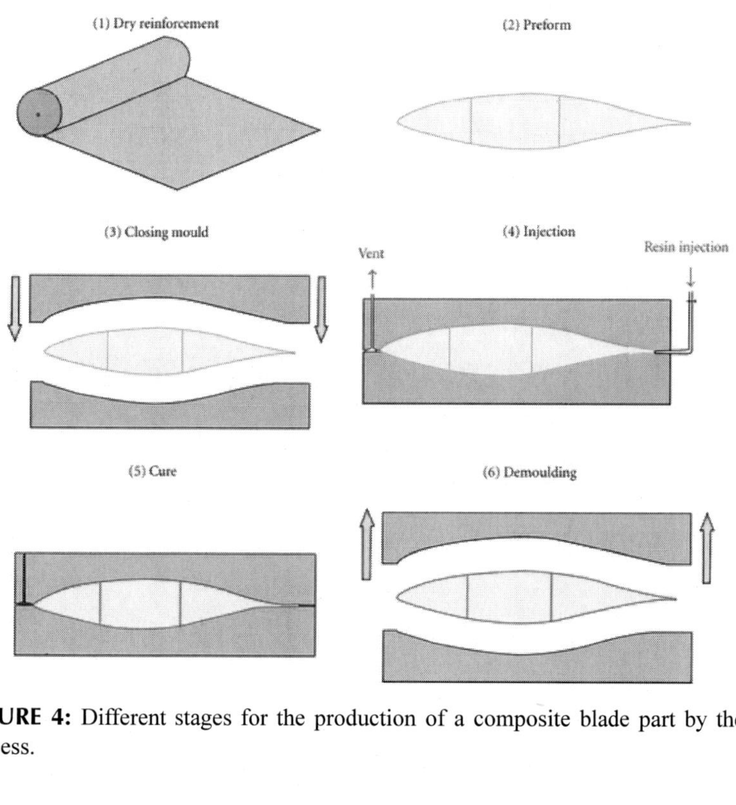

FIGURE 4: Different stages for the production of a composite blade part by the RTM process.

- Stage 4: injection of the resin, progressive flow of resin and impregnation of the fibre bed until filling.
- Stage 5: polymerisation process, drying and hardening of the resin (curing).
- Stage 6: opening the mould and demoulding the composite blade part.

Stage 4 appears to be an important step in the production process of composite blades. This step of injection and flow of a resin through the fibrous medium is based on the use of Darcy's law [13] which is mainly governed by the permeability value of the resin K, a physical characteristic representing the capacity of resin transfer through the fibrous material selected [14]. Further to that, this permeability depends on several factors such as the nature of the reinforcement, the direction and arrangement of fibres, the stacking sequence of plies, the temperature of the resin, the position of injection-vent ports, and so forth. Therefore, the simulation of flow behaviour in an anisotropic fibrous medium [15] must be studied carefully and the permeability values have to be correctly defined, because a minor error in the calculation of these values can lead to considerable variations that cannot be accepted in practice.

3.5 FORMULATION OF THE PERMEABILITY (DARCY'S LAW)

3.5.1 PRINCIPLE OF MEASURING PERMEABILITY (ONE-DIMENSIONAL FLOW 1D)

In 1856, Darcy has shown that for a Newtonian incompressible fluid in laminar flow, the speed at which the fluid behaves in a homogeneous isotropic medium is proportional to the pressure gradient and inversely proportional to its dynamic viscosity [13]:

$$v = \frac{Q}{s} = \frac{K}{\mu} \times \frac{\Delta P}{\Delta L} \tag{5a}$$

where, v is the fluid velocity ($m \cdot s^{-1}$); Q is the discharge rate ($m^3 \cdot s^{-1}$); S is the cross-sectional area to flow (m^2); K is the permeability of the medium (m^2); μ is the fluid viscosity (Pa·s); ΔP is the pressure difference (Pa); ΔL is the length of the porous medium (m).

Using the pressure gradient notation (i.e., ∇P = ΔP/ΔL) leads to

$$v = \frac{K}{\mu} \times \nabla P \quad (5b)$$

3.5.2 LONGITUDINAL AND TRANSVERSE PERMEABILITIES (THREE-DIMENSIONAL FLOW 3D)

The relation expressed by (5b) can be generalized in a three-dimensional system, as illustrated in Figure 5.

Consequently, in the three-dimensional resin flow (3D), the generalized Darcy's law can be written in the following compact form [16, 17]:

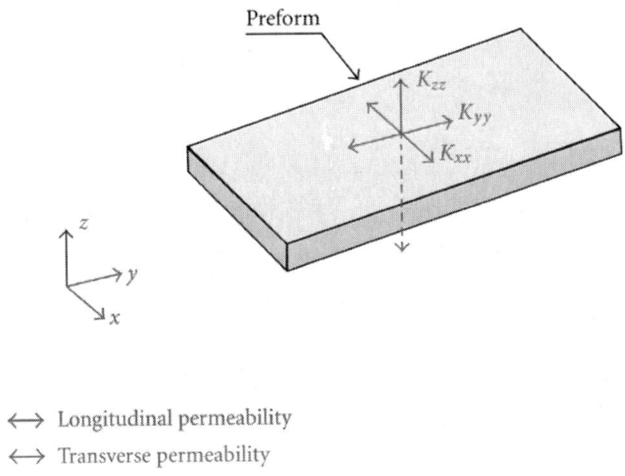

FIGURE 5: Longitudinal and transverse permeabilities in a 3-dimensional system.

$$\bar{v} = -\frac{1}{\mu}[K]\nabla P \tag{6a}$$

or in the following developed form:

$$\begin{Bmatrix} v_x \\ v_y \\ v_z \end{Bmatrix} = -\frac{1}{\mu}\begin{bmatrix} K_{xx} & K_{xy} & K_{xz} \\ K_{yx} & K_{yy} & K_{yz} \\ K_{zx} & K_{zy} & K_{zz} \end{bmatrix}\begin{Bmatrix} \frac{\delta P}{\delta x} \\ \frac{\delta P}{\delta y} \\ \frac{\delta P}{\delta z} \end{Bmatrix} \tag{6b}$$

where v is the velocity vector ($m \cdot s^{-1}$); [K] is the permeability tensor (m^2); ∇P is the pressure gradient ($Pa \cdot m^{-1}$).

In most cases, composite blades have thin laminated thicknesses in comparison to their other dimensions (length and width). Therefore, the transverse permeability through the preform thickness can be neglected. Based on this assumption, (6b) can be written in the two-dimensional flow system (2D) as

$$\begin{Bmatrix} v_x \\ v_y \end{Bmatrix} = -\frac{1}{\mu}\begin{bmatrix} K_{xx} & K_{xy} \\ K_{yx} & K_{yy} \end{bmatrix}\begin{Bmatrix} \frac{\delta P}{\delta x} \\ \frac{\delta P}{\delta y} \end{Bmatrix} \tag{7}$$

As the permeability tensor K depends on the angle of fibre orientation (as shown in Figure 6), it can therefore be written as [17].

1. In the (1, 2) principal coordinate system:

$$\begin{bmatrix} K_{xx} & K_{xy} \\ K_{yx} & K_{yy} \end{bmatrix} = \begin{bmatrix} K_{11} & 0 \\ 0 & K_{22} \end{bmatrix} \tag{8}$$

2. In the (x, y) general coordinate system:

$$\begin{bmatrix} K_{xx} & K_{xy} \\ K_{yx} & K_{yy} \end{bmatrix} = \begin{bmatrix} K_{11}C^2 + K_{22}S^2 & (-K_{11} + K_{22})CS \\ (-K_{11} + K_{22})CS & K_{11}S^2 + K_{22}C^2 \end{bmatrix} \tag{9}$$

where, C = cos(θ) and S = sin(θ).

Also, the permeability in (1, 2) system can be evaluated, from Carman-Kozeny equation [18], as follows:

$$K_{ij} = \frac{1}{K_{ij}} \frac{R_f^2}{4} \frac{\left(1 - V_f\right)^3}{V_f^2} \quad (i, j = 1,2) \tag{10}$$

where K_{ij} is Kozeny constant; R_f is the fibre radius; V_f is the fibre volume fraction.

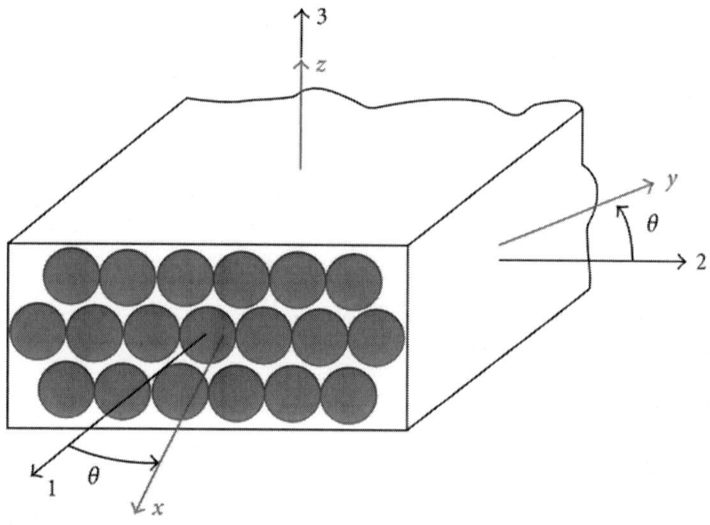

FIGURE 6: Principal and general coordinate systems of a fibrous porous medium.

On the other hand, the average permeability components for a preform composed of plies each of thickness h^I can be calculated according to the following rule of superposition [17]:

$$\overline{K}_{ij} = \frac{1}{H}\sum_{I=1}^{n} h^I K_{ij}^I \tag{11}$$

where H is the total thickness of the preform and h^I is the thickness of a ply .

Using a combination of Darcy's law and continuity equations yields the equation governing the pressure distribution, which can be written in compact form as

$$\nabla \cdot \left(\frac{K}{\mu} \nabla P\right) = 0 \tag{12a}$$

Or in fully developed form, (12a) can be written as

$$\frac{\partial}{\partial x}\left(\frac{K_{xx}\partial P}{\mu \partial x}\right) + \frac{\partial}{\partial x}\left(\frac{K_{xy}\partial P}{\mu \partial y}\right) + \frac{\partial}{\partial y}\left(\frac{K_{yx}\partial P}{\mu \partial x}\right) + \frac{\partial}{\partial y}\left(\frac{K_{yy}\partial P}{\mu \partial y}\right) = 0 \tag{12b}$$

The obtained system of equations can be solved by numerical approaches, where the corresponding boundary conditions of the system are generally defined as follows [18]:

1. at the injection port: $P = P_0$ (constant pressure);
2. at the flow front: $P = P_f$ (atmospheric pressure, i.e., 1013.25 hPa);
3. at the mould wall: $\delta P/\delta n|_{wall} = 0$.

A finite element method, employing a computer program, has been used in the current investigation.

It should be noted that this study is focused solely on a numerical analysis to give an idea about the behaviour of the resin flow in a flat anisotro-

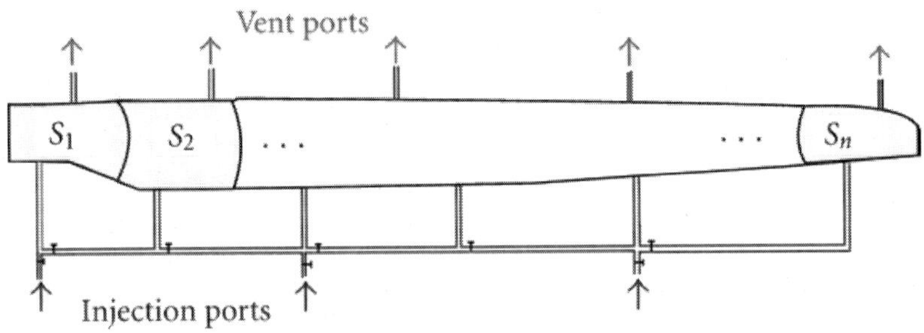

FIGURE 7: Progressive impregnation of fibrous preforms by RTM sequential injection process.

pic fibrous preform, characteristic of a wind turbine blade. It is clear that a particular inquiry should be paid to experimental study in order to conduct a test-calculation correlation. This issue will be investigated later and once the experimental results are available, their comment will be discussed in future publications.

3.6 RESULTS AND DISCUSSION

For large-scale composite wind turbine blades, designed mainly for off-shore applications, the resin injection is performed in a sequential manner [19]. In such RTM process simulation, the injection ports are located on the trailing edge, whereas the vent ports are located on the leading edge. Figure 7 shows the position of these ports and illustrates how the procedure is started. The injection process starts from the blade root, characterised by the section S_1. This latter corresponds to the most critical area, submitted during working conditions to high stress levels. Once the fibrous preform corresponding to section S_1 is saturated with resin, the injecting operation is then moved progressively to the next section S_2 and so on, until it reaches the last section S_n, corresponding to section relative to the free end of the wind turbine blade.

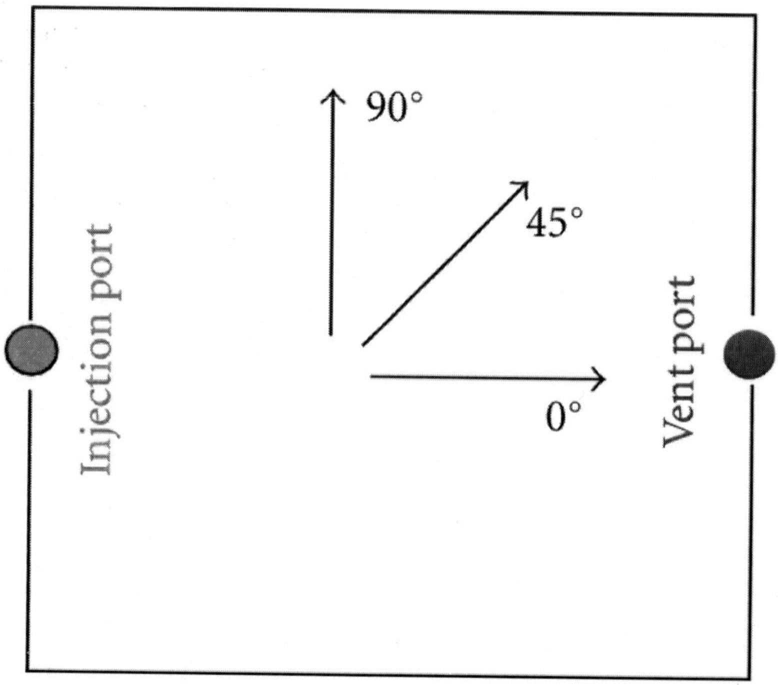

FIGURE 8: Numerical simulation of resin flow behaviour during mould filling stage for a single-layer fibrous preform.

To further generalize the current moulding technique and get an idea about the resin flow behaviour during the resin filling stage, two unidirectional fibrous preforms are considered in this analysis. The first one was made up of one-layer thickness of 9 mm composed of a certain number of unidirectional plies, whereas the second one was made up of two layers with different fibre orientations and the thickness of each layer was assumed to be equal to 4.5 mm. The fibrous preforms are in the form of square flat plates of dimensions 40 cm × 40 cm and are considered to be extracted from the original blade structure (i.e., upper or lower surfaces corresponding to zone B).

Figure 8(a) shows the positions of injection and vent ports; they are located at the midpoint of the mould edge and the opposite side, respectively.

The numerical simulation of resin flow behaviour through the fibrous preform during mould-filling stage is calculated using a finite element program based on (6a) and (6b). The various concentrations of pressure field are given in the form of different colours, as shown in Figures 8(b)–8(d).

3.6.1 SIMULATION OF FLOW RESIN BEHAVIOUR FOR THE CASE OF ONE UNIDIRECTIONAL LAYER

Three unidirectional fibre orientations (i.e., $\theta=0°$, $\theta=90°$, and $\theta=45°$) were considered in this analysis and the output results are illustrated in Figure 8. It can be seen that the flow of the resin along the fibre direction $\theta=0°$ (see Figure 8(b)) is more important than the other directions (Figures 8(c) and 8(d)). The reason for this is due to the presence of important volume fraction of pores in the longitudinal direction of fibres. These pores will provide the preferential paths of resin flow through the porous medium and will accelerate the process of impregnation. On the other hand, the flow rate is slow when fibres are orientated at $\theta = 90°$ (Figure 8(c)). This can be explained by the fact that fibres are perpendicular to the direction of resin movement, and this will create a sort of barrier which prevents the resin from spreading easily because of a low presence of pores in such direction. Therefore, the idea of a concentric flow of resin with regard to the position of single-point injection is not truly representative for orthotropic unidirectional fibre reinforcements.

3.6.2 SIMULATION OF FLOW RESIN BEHAVIOUR FOR THE CASE OF TWO UNIDIRECTIONAL LAYERS

For this case study, positions of injection and vent ports remain the same as the previous analysis and are illustrated in Figure 9(a). However, the number of layers forming the laminated fibrous preform is doubled and each layer is oriented at a specific angle. To this end, three case studies with different orientations of layers are considered in this analysis and are symbolised by the following staking sequences: [45°/90°], [45°/0°], [90°/0°], and [45°/–45°]. The output results of this investigation are presented in Figures 9(b)–9(d), from which it can be discerned that the resultant flow is dominant in the case where stacking arrangement presents a significant distribution of pores through the fibrous preform, which provides a better flow of resin (see Figure 9(c)). On the contrary, the drainage of resin is anisotropic, slower, and less important for the case shown in Figure 9(b). Further to the fibre direction, it should be pointed out that the permeability depends also on the stacking order of layers (mainly for the transverse permeability).

The choice of an appropriate stacking sequence is usually determined by a finite element structural analysis and the output numerical results must meet the criteria required by the new certification specifications put into effect. However, any change in the fibre orientation of layers may, in one hand, promote the process of drainage of the resin, but on the other hand, it may affect the mechanical properties of the material and therefore the stiffness and strength of the resulting blade product. The final choice of stacking sequence must meet simultaneously and favourably the conditions identified by the numerical calculations and those imposed by the principles governing the RTM process. This particular issue should be carefully studied before the implementation of the process.

It should be noted that the integration of exact values of permeability into simulation software for RTM process can yield an acceptable and reliable approach regarding the resin flow behaviour. In addition, curves representing the pressure field can be viewed for each ply constituting the preform during mould filling stage.

Future simulation software for RTM process should consider the ecological impacts discussed earlier in Section 1 and search for ways to promote green design; this is however not the case for some software and simulation codes.

Further to that, the shape of the blade structure, resin viscosity, temperature change, and location of injection-vent ports are other parameters that can influence the phenomenon of resin transfer and its flow behaviour. Other research and development studies are still needed to be performed on these parameters to better simulate the problem and get closer to the real case with a good test-analysis correlation.

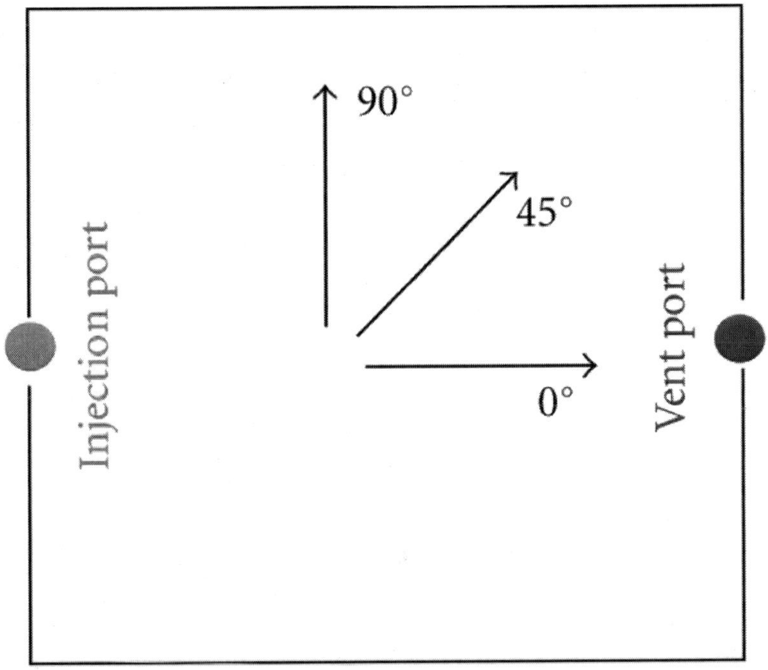

FIGURE 9: Numerical simulation of resin flow behaviour during mould filling stage for a double-layer fibrous preform.

3.7 CONCLUSION

Nowadays, quality assurance, health protection, and environmental preservation have become interdependent and interrelated aspects and are considered to be the primary factors that respond to the concept of sustainable development. In this context, the strategy to develop new generation of large-scale offshore wind turbines is an important issue providing a key role in fighting climate change. However, the methods used to manufacture the turbine components, particularly the blades, must be green and environmentally friendly.

The key benefit that can be made from this analysis is that RTM process has an industrial solution for the production of composite wind turbine blades with cost-effective consideration and improved production rate. In addition, it is a clean process, less polluting, and allows considerable time saving compared to traditional manufacturing techniques. Furthermore, the blade product is obtained in one shot with a total absence of bonding process of halfshells and has an excellent quality appearance on both sides and good mechanical properties. These advantages will undoubtedly attract the attention of relevant industrials and researchers and will boost innovation and creativity for the design of ultralarge wind turbine blades especially for future offshore applications.

Taking into account this ecological approach, the environmentally conscious designers, suppliers, and users will considerably encourage the progress and development of these manufacturing techniques, providing the industrial community with new methods and processes to be applied in modern technology of wind turbine blades.

The numerical analysis given in this paper reinforces the fact that numerical simulation of resin flow behaviour of complicated systems must not be dependent upon one analysis procedure only. Comprehensive modelling of a finite element solution from an experimental procedure should be undertaken before parameter studies are made.

REFERENCES

1. TPWind Secretariat, "2010–2012 Implementation Plan," Wind European Industrial Initiative Team, May 2010, http://setis.ec.europa.eu/activities/implementation-plans/Wind_EII_Implementation_Plan_final.pdf/view.
2. B. Attaf and L. Hollaway, "Vibrational analyses of glass-reinforced polyester composite plates reinforced by a minimum mass central stiffener," Composites, vol. 21, no. 5, pp. 425–430, 1990.
3. B. Attaf, "Generation of new eco-friendly composite materials via the integration of ecodesign coefficients," in Advances in Composite Materials-Ecodesign and Analysis, B. Attaf, Ed., pp. 1–20, Intech, Rijeka, Croatia, 2011.
4. B. Attaf, "Structural ecodesign of onshore and offshore composite wind turbine blades," in Proceedings of the 1ère Conférence Franco-Syrienne sur les Energies Renouvelables, Damascus, Syria, 2010.

5. B. Attaf, "Eco-conception et développement des pales d'éoliennes en matériaux composites," in Proceedings of the 1er Séminaire Méditerranéen sur l'Energie Eolienne, Algeria, 2010.
6. D. Cairns, J. Skramstad, and T. Ashwill, "Resin transfer molding and wind turbine blade construction," Technical Note SAND99-3047, Sandia National Laboratories, California, Calif, USA, 2000.
7. S. G. Advani, Flow and Rheology in Polymer Composites Manufacturing, Composite Materials Series, Elsevier Science, Amsterdam, The Netherlands, 1994.
8. B. Attaf, "Towards the optimisation of the ecodesign function for composites," JEC Composites Magazine, vol. 34, no. 42, pp. 58–60, 2007.
9. B. Attaf, "Probability approach in ecodesign of fibre-reinforced composite structures," in Proceedings of the Congrès Algérien de Mécanique (CAM '09), Biskra, Algeria, 2009.
10. S. M. Habali and I. A. Saleh, "Technical note: design and testing of small mixed airfoil wind turbine blades," Renewable Energy, vol. 6, no. 2, pp. 161–169, 1995. View at Scopus
11. K. M. Pillai, "Governing equations for unsaturated flow through woven fiber mats. Part 1. Isothermal flows," Composites A, vol. 33, no. 7, pp. 1007–1019, 2002.
12. C. Nardari, B. Ferret, and D. Gay, "Simultaneous engineering in design and manufacture using the RTM process," Composites A, vol. 33, no. 2, pp. 191–196, 2002.
13. H. Darcy and V. Dalmont, Les Fontaines Publiques de la Ville de Dijon, Paris, France, 1856.
14. Y. Luo, I. Verpoest, K. Hoes, M. Vanheule, H. Sol, and A. Cardon, "Permeability measurement of textile reinforcements with several test fluids," Composites A, vol. 32, no. 10, pp. 1497–1504, 2001.
15. A. Shojaei, S. R. Ghaffarian, and S. M. H. Karimian, "Three-dimensional process cycle simulation of composite parts manufactured by resin transfer molding," Composite Structures, vol. 65, no. 3-4, pp. 381–390, 2004.
16. K. Hoes, D. Dinescu, H. Sol et al., "New set-up for measurement of permeability properties of fibrous reinforcements for RTM," Composites A, vol. 33, no. 7, pp. 959–969, 2002.
17. C. H. Park, W. I. Lee, W. S. Han, and A. Vautrin, "Weight minimization of composite laminated plates with multiple constraints," Composites Science and Technology, vol. 63, no. 7, pp. 1015–1026, 2003.
18. H. Jinlian, L. Yi, and S. Xueming, "Study on void formation in multi-layer woven fabrics," Composites A, vol. 35, no. 5, pp. 595–603, 2004.
19. P. Desfilhes, "Composites—l'automatisation des grandes pieces," L'Usine Nouvelle, no. 2819, pp. 48–50, 2002.

CHAPTER 4

AERODYNAMIC SHAPE OPTIMIZATION OF A VERTICAL-AXIS WIND TURBINE USING DIFFERENTIAL EVOLUTION

TRAVIS J. CARRIGAN, BRIAN H. DENNIS, ZHEN X. HAN, AND BO P. WANG

4.1 INTRODUCTION

4.1.1 ALTERNATIVE ENERGY

As the world continues to use up nonrenewable energy resources, wind energy will continue to gain popularity. A new market in wind energy technology has emerged that has the means of efficiently transforming the energy available in the wind to a usable form of energy, such as electricity. The cornerstone of this new technology is the wind turbine.

A wind turbine is a type of turbomachine that transfers fluid energy to mechanical energy through the use of blades and a shaft and converts that form of energy to electricity through the use of a generator. Depending on whether the flow is parallel to the axis of rotation (axial flow) or perpendicular (radial flow) determines the classification of the wind turbine.

This chapter was originally published under the Creative Commons Attribution License. Carrigan TJ, Dennis BH, Han ZX, and Wang BP. Aerodynamic Shape Optimization of a Vertical-Axis Wind Turbine Using Differential Evolution. ISRN Renewable Energy ***2012*** *(2012). http://dx.doi.org/10.5402/2012/528418.*

4.1.2 WIND TURBINE TYPES

Two major types of wind turbines exist based on their blade configuration and operation. The first type is the horizontal-axis wind turbine (HAWT). This type of wind turbine is the most common and can often be seen littered across the landscape in areas of relatively level terrain with predictable year round wind conditions. HAWTs sit atop a large tower and have a set of blades that rotate about an axis parallel to the flow direction. These wind turbines have been the main subject of wind turbine research for decades, mainly because they share common operation and dynamics with rotary aircraft.

The second major type of wind turbine is the vertical axis wind turbine (VAWT). This type of wind turbine rotates about an axis that is perpendicular to the oncoming flow, hence, it can take wind from any direction. VAWTs consist of two major types, the Darrieus rotor and Savonius rotor. The Darrieus wind turbine is a VAWT that rotates around a central axis due to the lift produced by the rotating airfoils, whereas a Savonius rotor rotates due to the drag created by its blades. There is also a new type of VAWT emerging in the wind power industry which is a mixture between the Darrieus and Savonius designs.

4.1.2.1 VERTICAL-AXIS WIND TURBINES

Recently, VAWTs have been gaining popularity due to interest in personal green energy solutions. Small companies all over the world have been marketing these new devices such as Helix Wind, Urban Green Energy, and Windspire. VAWTs target individual homes, farms, or small residential areas as a way of providing local and personal wind energy. This reduces the target individual's dependence on external energy resources and opens up a whole new market in alternative energy technology. Because VAWTs are small, quiet, easy to install, can take wind from any direction, and operate efficiently in turbulent wind conditions, a new area in wind turbine research has opened up to meet the demands of individuals willing to take control and invest in small wind energy technology.

The device itself is relatively simple. With the major moving component being the rotor, the more complex parts like the gearbox and generator are located at the base of the wind turbine. This makes installing a VAWT a painless undertaking and can be accomplished quickly. Manufacturing a VAWT is much simpler than a HAWT due to the constant cross-section blades. Because of the VAWTs simple manufacturing process and installation, they are perfectly suited for residential applications.

The VAWT rotor, comprised of a number of constant cross-section blades, is designed to achieve good aerodynamic qualities at various angles of attack. Unlike the HAWT where the blades exert a constant torque about the shaft as they rotate, a VAWT rotates perpendicular to the flow, causing the blades to produce an oscillation in the torque about the axis of rotation. This is due to the fact that the local angle of attack for each blade is a function of its azimuthal location. Because each blade has a different angle of attack at any point in time, the average torque is typically sought as the objective function. Even though the HAWT blades must be designed with varying cross-sections and twist, they only have to operate at a single angle of attack throughout an entire rotation. However, VAWT blades are designed such that they exhibit good aerodynamic performance throughout an entire rotation at the various angles of attack they experience leading to high time averaged torque. The blades of a Darrieus VAWT (D-VAWT) accomplish this through the generation of lift, while the Savonius-type VAWTs (S-VAWTs) produce torque through drag.

4.1.3 COMPUTATIONAL MODELING

The majority of wind turbine research is focused on accurately predicting efficiency. Various computational models exist, each with their own strengths and weaknesses that attempt to accurately predict the performance of a wind turbine. Descriptions of the general set of equations that the methods solve can be found in Section 2. Being able to numerically predict wind turbine performance offers a tremendous benefit over classic experimental techniques, the major benefit being that computational studies are more economical than costly experiments.

A survey of aerodynamic models used for the prediction of VAWT performance was conducted by [1, 2]. While other approaches have been published, the three major models include momentum models, vortex models, and computational fluid dynamics (CFD) models. Each of the three models are based on the simple idea of being able to determine the relative velocity and, in turn, the tangential force component of the individual blades at various azimuthal locations.

4.1.3.1 COMPUTATIONAL FLUID DYNAMICS

Due to its flexibility, CFD has been gaining popularity for analyzing the complex, unsteady aerodynamics involved in the study of wind turbines [3, 4] and has demonstrated an ability to generate results that compare favorably with experimental data [5, 6]. Unlike other models, CFD has shown no problems predicting the performance of either high- or low-solidity wind turbines or for various tip speed ratios. However, it is important to note that predicting the performance of a wind turbine using CFD typically requires large computational domains with sliding interfaces and additional turbulence modeling to capture unsteady affects; therefore, CFD can be computationally expensive.

4.1.4 OBJECTIVES

The objective of the present work is to demonstrate a proof-of-concept optimization system and methodology similar to that which was introduced by [8], while aiming to maximize the torque, hence, the efficiency of a VAWT for a fixed tip speed ratio. To accomplish this, an appropriate model for predicting the performance of a VAWT is to be selected along with a robust optimization algorithm and flexible family of airfoil geometries.

Recent research has been conducted coupling models used for performance prediction with optimization algorithms. Authors in [9] used CFD coupled with a design of experiments/response surface method approach, focusing on only symmetric blade profiles in two dimensions using a seven-control-point Bezier curve. Bourguet only simulated one blade with a low solidity as to avoid undesirable unsteady effects. He found that when there exists a possibility of several local optima, stochastic optimization algorithms are better suited for the job as they tend to be more efficient than gradient-based algorithms. Authors of [10] and [11] coupled-low order performance prediction methods with optimization algorithms in a multicriteria optimization routine. Both of their approaches focused on HAWTs rather than VAWTs. Research has also led to patented blade designs using CFD coupled with optimization [12]. Other than using optimization techniques, inverse design methods can also be used to find an optimum design for a fixed tip speed ratio that satisfied the specified design performance characteristics. However, inverse design techniques require experience and intuition in order to specify desired performance, whereas optimization allows for designs to be generated that are more often than not beyond the intuition of a designer. After reviewing the available models and recent research efforts, CFD was chosen as the appropriate tool for predicting the performance of a VAWT because of its flexibility and accuracy. Due to the possibility of local optima, and the requirement for floating-point optimization for geometric flexibility, a parallel stochastic differential evolution algorithm was chosen for the optimization. The NACA 4-series family of wing sections was chosen as the geometry to be parameterized for the optimization, allowing either symmetric or cambered airfoil shapes to be generated. What separates this approach from all previous work is the consideration of both symmetric and cambered airfoil geometries, along with a full two-dimensional, unsteady simulation for a three-bladed wind turbine for various design points.

4.2 VERTICAL AXIS WIND TURBINE PERFORMANCE

4.2.1 WIND SPEED AND TIP SPEED RATIO

According to the National Climatic Data Center, the average annual wind speed in the United States is approximately 4 m/s [13]. Realizing that the majority of wind turbines that have been developed to this day typically start producing power in winds as low as 3 m/s, the standard rated wind speed is still as high as 12 m/s. Determining the wind speed at which a wind turbine will operate is the most important step in predicting its performance and even aids in defining the initial size of the wind turbine. Once the operating wind speed of the turbine has been decided upon, the first step in wind turbine design is to select a operating tip speed ratio [14] which can be expressed by

$$\lambda = \frac{\omega r}{V_\infty} \tag{1}$$

or the ratio of the rotational velocity of the wind turbine ωr and the freestream velocity component (wind speed) V_∞.

4.2.2 GEOMETRY DEFINITION

Once λ has been chosen, the geometry of the VAWT can be defined through a dimensionless parameter known as the solidity

$$\sigma = \frac{Nc}{d} \tag{2}$$

which is a function of the number of blades N, the chord length of the blades c, and the diameter of the rotor d. The solidity represents the fraction of the frontal swept area of the wind turbine that is covered by the blades.

4.2.3 PERFORMANCE PREDICTION

With λ chosen and the basic geometry of the VAWT defined, the next step is to predict the actual performance of the wind turbine. To do this, it is important to determine the forces acting on each blade. This is governed by the relative wind component W and the angle of attack α seen in the snapshot of a D-VAWT blade cross-section in Figure 1. As the blade ro-

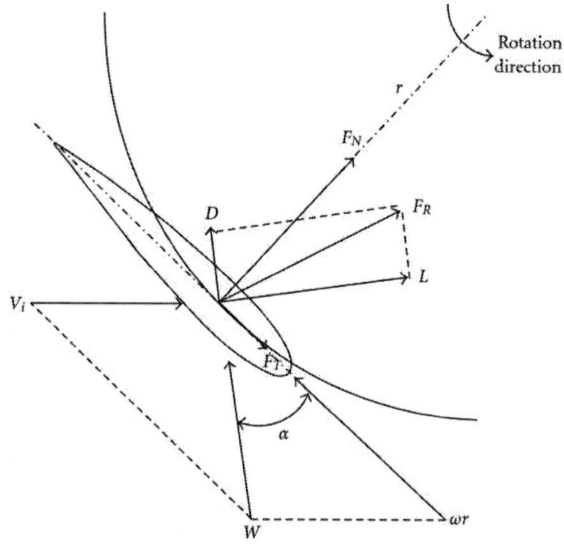

FIGURE 1: Velocity and force components for a Darrieus-type VAWT.

tates, the local angle of attack α for that blade changes due to the variation of the relative velocity W. The induced velocity V_i and the rotating velocity ωr of the blade govern the orientation and magnitude of the relative velocity. This in turn changes the lift L and the drag D forces acting on the blade. As the lift and drag change both their magnitude and orientation, the resultant force F_R changes. The resultant force can be decomposed into both a normal component F_N and a tangential component F_T. It is this tangential force component that drives the rotation of the wind turbine and produces the torque necessary to generate electricity.

4.2.3.1 AVERAGE TORQUE

Close inspection of the underlying physics involved in wind turbine aerodynamics reveals that α is governed by the tip speed ratio λ and, once determined, L and D can be found using empirical data or calculated using

CFD. L and D are then nondimensionalized by dividing through by the dynamic pressure to obtain the coefficient of lift C_l and the coefficient of drag C_d. These coefficients are used to calculate the tangential force coefficient

$$C_r = C_{;} \sin\alpha - C_d \cos\alpha \tag{3}$$

To retrieve the actual tangential force, C_t is multiplied by the dynamic pressure

$$F_T = \frac{1}{2} C_t \rho c h W^2 \tag{4}$$

where ρ is the air density and h is the height of the wind turbine. It is important to note that (4) represents the tangential force at only a single azimuthal position. Therefore, the process of determining α, C_t, and F_T must be repeated at all azimuthal locations before the torque can be calculated.

Because F_T is calculated at all azimuthal locations, it is said to be a function of θ and the average tangential force for a single rotation of one blade is

$$F_{Tavg} = \frac{1}{2\pi} \int_0^{2\pi} F_T(\theta) d\theta \tag{5}$$

where the average torque for N blades located at radius r from the axis of rotation is given by

$$\tau = N F_{Tavg} r \tag{6}$$

4.2.3.2 POWER AND EFFICIENCY

The final step in predicting the performance of the wind turbine is determining the power it is able to extract from the wind and how efficiently it can accomplish that task. The amount of power the wind turbine is able to draw from the wind is given by

$$P_T = \tau\omega \tag{7}$$

Therefore, the efficiency of the wind turbine is simply the ratio of the power produced by the wind turbine and the power available in the wind given by the expression

$$\text{COP} = \frac{P_T}{P_W} = \frac{\tau\omega}{1/2\rho d h V_\infty^3} \tag{8}$$

Equation (8) is significant in this work because it represents a non-dimensional coefficient of performance (COP) that is a function of the torque to be used as the objective function for the aerodynamic shape optimization.

It should be mentioned that the goal in designing a wind turbine is to do so in such a way to extract as much energy as possible. Analyzing (5) and (8) reveals that, while an increase in the height of the wind turbine would increase F_T, hence τ, theoretically COP would remain unaffected. However, if an increase in P_T is all that is desired, the height of the wind turbine could be increased. In order to increase the efficiency of the wind turbine for a given λ, the blade shape and σ would have to be adjusted. Equation (5) is a function of C_l and c, where C_l is a function of the blade shape and c is a function of σ. Because the shape of the blade, σ, and C_l are tightly coupled, it makes it difficult to select a geometry that maximizes the efficiency. Therefore, accomplishing this task is not straightforward and requires an iterative approach and the implementation of a simple, automated optimization methodology.

4.3 METHODOLOGY

4.3.1 REQUIREMENTS

For the objectives of the current study to be feasible, the requirement for a straightforward, modular, and automated design framework became realized. Successfully taking a physical system, such as a wind turbine, and attempting to adjust, analyze, and optimize the design to satisfy an objective, or multiple objectives, required more than a few bundled files and programs requiring user input. In fact, it was this realization that sparked the idea of a simple, automated optimization methodology. The optimization methodology proposed is a unique and modular system aimed at relaxing the ties between the computer and operator and simplifying the

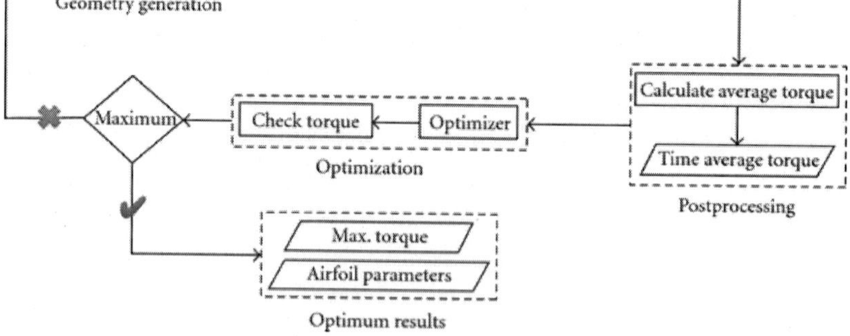

FIGURE 2: VAWT optimization methodology.

design process so more time can be spent analyzing a solution and understanding the physics of the problem.

4.3.2 UNIQUE MODULAR DESIGN

A modular system is one in which entire parts of the system can be removed and replaced without compromising the process flows within the system. Therefore, for a module to be removed and replaced, it must be substituted with a module of equivalent functionality. Figure 2 illustrates the concept as it applies to wind turbine optimization and the methodology used in this work. The first step in the optimization process is generating the geometry. This geometry is described as a set of cartesian coordinates and is passed to the mesh generation module. This tool is used to discretize the fluid domain and output a specific file to the CFD solver module. This module calculates a solution and passes information to the postprocessing module. The postprocessing tools manipulate the data, calculate the objective function value, and pass it to the optimizer. If the objective function is considered a maximum value, the optimization terminates. If not, the process starts over. Details pertaining to each of the modules used in this work will be discussed in the next section.

4.4 TOOLBOX

4.4.1 GEOMETRY GENERATION

The objective of the optimization was to find an aerodynamic shape that for a fixed tip speed ratio would maximize the efficiency of the wind turbine. The first step was to select a suitable shape, or series of shapes, that could be adjusted throughout the optimization process. An obvious choice was the NACA 4-series airfoil. The majority of VAWTs utilize NACA airfoil sections because they are easy to manufacture and their characteristics are widely available.

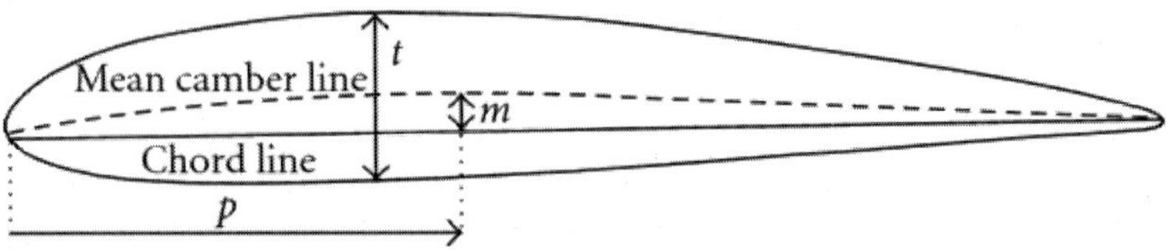

FIGURE 3: NACA 4424 4-series airfoil.

4.4.1.1 NACA 4-SERIES AIRFOILS

The NACA 4-series airfoil sections are defined by a mean camber line and a thickness distribution. In Figure 3, the mean camber line is the dashed line that splits the airfoil in half. The chord line is simply a straight line connecting the leading edge to the trailing edge of the airfoil whose length is defined as the chord length. The maximum thickness t is located at 30% of the chord for NACA 4-series airfoil sections. The maximum camber m, or maximum ordinate of the mean camber line, is located a distance p from the leading edge of the airfoil. The values of m, p, and t are expressed as percentages of the chord length and represent the four digits defining the NACA 4-series airfoil and are the parameters used in the optimization.

Reference [15] introduced the equations used to define the shape of a NACA 4-series airfoil. The mean camber line of the airfoil was described as an analytically defined curve which was the combination of two parabolic arcs that are tangent at the point of maximum camber. For an x-coordinate, the ordinate of the mean camber line can be expressed as

$$y_c = \begin{cases} \dfrac{m}{p^2}(2px - x^2) \\ \text{forward of maximum ordinate,} \\ \dfrac{m}{(1-p)^2}[(1-2p) + 2px - x^2] \\ \text{aft of maximum ordinate} \end{cases} \tag{9}$$

where m is the maximum camber and p is the chordwise location of the maximum camber. Once the camber line has been defined, the thickness distribution can be found by the following equation:

$$\pm y_t = \frac{t}{0.20}\left(0.29690\sqrt{x} - 0.12600x - 0.31560x^2 + 0.28430x^3 - 0.10140x^4\right) \tag{10}$$

where t is the maximum thickness of the airfoil located at 30% of the chord. After the camber and thickness distribution have been defined for various x locations (typically ranging from 0 to 1), the coordinates of the upper and lower airfoil surfaces can be obtained.

4.4.1.2 AIRFOIL CONSTRAINTS

For the purposes of maintaining high cell quality during the grid generation process and a converged CFD solution, constraints were placed on the parameters defining the airfoils that could be generated for the optimization and were normalized from 0 to 1 for the optimization. The idea was to avoid airfoil geometries with large leading and trailing edge camber leading to local boundary layer cell collisions during the grid generation procedure. While placing constraints on the airfoils to be generated leads to a smaller solution space, it was done so after numerous tests to ensure that optimized geometries were found in the solution space and not on the boundaries. While this may leads one to believe that a smaller solution space leads to less feasible designs, because the optimization algorithm chosen used floating-point values to define the parameters, essentially an infinite number of airfoil designs were attainable.

4.4.2 GRID GENERATION

After the airfoil geometry for the VAWT had been defined, the next step was to discretize the computational domain as a preprocessing step in the

CFD process. The act of discretizing the domain is termed grid generation and is one of the most important steps in the CFD process. For simple geometries where the direction of the flow is known beforehand, creating the grid is usually straightforward. For flows such as this, high-quality structured grids can be used that can accurately capture the flow physics. However, as geometry becomes complex and the flows more difficult to predict with the onset of turbulence and separation, grid generation is no longer a trivial task. For flows such as this, unstructured grids consisting of triangles and tetrahedra provide increased flexibility and are often used.

4.4.2.1 GRID CONSIDERATIONS

Because either structured or unstructured techniques can be used to discretize a computational domain, it is important to exercise the capabilities of the solver to determine its sensitivity to the varying cell types. A good rule of thumb proposed by [7] can be seen in Figure 4. From the figure, a

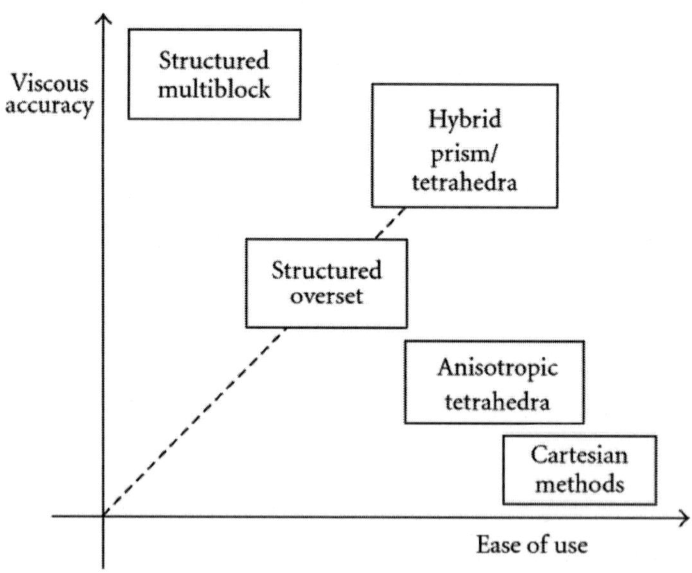

FIGURE 4: Grid-type accuracy versus ease of use [7].

multiblock structured grid is said to provide the highest level of viscous accuracy; yet, it also suggests that a hybrid grid topology would provide a balanced level of accuracy and automation, an important characteristic for the optimization process.

Before a final decision was to be made on the type of grid used for the VAWT simulation, a comprehensive grid dependency study was conducted to find a grid independent solution. For this work, a family of multiblock structured grids were created alongside a family of equivalent hybrid grids. The torque was calculated for each of the grids, and a grid-independent solution was found. Details regarding the grid generation and dependency studies will be discussed further in Section 5.

As a result of the grid dependency study and the extensive work done in the areas of aerodynamic design and optimization using unstructured grid generation techniques [16–19], a hybrid grid was chosen as the most appropriate for this work. The hybrid grid consists of a structured boundary layer transitioning to isotropic triangles in the far field and can be seen for the leading edge of a VAWT blade in Figure 5. This choice provided

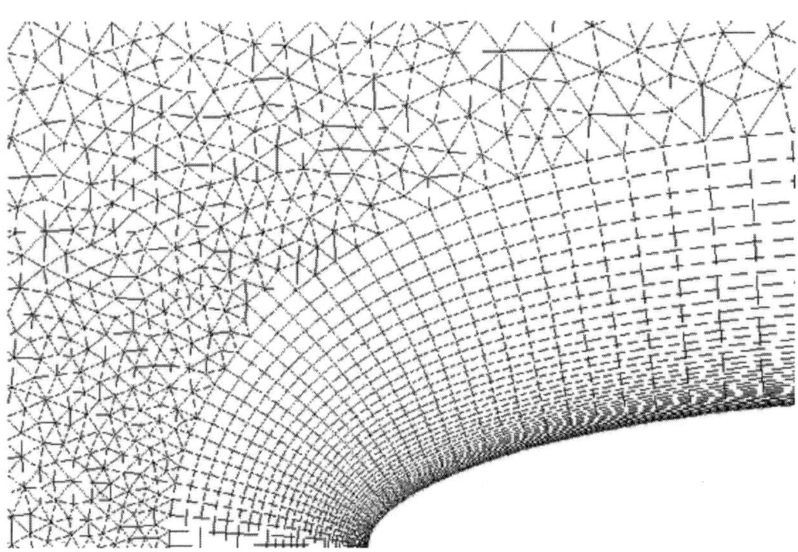

FIGURE 5: Leading edge boundary layer grid for blade geometry.

a flexible and completely automated approach to the grid generation of numerous VAWT geometries.

4.4.2.2 POINTWISE

Pointwise V16.02 was used to generate the grids used for the VAWT study. For the grid dependency study, structured grids were constructed manually, while automated grid generation techniques were used to construct the hybrid grids. The far field was split into a rotating and nonrotating zone and was discretized using either structured or unstructured elements. The scripting capabilities of Pointwise were exercised while constructing the hybrid grids and allowed for the grid generation of the airfoil geometries to easily be integrated into the optimization process. A Pointwise script was written in Glyph2, based on Tcl, that imported the airfoil geometry as a list of x, y coordinates and constructed the hybrid grid based on several user-defined parameters such as the initial cell height in the boundary layer and the solidity of the wind turbine. The automated script also set up the appropriate boundary conditions and exported the file for the solver.

4.4.3 SOLVER

Once the computational domain had been discretized, the equations governing fluid flow were solved using an appropriate discretization technique in order to calculate the torque. The commercial solver FLUENT v6.3 was used for this work [20]. FLUENT uses the finite volume method to discretize the integral form of the governing equations.

4.4.3.1 NUMERICAL METHOD

For the simulation, a pressure-based segregated solver was chosen where the SIMPLE algorithm was used to handle the pressure-velocity coupling that exists. A 2nd-order interpolation scheme for pressure was used along with a 2nd-order upwind discretization scheme for the momentum equation and modified turbulent viscosity. The gradients required for the discretization of the convective and diffusive fluxes were computed using a cell-based approach. Because the simulation was time dependent, a 2nd-order implicit time integration was chosen for the temporal discretization. A time step was chosen small enough to reduce the number of iterations per time step and to properly model the transient phenomena.

Turbulence modeling was accomplished through the use of the Spalart-Allmaras one-equation turbulence model where a transport equation is solved for the eddy viscosity [21]. The y^+ for the blades varied at different azimuthal locations, but consistently placed the first cell centroid of the wall-adjacent cells inside the viscous sublayer ($y^+ < 5$) of the boundary layer. Therefore, because the grid was fine enough to resolve the viscous sublayer, the laminar stress-strain relationship $u^+ = y^+$ was used to determine the wall shear stress.

The system of equations resulting from the discretization and linearization of the governing integral equations were solved using an algebraic multigrid (AMG) method coupled with a point implicit Gauss-Seidel solver [22]. Due to the size and unsteady nature of the problem, the overall average computation time to achieve a quasisteady state took approximately 2.5 hours on a 2.83 GHz Intel Core2Quad processor.

4.4.3.2 COMPUTATIONAL DOMAIN AND BOUNDARY CONDITIONS

The interior domain containing the wind turbine blades was considered as a moving mesh, while the outer domain was stationary. The interior sliding domain rotated with a given rotational velocity for a specified λ. The inlet to the computational domain was defined as a velocity inlet with a uniform velocity component and a modified turbulent viscosity v equal to 5v, where v is the molecular kinematic viscosity of air. The outlet was marked as a pressure outlet with the gauge pressure set to zero.

4.4.4 POSTPROCESSING

Once the solution had been calculated using FLUENT and all relevant data had been written to a file, the average torque could then be determined. A small script parsed through the output file and saved only the torque values that were recorded every 15 time steps. This file then contained torque as a function of time. A graph of the torque versus time can be seen in Figure 6. At a certain point, the flow became quasi-steady, and the oscillations were more uniform. One single rotation of the wind turbine has been outlined in the figure. The three peaks in the torque represent the times at which each blade passed around the front of the wind turbine, while the three valleys represent the times at which each blade moved around the back of the wind turbine. Therefore, more blades would result in a higher frequency oscillation for the same rotation speed. In order to calculate a single scalar value of the torque for the optimizer, the oscillating torque was averaged.

4.4.4.1 AVERAGE TORQUE

In Section 2, the tangential force component driving the wind turbine, and also used to compute the torque, was a function of azimuthal location.

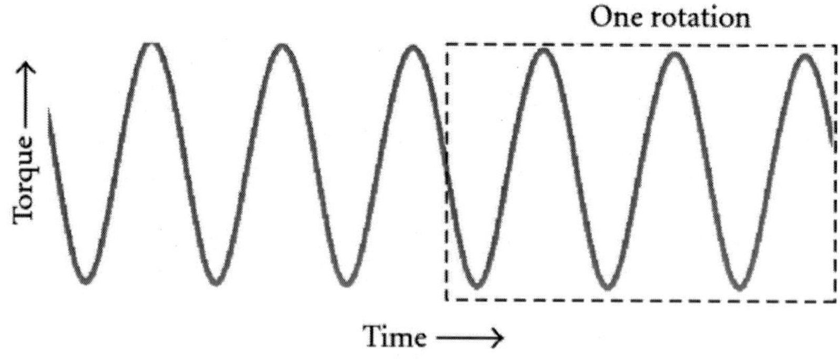

FIGURE 6: Variation of torque as a function of time.

During the simulation process, the torque was recorded as a function of time; therefore, it is important to introduce the average value of a function f(t) over the interval [a, b] as

$$f_{avg} = \frac{1}{b-a}\int_a^b f(t)dt \tag{11}$$

where a would represent the time at the beginning of a single rotation and b is the time at the end of a single rotation. This equation states that the average value of the function f(t) is equal to the integral of that function for a single rotation divided by the time required to complete a single rotation. Using the trapezoidal rule, the definite integral can be expressed by

$$\int_a^b f(t)dt = \frac{b-a}{2n}\left[f(t_0) + 2\sum_{i=1}^{n-1} f(t_i) + f(t_n)\right] \tag{12}$$

where n is the number of segments used to split the interval of integration. Using (11) and (12) and replacing n by $(t_n - t_0)/\Delta t$, the average value of the torque for a single rotation of the wind turbine is defined as

$$\tau_{avg} = \frac{\Delta t}{2(t_n - t_0)}\left[\tau(t_0) + 2\sum_{i=1}^{n-1} \tau(t_1) + \tau(t_n)\right] \tag{13}$$

where t_0 is the time at the beginning of a rotation, t_n is the time at the end of the rotation, and Δt is the time step used when recording the torque in FLUENT. Using (13), the average torque for the final rotation of the wind turbine was calculated and used as the objective function value driving the optimization algorithm.

4.4.5 OPTIMIZATION

In order to maximize the average torque of the wind turbine given the NACA 4-series airfoil design parameters (Section 4.1) and the solidity and tip speed ratio design constraints, a simple and robust optimization algorithm was required. This act of searching for the minimum or maximum value of a function while varying the parameters, or values of that function, and incorporating any constraints is called optimization. In optimization, the function is often termed the objective function or cost function, and it is the goal of the optimization algorithm to find the true minimum or maximum of that objective function as efficiently as possible. However, in design the objective function may be a rather complex, nonlinear, or non-differentiable function that is under the influence of many parameters and design constraints. This possibility rules out any simple, gradient-based optimization algorithms such as the method of steepest descent or Newton's method, as these algorithms require the objective function to be differentiable and are only efficient at finding local minimum or maximum values. Therefore, global optimization algorithms are favored for design optimization.

4.4.5.1 DIFFERENTIAL EVOLUTION

The differential evolution (DE) algorithm is a global, stochastic direct search method aimed at minimizing or maximizing an objective function based on constraints that are represented by floating-point values rather than binary strings like most evolutionary algorithms [23–25]. The DE algorithm is robust, fast, simple, and easy to use as it requires very little user input. These traits lead to the choice of DE as the algorithm used in the current study.

4.4.5.2 INITIALIZATION

In order to determine the maximum value of the objective function, the DE algorithm starts with a randomly populated initial generation of NP

D-dimensional parameter vectors, where NP is the number of parents in a population and D is the number of parameters. For this work two optimizations were conducted. A 3-parameter optimization (D = 3) for a fixed tip speed ratio and solidity, as well as, a 4-parameter optimization (D = 4) where the solidity became a parameter, providing complete geometric flexibility. For both cases NP = 14.

4.4.5.3 MUTATION

After initializing the population, each target vector $X_{i,\,G}$ in that generation undergoes a mutation operation given by

$$\vec{\upsilon}_{i,G+1} = \vec{x}_{r1,G} + F\left(\vec{x}_{r2,G} - \vec{x}_{r3,G}\right) \tag{14}$$

where the index r represents a random population member in the current generation, F is a scaling factor $\in [0, 2]$ dictating the amplification of the difference vector, and the result is called the mutant vector. A scaling factor F = 0.8 was selected for this work. This mutant operation is a characteristic of a variant of DE that utilizes a single difference operation; therefore, NP $\geq$ 4 such that the index i is different than the randomly chosen values of r1 , r2 , r3.

Other variants of DE exist that utilize more difference operations to determine the mutant vector. The DE strategy used in this work DE/best/2/exp utilizes two difference vectors. The idea is that by using two difference vectors the diversity of large populations can be improved, increasing the possibility that members of a population span the entire solution space and reducing the risk of premature convergence. The mutation operation for the DE variant used in this work is given by

$$\vec{\upsilon}_{i,G+1} = \vec{x}_{best,G} + F\left(\vec{x}_{r1,G} + \vec{x}_{r2,G} - \vec{x}_{r3,G} - \vec{x}_{r4,G}\right) \tag{15}$$

where $x_{best,\,G}$ represents the best performing parameter vector from the current population. This is different than the previous strategy that utilized a random population member to perform the mutation operation. The hope is that by using the best parameter vector in the population, the number of generations required for convergence will decrease.

4.4.5.4 CROSSOVER

The crossover operation generates a trial vector by selecting pieces of the target vector and mutant vector. The trial vector is determined by

$$\vec{u}_{ji,G+1} = \begin{cases} \vec{v}_{ji,G+1} & \text{if (randb(j)} \leq \text{CR) or j} = \text{rnbr(i)} \\ \vec{x}_{ji,G} & \text{if (randb (j)} > \text{CR) and j} \neq \text{rnbr(i)} \end{cases} \quad (16)$$

where CR is the crossover constant, or crossover probability ∈ [0, 1], and randb(j) is a randomly chosen number ∈ [0, 1] evaluated during the jth evaluation, where j = 1,2,3,…D,. If the value of randb(j) happens to be less than or equal to CR, the trial vector gets populated with a parameter from the mutant vector. However, if the random number that has been generated happens to be larger than CR, the trial vector gets a parameter from the target vector. To ensure that at least one parameter value is chosen from the mutant vector, a random value ∈ 1, 2, 3,…,D is chosen as rnbr(i). If CR = 1, all trial vector parameters will come from the mutant vector. This illustrates that the choice in CR works to control the crossover probability. In this work, CR = 0 . 6.

4.4.5.5 SELECTION

The last step in the DE algorithm is selection. Once the trial vector has been formed, it must be decided whether or not it should move to the next generation. Therefore, in the selection process, if the trial vector performs better than the target vector, resulting in a larger objective function value, the trial vector moves on to the next generation. However, if the newly generated trial vector is outperformed by the original target vector, the target vector remains a population member in the next generation.

In this work, the DE code generated new airfoil parameters for the first case, and new airfoil parameters and solidities for the second case of each generation through mutation, crossover, and selection operations. Each new set of parameters was used to generate the airfoils of the VAWT for which the torque could then be calculated using the FLUENT solver. The torque was then averaged by the postprocessing module and used as the objective function value driving the DE algorithm.

4.5 RESULTS

The overall objective of the work was to successfully demonstrate a proof-of-concept optimization system capable of maximizing the efficiency of a three-bladed VAWT. Two test cases were conducted to demonstrate the robustness of the optimization system. The first test case was a 3-parameter optimization where the both the solidity and tip speed ratio were fixed. The second test case was a 4-parameter optimization for a fixed tip speed ratio. Before the final results of the optimization are presented, an overview of the grid dependency studies will be introduced. Next, the performance of a baseline geometry will be presented. Finally, the results of the two optimization test cases will be introduced and compared with the performance of the baseline geometry.

4.5.1 GRID DEPENDENCY STUDIES

For this work, a family of structured and equivalent hybrid grids were created in hope to find a grid that provided adequate resolution of the unsteady phenomena while the construction of the grid would remain highly automated for the optimization process.

To begin, a simple blade shape was used for the grid study. The VAWT consisted of three 60 degree semicircular blades with a constant thickness of 0.025 m giving the rotor a solidity $\sigma = 1.5$. Each blade was separated by 60 degrees at a radius of 1 m from the axis of rotation, providing a simple geometry with which to define the initial topology. Because the blades had to spin in the simulation, an interior sliding domain was to be constructed with a radius of 25 m. The outer stationary domain, and the extent of the far field, was defined to be 50 m. The far field domain was large enough such that the unsteady flow characteristics would develop and dissipate inside the domain, eliminating the concern for reverse flow.

4.5.1.1 STRUCTURED AND HYBRID GRIDS

Both structured and hybrid grid families were constructed for the grid dependency study. Structured grids were constructed using quadrilateral elements; therefore, opposing grid lines must contain the same number of points to construct a domain consisting of purely quadrilateral cells. A characteristic, and even a disadvantage of the structured grid topology, is that the local blade resolution used to resolve the boundary layer is propagated into the far field. This tends to lead to larger cell counts when using structured grids.

The hybrid grid topology used for this study consisted of a structured boundary layer transitioning to unstructured triangles. Unlike the structured grid, the hybrid grid topology was easy to construct and automate. The boundary layer was constructed using a normal hyperbolic extrusion technique in Pointwise [26]. The user need only to specify the initial cell height, growth rate, and the number of layers for the extrusion. A benefit from using the hybrid topology was that appropriate boundary layer resolution was obtained while maintaining a low cell count in the far field. Unlike the structured grids, the far field and boundary layer were almost entirely decoupled, resulting in a much lower cell count.

A comparison of the structured and hybrid grid families can be seen in Figure 7. The local blade resolution was preserved using the normal hyperbolic extrusion technique during the construction of the hybrid grids. As was mentioned earlier, the resolution and spacing constraints placed on the structured grid near the blade can be seen propagating away from the blade itself, whereas for the hybrid case there is a clear boundary that separates the boundary layer grid from the rest of the far field. For instance, while the coarse grids contain 50,000 cells for the same local blade resolution, once the spacing was adjusted to achieve higher resolution, the structured grid contained 100,000 cells as opposed to the hybrid grid

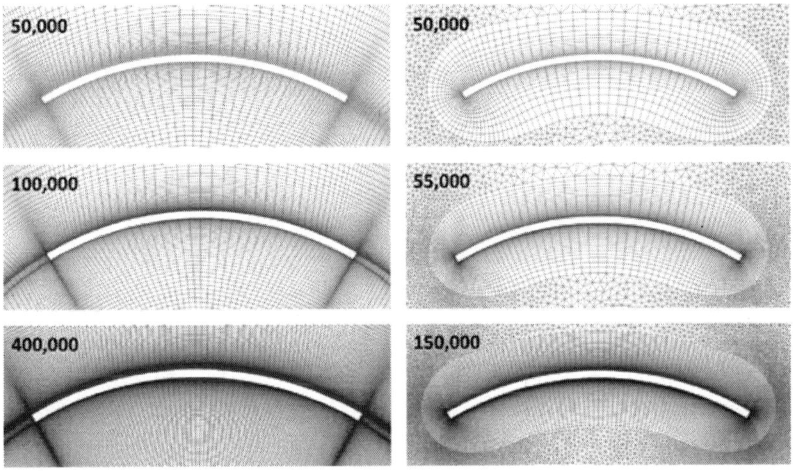

FIGURE 7: Structured and hybrid grid family comparison.

containing only 55,000 cells. In this case, the local blade resolution that was enforced for the structured grid propagated into the far field. However, while the local blade resolution changed for the hybrid grid, the far field remained unaffected.

4.5.1.2 GRID-INDEPENDENT SOLUTION

The torque was calculated for each grid using the FLUENT solver, the settings of which were discussed in Section 4. A time step of $\Delta t = 2\pi/\omega N$ was used where ω is the rotation rate, and N is the number of cells in the circumferential direction. This was calculated for the 100,000 cell structured mesh with $\omega = 10$ rad/s to be approximately 0.001 s, the time step that was used for all simulations. This represents the amount of time for the sliding domain to move one grid point in the circumferential direction and was found adequate for the simulation.

Convergence was monitored by observing the residuals as well as the torque. In the ideal case, the residuals should converge to true zero. However, a more relaxed convergence criteria of 1e-5 was enforced for continuity, momentum, and modified turbulent viscosity. The residuals were monitored every time step, while the torque was recorded every 15 time steps. The solution consistently became quasi-steady after 5 rotations, approximately 3150 time steps. The time step used for the simulation allowed the solution to converge after 30 iterations per time step, resulting in nearly 100,000 iterations to achieve a quasi-steady state.

The average torque was calculated for the last rotation of the wind turbine for each of the grids. From this grid dependency study, it was found that the 100,000 cell structured grid and 55,000 cell hybrid grid seem to exhibit grid convergence. However, due to the complexity of the topology required to construct the structured grid and the difficulty of applying this topology to varying geometries, the 55,000 cell hybrid grid topology was chosen for the optimization.

To demonstrate the automation and quality of the hybrid grid topology for arbitrary blade geometries, a hybrid grid was constructed for a high-solidity VAWT geometry and a low-solidity geometry seen in Figure 8. The normal hyperbolic extrusion created layers of quads that marched smoothly away from the blade, transitioning to isotropic triangles. Utilizing this

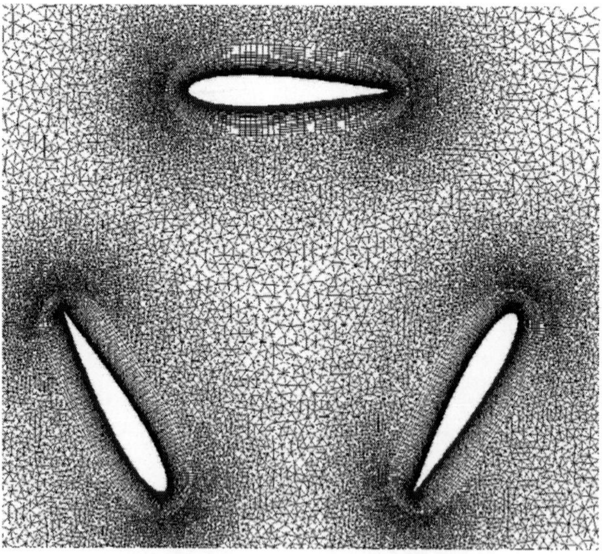

FIGURE 8: Hybrid grids for VAWT geometry, $\sigma = 1.5$ (a) and $\sigma = 0.4$ (b).

technique resulted in high-quality, automated hybrid grid generation for all airfoil geometries analyzed throughout the optimization process.

4.5.2 BASELINE GEOMETRY

A baseline VAWT geometry was selected with which the results of the optimization could be compared. The idea was to select a typical VAWT airfoil cross-section. Therefore, the NACA 0015 was selected as the baseline airfoil cross-section simply due to the fact that a number of researchers attribute this geometry with good overall aerodynamic performance [3–5]. The NACA 0015 airfoil cross-section can be seen in Figure 9.

4.5.2.1 BASELINE PERFORMANCE

The performance of the baseline three-bladed VAWT utilizing NACA 0015 airfoil cross-sections was evaluated for $\sigma = 1.5$ and $\lambda = [0.5, 1.5]$. By keeping ω constant at 10 rad/s for $\sigma = 1.5$, V_∞ was adjusted to control λ. This provided relevant performance data surrounding $\lambda = 1$, the tip speed ratio design constraint for the optimization. A total of 5 simulations were

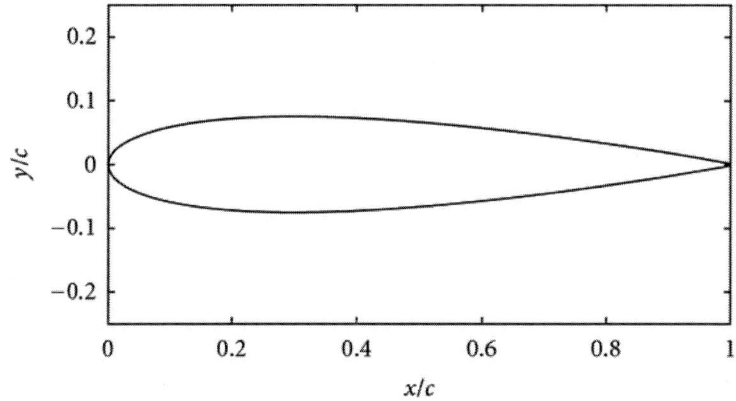

FIGURE 9: NACA 0015 baseline geometry.

run to build up a performance envelope for the baseline geometry. The average torque was calculated for each simulation and was used to determine the coefficient of performance. The results of the analysis can be seen in Figure 10.

Figure 10 defines the performance envelope for a VAWT utilizing the NACA 0015 airfoil for $\sigma = 1.5$. It can be seen that there exists a point at which the efficiency is highest ($\lambda \approx 1.2$) and can be described as the optimum tip speed ratio for the geometry. As expected, as the wind speed changes, driving the tip speed ratio away from the optimum, the efficiency decreases. From this figure, it can be deduced that, in order for the baseline wind turbine design to perform optimally at $\lambda = 1$, the solidity of the rotor would have to be changed while retaining the NACA 0015 airfoil cross-section. This would give the wind turbine even more geometric flexibility and lead to the decision to allow the solidity to become a design parameter in the 4-parameter optimization test case. However, in order to compare the results of the NACA 0015 with the optimization test cases and demonstrate how VAWT design can benefit from using optimization, the solidity of the baseline geometry was not adjusted.

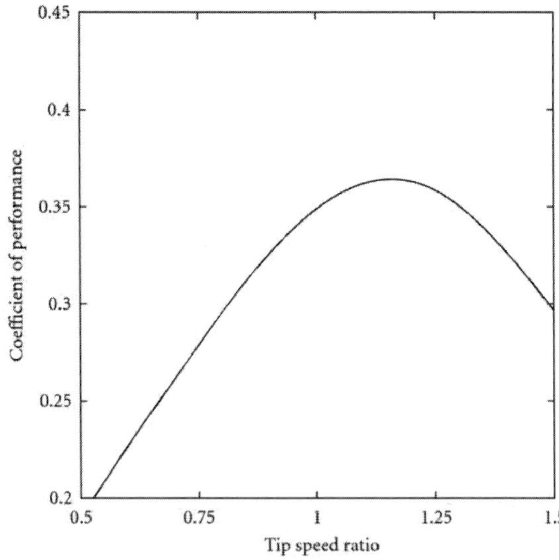

FIGURE 10: NACA 0015 performance envelope, $\sigma = 1.5$.

4.5.3 CASE 1: 3-PARAMETER OPTIMIZATION

The first test case to run through the optimization system was the 3-parameter case. The idea was to maximize the torque of the VAWT for a fixed solidity and tip speed ratio. The case ran for approximately 1 week on the cluster described in Section 4, after which the maximum number of user specified generations was reached (G = 11). Because there was no guarantee that the optimization algorithm would find the optimum design, the goal was to obtain an improved design that was able to achieve a higher efficiency than the baseline geometry.

To demonstrate the capabilities of the optimization system and show that 1 week was enough time to achieve an optimized geometry, 2 unique initial populations that were randomly generated by the DE code were run through the optimization system. The results of the 2 unique runs will be presented and compared with the baseline geometry. The optimization is said to have been successful if the VAWT utilizing the optimized airfoil cross-section achieved a higher efficiency than the baseline geometry at the design tip speed ratio ($\lambda = 1$).

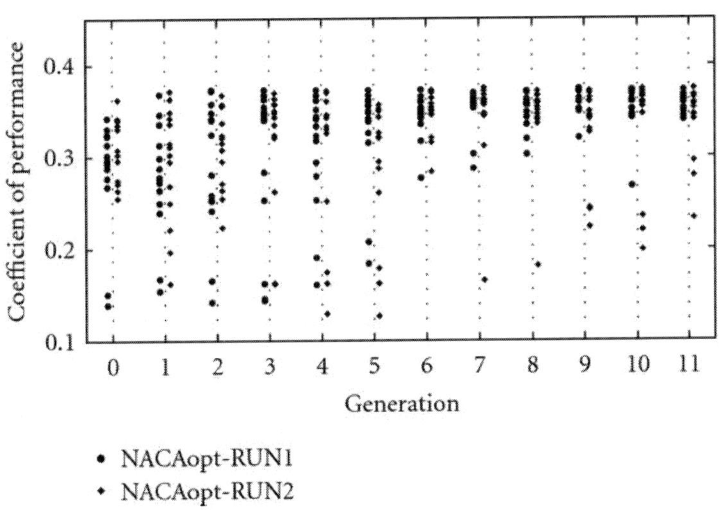

FIGURE 11: COP versus generation for all population members, 1st test case.

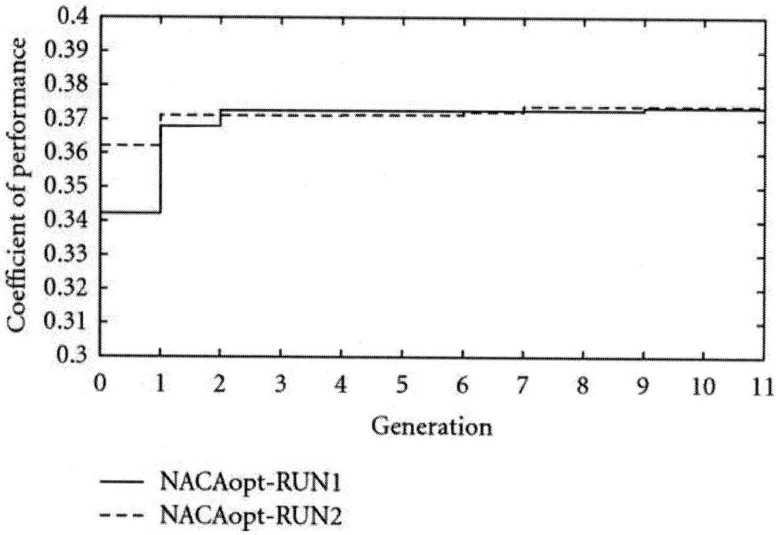

FIGURE 12: Max COP versus generation, 1st test case.

4.5.3.1 OPTIMIZATION RESULTS

Due to the nature of the DE algorithm, the initial population is random and completely different for the 2 runs conducted. The reason for starting with 2 different initial populations was to ensure that 11 generations was a sufficient amount time to find an optimized design while avoiding premature convergence or stagnation.

The diversity of the population for all generations can seen in Figure 11. This figure illustrates how the COP varies with generation. NACAopt-RUN1 and NACAopt-RUN2 refer to the 2 unique runs conducted for the 1st test case. It can be seen that the populations for each of the first 5 generations are quite diverse. However, after the 5th generation the populations begin to converge while still remaining somewhat diverse, a characteristic of the stochastic nature of the DE algorithm.

While Figure 11 illustrates the diversity of the population for each generation, Figure 12 provides a history of the best overall objective function value throughout the optimization. If the COP at the current generation happens to be higher than the previous maximum, it is replaced and the new airfoil design parameters are used to generate the next population. After 11 generations NACAopt-RUN1 and NACAopt-RUN2 were able to achieve a maximum COP of 0.373 and 0.374, respectively, despite the fact that each run was initialized from a different initial population.

The optimized geometry for both runs can be seen in Figure 13 compared with the NACA 0015 cross-section. The NACAopt-RUN1 airfoil has a maximum camber of 0.0094c, a maximum camber location of 0.599c, and a maximum thickness of 0.177c, where c is the chord length of the airfoil. The choice in a cambered airfoil geometry over a symmetric cross-section could be an indication that slight camber increases the efficiency of high-solidity rotors that experience undesirable blade vortex interactions. The fact that the maximum COP and the optimized airfoil cross-section for both runs are indistinguishable indicates that 11 generations is sufficient. Therefore, it is unnecessary to discuss the performance of both VAWTs and only the performance of the NACAopt-RUN1 will be presented.

The performance envelope for the VAWT using the NACAopt airfoil cross-section can be seen in Figure 14. Because the optimization was run for $\lambda = 1$, the blade shape was tailored to perform as best as possible at this value. Therefore, the optimum tip speed ratio is much closer to 1, signifying that the solidity of the rotor would have to be adjusted to achieve maximum efficiency at $\lambda = 1$.

4.5.3.2 BASELINE COMPARISON

While the optimization algorithm was able to find an optimized NACA 4-series geometry for $\sigma = 1.5$ and $\lambda = 1$ with very little user input and little or no designer intuition or experience, it had to be compared with the baseline geometry to quantify the performance gained by using such approach. The performance envelopes for the NACAopt and NACA 0015 VAWT designs are shown in Figure 15. For the design tip speed ratio $\lambda = 1$, the NACAopt design has a COP = 0.373, 2.4% higher than the NACA 0015 baseline geometry, which over the lifetime of the VAWT is considered a significant improvement.

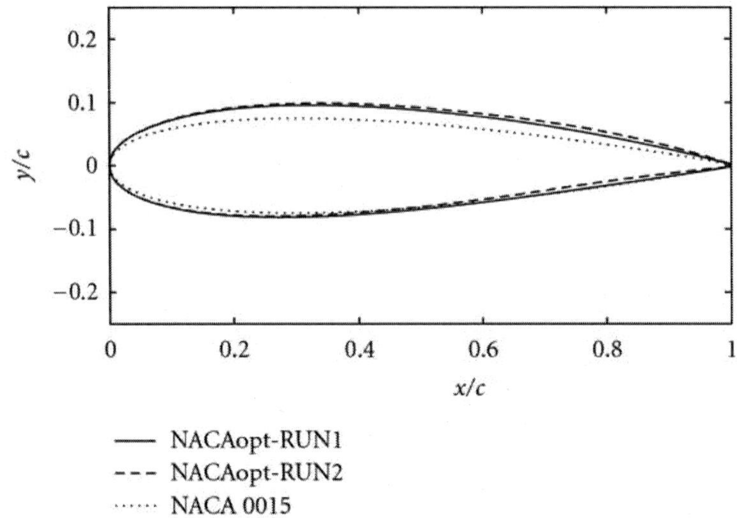

FIGURE 13: Optimized NACA 4-series airfoil geometry, 1st test case.

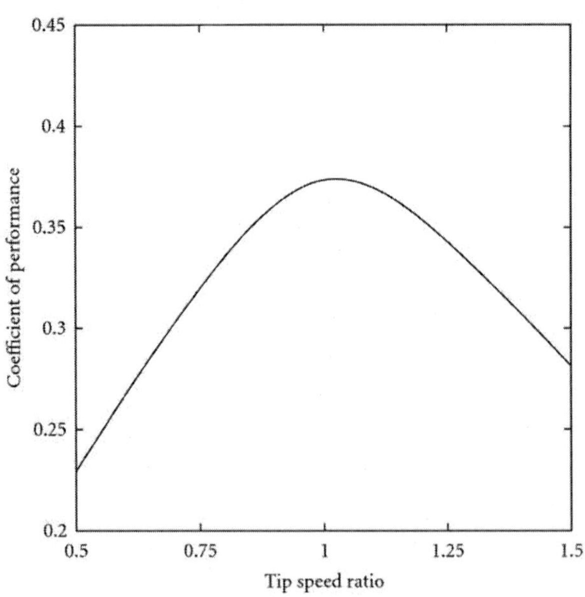

FIGURE 14: NACAopt performance envelope, 1st test case.

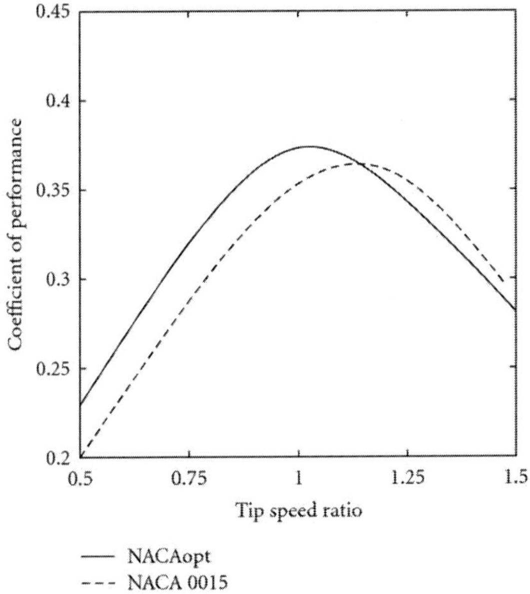

FIGURE 15: NACAopt versus NACA 0015 performance, 1st test case.

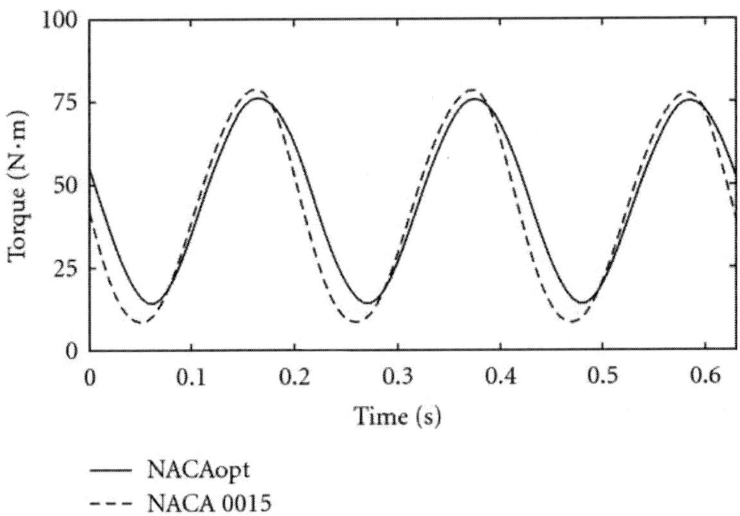

FIGURE 16: NACAopt versus NACA 0015 torque for $\lambda = 1$, 1st test case.

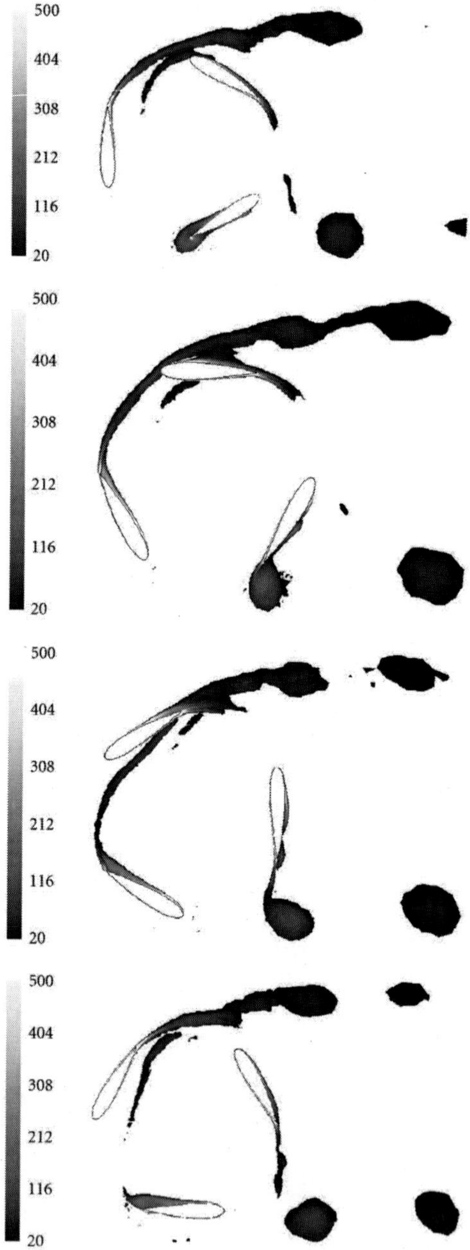

FIGURE 17: NACAopt (a) and NACA 0015 (b) vorticity contours, 1st test case.

In order to understand the mechanism for improved efficiency over the baseline geometry, the torque for a single rotation was observed, seen in Figure 16. While the frequency of the oscillation in the torque is the same for both geometries, the peak-to-peak amplitude for the NACA 0015 is higher than that of the NACAopt geometry. The higher thickness of the NACAopt geometry allows for such a cross-section to achieve a slightly higher angle of attack before stall than that of the NACA 0015 airfoil. Therefore, due to the increase in drag associated with the dynamic stall of the NACA 0015, a higher cyclic loading is observed. Not only did the NACAopt obtain a higher efficiency, but also a reduction in cyclic loading which could lead to a longer lifespan than the NACA 0015 geometry.

Interesting flow field phenomena were captured when visualizing the vorticity seen in Figure 17. The image clearly reveals that the wake of one blade actually interacts with the trailing blade, a characteristic typical of high-solidity rotors. This interaction disturbs the flow, altering the velocity field around the trailing blade, and is most likely the reason a cambered airfoil was chosen for this high-solidity geometry. In the pair of images labeled b, a leading edge separation bubble can be seen forming on the lower left blade for the NACA 0015 geometry. However, the same phenomena is not observed for the NACAopt geometry. In c and d as the blade continues to rotate counterclockwise the separation bubble becomes larger and eventually separates, contributing the trailing vortex and increasing its strength. The increase in the efficiency of the NACAopt geometry can be attributed to the airfoil cross-section's favorable characteristics at higher angles of attack, leading to the elimination of the leading edge separation bubble and a reduction in cyclic loading.

4.5.4 CASE 2: 4-PARAMETER OPTIMIZATION

The second test case to run through the optimization system was the 4-parameter case. For this case, the idea was to maximize the torque of the VAWT for a fixed tip speed ratio and let the solidity of the rotor become a design variable. Allowing the solidity to become a parameter gave the wind turbine complete geometric flexibility. Not only was the blade shape allowed to change, but also the size of the blade. The case ran for approximately

10 days on the cluster described in Section 4, after which the maximum number of user specified generations was reached (G = 20). The goal for this case was to demonstrate that, with increased geometric flexibility, a VAWT could be designed that outperformed the baseline NACA 0015 geometry, providing a solution that was beyond the intuition of the designer. Similar to the first case, the optimization was run for $\lambda = 1$.

4.5.4.1 OPTIMIZATION RESULTS

The objective function value, COP, can be seen for each generation in Figure 18. Similar to the first case, this figure illustrates how the COP varies with generation. For the first 8 generations, the stochastic nature of the DE algorithm is evident. However, after the 8th generation the populations begin to converge and lose their diversity.

The history of the maximum COP throughout the optimization is shown in Figure 19. After just the 2nd generation, the maximum COP does not change for 9 generations, signifying the possibility of premature convergence. However, looking back at Figure 18, the population has not lost its diversity, an indication that the algorithm did not converge prematurely. After the 9th generation the maximum COP began changing every couple of generations and eventually reached a COP of 0.409 after the 20th generation.

The optimized airfoil cross-section can be seen in Figure 20. The NACAopt airfoil is symmetric with a maximum thickness of 0.237c and a rotor solidity of 0.883. The blade is 58% thicker than the NACA 0015 and the solidity has been reduced by 40%. The choice in a symmetric airfoil is significant. Because low-solidity rotors do not experience strong blade vortex interactions, the positive and negative angles of attack that the blades experience are of the same magnitude; therefore, symmetric airfoils are typically used. Compared with the 3-parameter optimization this dramatic change in geometry indicates that, when given the opportunity, the optimization tends to seek out symmetric airfoil cross-sections. In the previous case, a slightly cambered geometry was chosen; this was most likely the result of the smaller design space associated with the 3-parameter optimization.

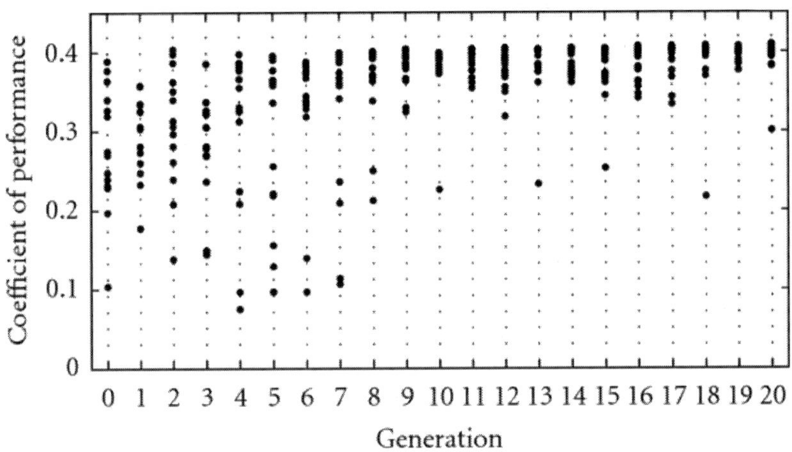

FIGURE 18: COP versus generation for all population members, 2nd test case.

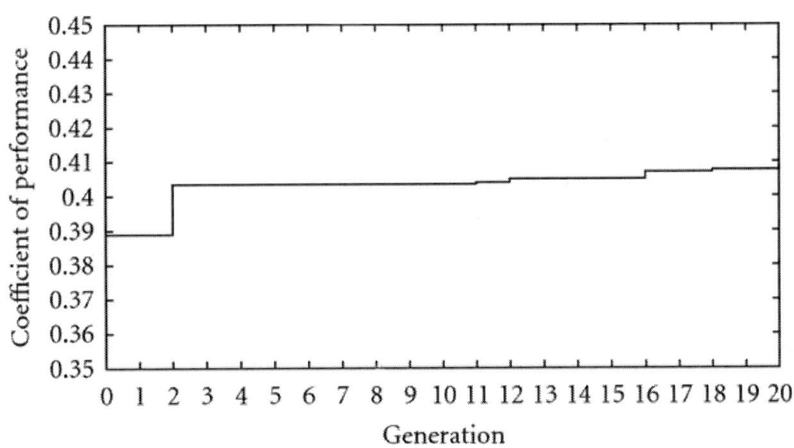

FIGURE 19: Max COP versus generation, 2nd test case.

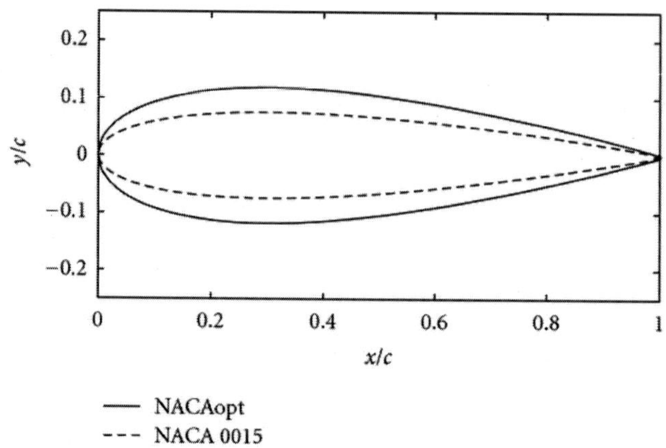

FIGURE 20: Optimized NACA 4-series airfoil geometry (σ = 0.883), 2nd test case.

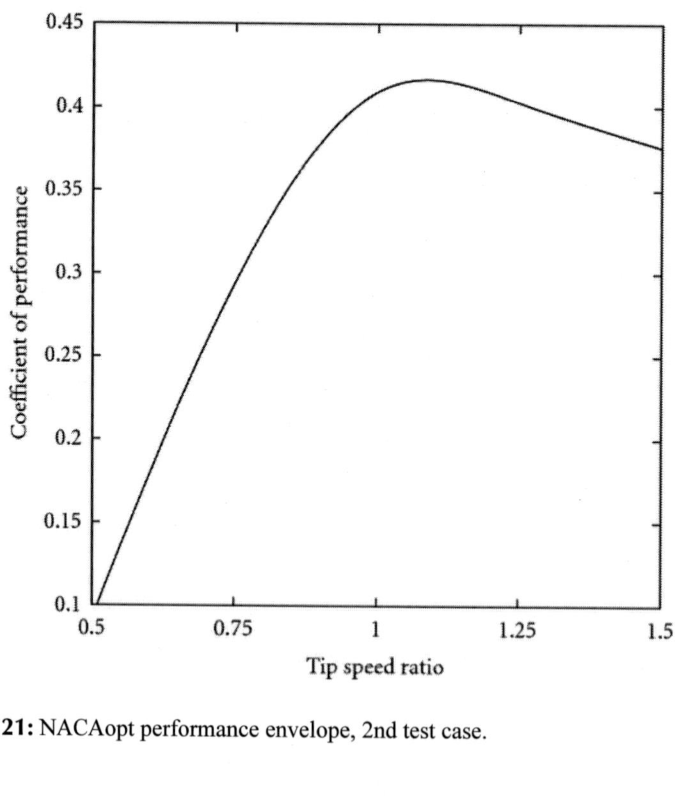

FIGURE 21: NACAopt performance envelope, 2nd test case.

The performance envelope for the NACAopt geometry can be seen in Figure 21. Allowing the solidity to become a design parameter improved the peak performance over both the baseline geometry and the 3-parameter optimization. However, contrary to initial belief, the optimum tip speed ratio is not equivalent to the design tip speed ratio. While the 4-parameter optimization allowed the entire geometry to adjust for best performance, this was accomplished only for a single tip speed ratio, the design tip speed ratio. Therefore, there was no guarantee that the optimum tip speed ratio and design tip speed ratio would coincide, a claim that has been considered a topic for future research.

4.5.4.2 COMPARISON

The optimization algorithm was able to find an optimized NACA 4-series airfoil cross-section with $\sigma = 0.883$ for $\lambda = 1$ in 20 generations, the performance of which was compared with the baseline NACA 0015 geometry shown in Figure 22. The NACAopt design was able to achieve a COP = 0.409 at $\lambda = 1$, ultimately resulting in a 6% increase in efficiency over the baseline NACA 0015 geometry and even a 3.6% increase in efficiency when compared with the 3-parameter optimization. This case successfully demonstrated that allowing the solidity to become a parameter, and hence providing complete geometric flexibility, resulted in a significant increase in the efficiency.

In an attempt to determine the reason for the higher efficiency associated with the NACAopt geometry, the torque for a single rotation of the optimized design was compared with the baseline geometry, shown in Figure 23. While the frequency of the oscillation is the same because both designs operate at $\lambda = 1$, there is an obvious phase shift in the torque oscillations resulting in the maximum performance of the NACAopt design occurring slightly earlier than the NACA 0015 rotor. The NACAopt designs 40% reduction in solidity coupled with the 58% increase in thickness allowed for such a cross-section to achieve a higher overall peak performance when compared with the 15% thick NACA 0015 geometry.

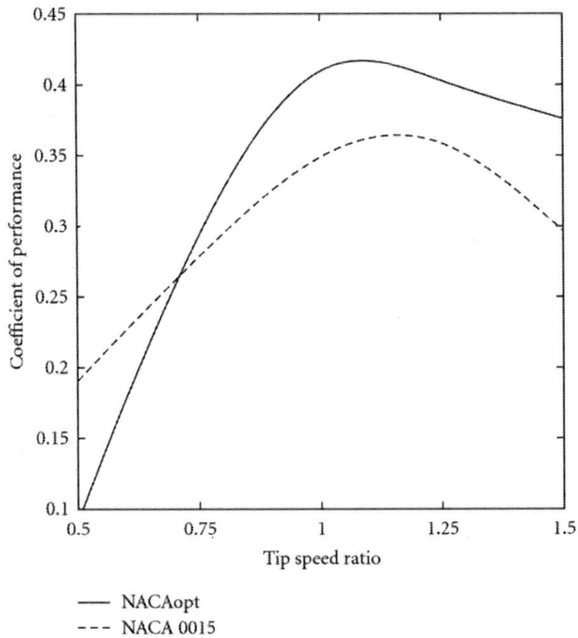

FIGURE 22: NACAopt versus NACA 0015 performance, 2nd test case.

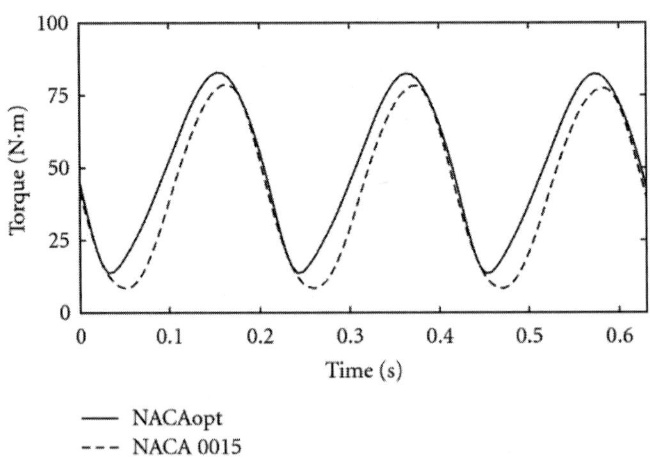

FIGURE 23: NACAopt versus NACA 0015 torque for $\lambda = 1$, 2nd test case.

4.6 CONCLUSIONS

This work successfully demonstrated a fully automated process for optimizing the airfoil cross-section of a VAWT. The generation of NACA airfoil geometries, hybrid mesh generation, and unsteady CFD were coupled with the DE algorithm subject to tip speed ratio, solidity, and blade profile design constraints. The optimization system was then used to obtain an optimized blade cross-section for 2 test cases, resulting in designs that achieved higher efficiency than the baseline geometry. The optimized design for the 1st test case achieved an efficiency 2.4% higher than the baseline geometry. The increase in efficiency of the optimized geometry was attributed to the elimination of a leading edge separation bubble that was causing a reduction in efficiency and an increase in cyclic loading. For the 2nd test case, the VAWT was given complete geometric flexibility as both the blade shape and rotor solidity were allowed to change during the optimization process. This resulted in a geometry that achieved an efficiency 6% higher than the baseline NACA 0015 geometry. This increase in efficiency was a result of the 40% decrease in solidity coupled with the 58% increase in thickness, leading to a slight phase shift in the torque and higher overall peak performance. While this study is significant, it represents an initial step towards the development of an operational VAWT utilizing an optimized blade cross-section and requires further research and development.

REFERENCES

1. M. Islam, D. S. K. Ting, and A. Fartaj, "Aerodynamic models for Darrieus-type straight-bladed vertical axis wind turbines," Renewable and Sustainable Energy Reviews, vol. 12, no. 4, pp. 1087–1109, 2008.
2. I. Paraschivoiu, F. Saeed, and V. Desobry, "Prediction capabilities in vertical-axis wind turbine aerodynamics," in Proceedings of the World Wind Energy Conference and Exhibition, Berlin, Germany, 2002.
3. C. J. Ferreira, H. Bijl, G. van Bussel, and G. van Kuik, "Simulating Dynamic Stall in a 2D VAWT: modeling strategy, verification and validation with Particle Image Velocimetry data," Journal of Physics, vol. 75, no. 1, Article ID 012023, 2007.
4. J. C. Vassberg, A. K. Gopinath, and A. Jameson, "Revisiting the vertical-axis wind-turbine design using advanced computational fluid dynamics," in Proceedings of the

43rd AIAA Aerospace Sciences Meeting and Exhibit, pp. 12783–12805, Reno, Nev, USA, January 2005.

5. J. Edwards, N. Durrani, R. Howell, and N. Qin, "Wind tunnel and numerical study of a small vertical axis wind turbine," in Proceedings of the 46th AIAA Aerospace Sciences Meeting and Exhibit, Reno, Nev, USA, January 2008.
6. M. Torresi, S. M. Camporeale, P. D. Strippoli, and G. Pascazio, "Accurate numerical simulation of a high solidity Wells turbine," Renewable Energy, vol. 33, no. 4, pp. 735–747, 2008.
7. T. J. Baker, "Mesh generation: art or science?" Progress in Aerospace Sciences, vol. 41, no. 1, pp. 29–63, 2005.
8. A. Ueno and B. Dennis, "Optimization of apping airfoil motion with computational uid dynamics," The International Review of Aerospace Engineering, vol. 2, no. 2, pp. 104–111, 2009.
9. R. Bourguet, G. Martinat, G. Harran, and M. Braza, "Aerodynamic multi-criteria shape optimization ofvawt blade profile by viscous approach," Wind Energy, pp. 215–219, 2007.
10. M. Jureczko, M. Pawlak, and A. Mężyk, "Optimisation of wind turbine blades," Journal of Materials Processing Technology, vol. 167, no. 2-3, pp. 463–471, 2005.
11. P. Fuglsang and H. A. Madsen, "Optimization method for wind turbine rotors," Journal of Wind Engineering and Industrial Aerodynamics, vol. 80, no. 1-2, pp. 191–206, 1999.
12. H. Rahai and H. Hefazi, "Vertical axis wind turbine with optimized blade profile," Tech. Rep. 7,393,177 B2, July 2008.
13. D. Dellinger, "Wind - average wind speed," 2008, http://www.ncdc.noaa.gov/oa/climate/online/ccd/avgwind.html.
14. N. S. Çetin, M. A. Yurdusev, R. Ata, and A. Özdemir, "Assessment of optimum tip speed ratio of wind turbines," Mathematical and Computational Applications, vol. 10, no. 1, pp. 147–154, 2005.
15. I. Abbott and A. von Doenhoff, Theory of Wing Sections Including a Summary of Airfoil Data, Dover, New York, NY, USA, 1959.
16. W. Anderson and D. Bonhaus, "Aerodynamic design on unstructured grids for turbulent ows," Tech. Rep. 112867, National Aeronautics and Space Administration Langley Research Center, Hampton, Va, USA, 1997.
17. J. Elliott and J. Peraire, "Practical three-dimensional aerodynamic design and optimization using unstructured meshes," AIAA Journal, vol. 35, no. 9, pp. 1479–1485, 1997.
18. M. Giles, "Aerodynamic design optimisation for complex geometries using unstructured grids," Tech. Rep. 97/08, Oxford University Computing Laboratory Numerical Analysis Group, Oxford, UK, 2000.
19. E. J. Nielsen and W. K. Anderson, "Aerodynamic design optimization on unstructured meshes using the Navier-Stokes equations," AIAA Journal, 1998, AIAA-98-4809.
20. Fluent, "Fluent 6.3 user's guide," Tech. Rep., Fluent Inc., Lebanon, NH, USA, 2006.
21. P. Spalart and S. Allmaras, "A one-equation turbulence model for aerodynamic ows," in Proceedings of the 30th AerospaceSciences Meeting and Exhibit, Reno, Nev, USA, 1992, 92-0439.

22. J. Ferziger and M. Peric, Computational Methods for Fluid Dynamics, Springer, New York, NY, USA, 3rd edition, 2002.
23. K. V. Price, "Differential evolution: a fast and simple numerical optimizer," in Proceedings of the Biennial Conference of the North American Fuzzy Information Processing Society (NAFIPS '96), pp. 524–527, June 1996.
24. R. Storn and K. Price, "Differential evolution—a simple and efficient adaptive scheme for global optimizationover continuous spcaes," Tech. Rep. TR-95-012, ICSI, March 1995.
25. R. Storn and K. Price, "Differential evolution—a simple and efficient heuristic for global optimization over continuous spaces," Journal of Global Optimization, vol. 11, no. 4, pp. 341–359, 1997.
26. J. Steinbrenner, N. Wyman, and J. Chawner, "Development and implementation of gridgen's hyperbolicpde and extrusion methods," in Proceedings of the 38th AIAA Aerospace Sciences Meeting and Exhibit, Reno, Nev, USA, 2000.

PART II

GENERATORS AND GEAR SYSTEMS

CHAPTER 5

PERFORMANCE EVALUATION OF AN INDUCTION MACHINE WITH AUXILIARY WINDING FOR WIND TURBINE POWER

RIADH W. Y. HABASH, QIANJUN TANG, PIERRE GUILLEMETTE, AND NAZISH IRFAN

5.1 INTRODUCTION

Wind energy has been shown to be one of the most feasible sources of renewable energy. It presents attractive opportunities to a wide range of people, including investors, entrepreneurs, and users. Wind along with other renewable energy sources such as bio and hydro require electromechanical systems to convert naturally available energy sources to rotation through prime movers and then to electricity through electric generators. The prime movers and generators are critical components of such systems that must be affordable, reliable, environmentally safe, and user-friendly.

Self-excited induction generators (SEIG) (squirrel cage and/or wound rotor) are strong candidate for such applications. The fact that they are not yet widely used in the field reflects a major gap in knowledge. An attrac-

This chapter was originally published under the Creative Commons Attribution License. Habash RWY, Tang Q, Guillemette P, and Irfan N. Performance Evaluation of an Induction Machine with Auxiliary Winding for Wind Turbine Power. ISRN Renewable Energy ***2012*** *(2012). http://dx.doi.org/10.5402/2012/167192.*

tive option is to take an "off-the-shelve" induction machine and modify it suitably to provide optimized performance in terms of efficiency, suppressed signal distortion and harmonics, resistive losses and overheating, and power factor.

In the 1935s, Bassett and Potter [1] demonstrated the possibility of using an induction machine, in the self-excited mode. Since then, the use of induction machines as generators is becoming more popular for the renewable sources [2–5]. The simplicity and flexibility exhibited by the induction machine in providing electromechanical energy conversion make it the favoured choice for wind systems operating with an existing utility grid. Induction generators in general have many advantages: simple, cheap, reliable, brushless (squirrel cage rotor), no synchronizing equipment, absence of DC power supply for excitation, good over-speed capability, inherent protection against short circuit, easy to control, not producing sparks like DC motors, and require very little maintenance [6–8]. The induction machine, however, is not without its drawbacks including the need for a high starting current, reactive power for operation, and poor voltage regulation under varying speeds. Thus its power factor is inherently poor, and it is worse especially at starting and when running with light loads or when operating with power electronics converters. At starting, the input power to an induction motor is mainly reactive. It draws up to 6 times of its rated current at about 0.2 power factor and takes some time to come to its rated speed, where the power factor improves significantly to above 0.6 depending on the load. This high starting current at a poor power factor usually affects the loads and limits the application range of the machine; accordingly, new techniques should be developed to enhance its performance.

In the literature, several techniques to improve the power factor and accordingly the performance of induction machines have been suggested, including the synchronous compensation, fixed capacitors, fixed capacitors with switched inductor, solid-state power factor controller, and switched capacitors [9–13]. A three-phase induction motor equipped with a three-phase auxiliary winding in delta configuration, which is magnetically coupled to the main winding connected in a star configuration, has recently been proposed as well [9–11]. This scheme uses thyristor switched capacitors connected in parallel to each phase of the auxiliary winding. A three-phase asynchronous machine which employs an auxiliary three-phase winding in wye configuration together with a pulse width modulation (PWM) inverter to supply the excitation to the machine has also been suggested [9–11, 13]. However, these techniques suffer several drawbacks. The synchronous compensation technique is complex and not cost effective. Other techniques incorporate directly the connection of capacitor and lead to the problems of voltage regeneration and over voltages and a very high current inrush during starting. In addition, techniques incorporating controlled switches in the stator winding circuit generate large harmonic current in the machine and in the line.

In this paper, an enhanced squirrel cage induction generator (SCIG) model with an auxiliary winding is proposed, analyzed, and verified experimentally. A simple and low-cost scheme where resonance can be achieved without connection to the terminals is proposed. This may be achieved by using an LC resonant circuit as an auxiliary winding which is only magnetically coupled to the stator main winding to supply leading reactive power to the machine. Due to its high improved characteristics, this generator can enhance the performance of the SWEC.

5.2 INDUCTION GENERATOR FOR WIND POWER

An induction machine operates as a generator if a supply of reactive power is available to provide the machine's excitation. A SEIG, although known for more than a half century, is still a subject of considerable attention. The interest in this topic is primarily due to the application of SEIG in isolated power systems. When an induction machine is driven at a speed greater than the synchronous speed (negative slip) by means of an external prime mover, the direction of induced torque is reversed and theoretically it starts working as an induction generator [14]. Self-excitation in an induction machine occurs when the rotor is driven by a prime mover and a suitable capacitance is connected across the stator terminals, allowing the induction machine to be used as a standalone generator [15]. An induction generator does not develop reactive power but it consumes it, so it is required to connect a capacitor with the auxiliary winding for self-excitation. This capacitor develops the required reactive power needed by both generator and load, and any reactive power diverted to the load causes a major drop in the generator voltage. Nonetheless, because of its inherently poor voltage regulation and efficiency, the single-phase induction generator has had few applications in a wind generation. One attempt at addressing the voltage regulation weakness is a self-regulated self-excited single-phase induction generator which uses two capacitors connected in shunt and in series with the main and the auxiliary winding of the machine, respectively [16, 17]. On the other hand, incorporation of copper for the rotor bars and end rings in place of aluminum would result in improvements in motor energy efficiency [18, 19].

The induction generator can work in two modes (e.g., grid connected and isolated mode). In case of a grid-connected mode, the induction generator can draw reactive power either from the grid but it will place a burden on the grid or by connecting a capacitor bank across the generator terminals [20].

The main factor which characterizes the induction machine is its power curve. The shaft power from the electric generator is calculated using loss separation as follows:

$$P_{shaft} = P_{output} + P_{ohmic} + P_{core} + P_{friction} \quad (1)$$

The output power (P_{output}) is measured using a power analyser. The analyser determines the power, electrical frequency, and stator currents from the generator to a variable resistive load bank. The load bank is used to vary the load on the generator, at a particular incident wind speed, in order to determine the maximum power point. The shaft power (P_{shaft}) is then determined by incorporating resistive losses (P_{ohmic}) associated with power loss in the stator resistance, core loss (P_{core}) associated with hysteresis and eddy-current losses in the iron core of the machine, and friction and windage losses in the generator ($P_{friction}$).

The emergence of new grid codes will pose wind turbine developers to new challenges, mainly with a high penetration of wind power in the network, the wind turbines should be able to continuously supply the network during voltage sags. These new grid codes which are being proposed in Norway [21] and other countries will most likely influence the topol-

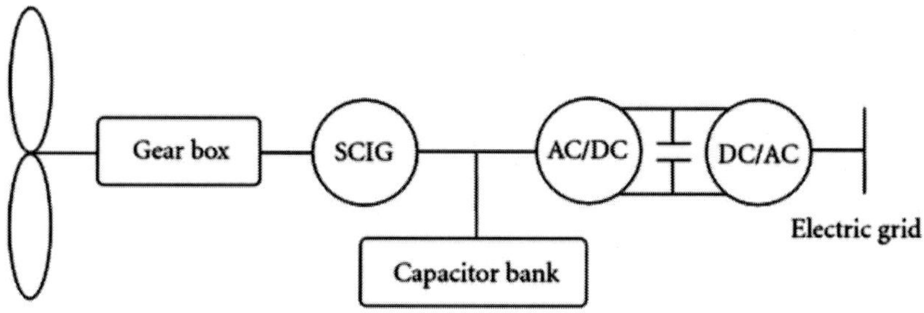

FIGURE 1: Grid connection scheme for a wind turbine.

ogy of the electrical system (generator and network interface) of future wind turbines. To cope with these new challenges, several industries have already directed research efforts to the development of machines through capability. Among the technology choices, SCIGs are a very attractive for wind power generation because they are robust, inexpensive, and have low cost and maintenance requirement.

Since the SCIG draws reactive power from the grid, this concept was extended with a capacitor bank for reactive power compensation. Smoother grid connection was also achieved by incorporating a soft starter. Because the generator operation is only stable in the narrow range around the synchronous speed, the wind turbine equipped with this type of generator is often called fixed-speed system. The grid connection scheme of a fixed speed wind turbine with SCIG is shown in Figure 1.

The need for reactive power support and poor power factor are the two major drawbacks of induction generators. Induction generators as well as the load, which are generally inductive in nature, require the supply of reactive power. Unbalanced reactive power operation results in voltage variation. Reactive power control by using VAR compensator (SVC) [22], or static-synchronous compensator (STATCOM) [23], work well but they may add harmonics to the electrical network while compensating reactive power continuously and may not be able to provide the adequate amount of reactive power under varying input and/or load conditions such as wind energy sources which fluctuate highly in nature. On the other hand, several techniques to improve the power factor of induction machines have been suggested, namely, capacitors, capacitors with switched inductor, and solid-state power factor controllers [10, 11]. The initiation of the induction machine excitation can be viewed as the response of a resonant circuit, comprising the machine and the capacitance connected to its terminals. Once resonance is approached, the generated voltage will grow [24].

5.3 PROPOSED TECHNIQUE

In this paper, a passive technique is proposed to overcome most of the drawbacks noted above. The proposed technique makes use of an auxiliary winding connected in wye configuration (with capacitors) as shown in Figure 2. It is only magnetically coupled to the main winding. Therefore, the performance can be increased without any additional active mass. This method uses combined (two three-phase) windings on the stator similar to the scheme used in delta-star connected three-phase transformer (neglecting the rotor effect). The main stator winding is the primary connected in

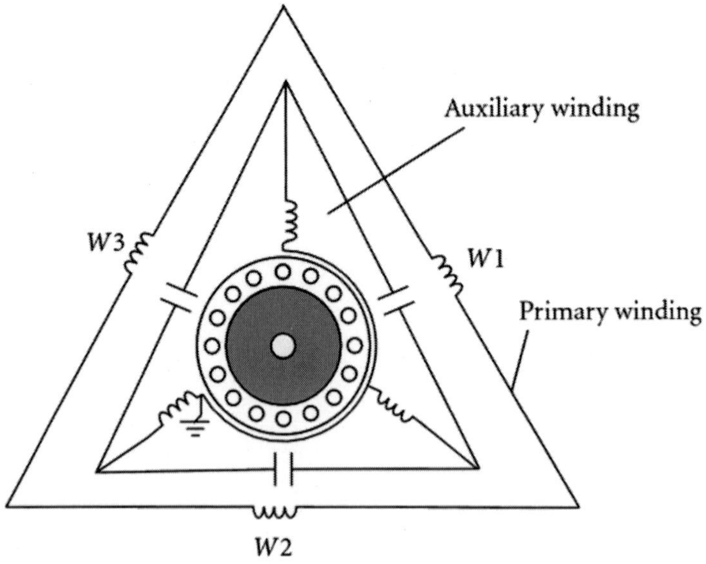

FIGURE 2: A three-phase generator with auxiliary winding.

delta to the source and the auxiliary winding is the secondary in wye. It means that the third harmonics component would be short circuited by the delta side with the result that there will be no third harmonic voltage across the lines. In addition, the above two sets of windings have the same poles, so they share the same operating frequency. Basing on delta-wye transformation of the auxiliary windings and on transformer approach of the induction machine, the electric model per phase of the proposed strategy is shown in Figure 3. In the proposed scheme, a three phase induction machine with a dual stator winding is employed. One set of the three phase windings (main) is directly connected to the supply while the other set of the three phase windings (auxiliary) is connected to a capacitor. Both windings (main and auxiliary) are magnetically coupled but electrically isolated. The main idea of the proposed scheme is to connect suitable capacitor in auxiliary windings such that the main winding will carry mainly active power while the auxiliary winding will carry mainly reactive power.

The couplings between the elements of the machine are presented as ideal transformers with N_a: the turn's ratio between auxiliary winding and stator (N_a less than 1); N_r: the turn's ratio between rotor and stator (N_r less than 1); N_{ra}: the turn's ratio between rotor and auxiliary winding (N_{ra} less than 1). Because of no electric connection between the two sets of windings and the usage of the properly designed windings, the electromagnetic compatibility (EMC) of the machine is improved significantly.

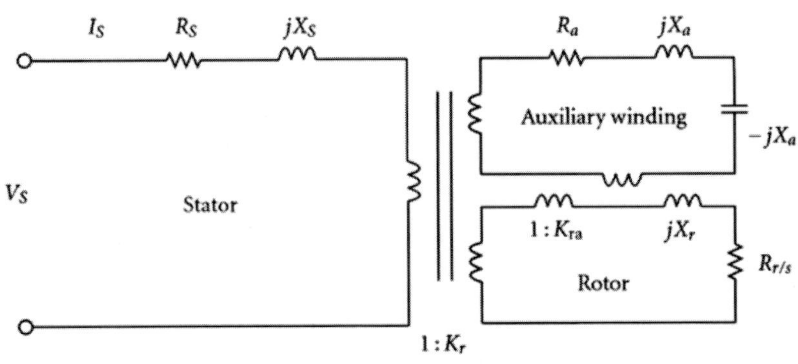

FIGURE 3: Model per phase of the proposed strategy.

With sufficient ampere-turn capability of the auxiliary winding, it is possible to obtain nearly unity power factor operation at the terminals of the main winding over a range of load conditions including a rated load. The auxiliary winding gives priority to the harmonic suppression, and also has the function of a reactive compensation which provides the means for maximum energy conversion and efficiency.

The winding geometry of the modified generator (Trias) combines inductive and capacitive effects into the machine, thereby creating an effect comparable to a resistive load as shown in Figure 4. To compute the reactance needed for power correction of a typical induction machine, we need to estimate the negative reactance power and therefore the capacitance along the operating conditions of the machine. It is important therefore to determine the capacitor value for a minimum and maximum compensation of the power factor and also to take into consideration the value of the current that flows in the auxiliary winding as the size of the wire depends strongly on it. Usually, the current in auxiliary winding is leading over the stator current but it is lower in magnitude compared to the stator current. This is a must situation during operation as the auxiliary winding has smaller wire size in order to be accommodated in the same slots with the main winding Consider.

$$X_{ceq} = \frac{|V|^2}{Q_c}$$

$$C = -\frac{1}{\omega X_{ceq}} \qquad (2)$$

where X_{ceq} is the reactive impedance, V is the rms voltage across the load, Q_c is the capacitive reactive power, and ω is the angular frequency. As an induction motor, all the energy supplied by the power utility goes into creating real work (kW). In doing so, the machine will operate at near unity power factor, almost with all kinds of loads. Also, the machine has the same characteristic when operating as a generator.

Stable operating points for the SEIG under balanced conditions may be determined from a standard equivalent circuit by simply balancing the

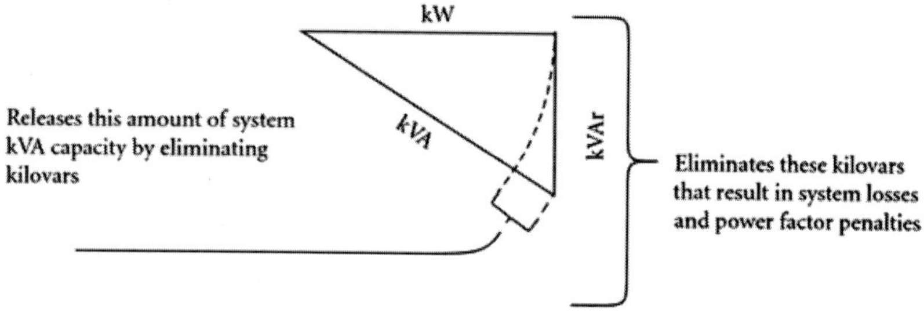

FIGURE 4: Power triangle of an induction machine.

real- and reactive-power flow between the machine, the excitation capacitance, and load. One method for solving at these operating points has been presented in [25]. The amount of inductance and capacitance required to maintain the generated voltage at a rated value can therefore be determined for a range of operating conditions. To determine operating points when the loading on the generator is unbalanced, it is necessary to use generalised electric machine theory.

Since both the windings (main and auxiliary) occupy the same slots and are therefore mutually coupled by their leakage flux, they can be modeled by two branches each having separate leakage reactance and resistance with a common mutual inductance. The effect of capacitor in auxiliary winding is represented by X_{ceq}. For a 920 hp, 460 V, 6 poles, and 60 Hz induction motor, Figure 5 shows the variation of imaginary part of the impedance (Z) with respect to X_{ceq} for different values of slip and also demonstrates that a unity power factor can be obtained at different values of the slip. It can be observed that for a particular slip, a unity power factor can be obtained at two different values of X_{ceq}. The larger value of X_{ceq} (smaller capacitance) corresponds to a small value of current and a smaller value of X_{ceq} (larger capacitance) corresponds to a higher current. It may also be concluded from Figure 5 that to obtain a unity power factor at higher load requires smaller value of X_{ceq} than that required for lighter load.

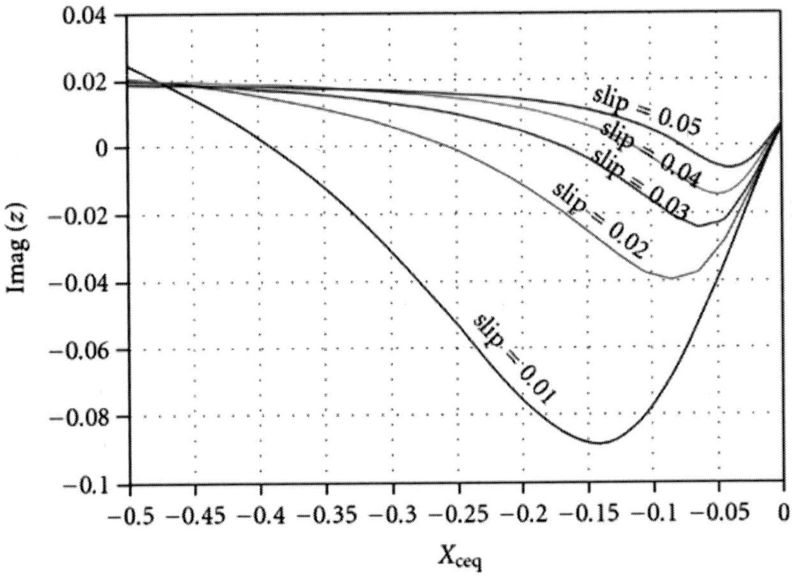

FIGURE 5: Imaginary part of the total impedance Z as a function of X_{ceq} for different values of the slip.

5.4 EXPERIMENTAL RESULTS

There exist several standards for testing electric machinery. For induction machines, the three most important ones are IEEE Standard 112, currently in use in USA and some parts of the world; JEC 37, in Japan; IEC 34-2, in use in most European countries. In Canada, the standard specified in the Energy Efficiency Regulations is "Method for Determining Energy Performance of Three-phase Induction Motors: CSA C390-98." This Standard is equivalent to the well-recognized standard "IEEE 112-1996, Method B: Test Procedure for Poly-phase Induction Motors and Generators."

A typical experimental test to compare a standard SCIG with the proposed one (standard SCIG with a passive auxiliary winding: Trias) is shown in Figure 6. A DC motor is connected to the shaft of the two induction machines as a drive. By varying the load from 10% up to 125% of the full load, different values of input power, power factor, reactive power, and apparent power are, respectively, obtained. The experimental results recorded during the experimental tests are given in Table 1 and Figures 7 and 8. It is shown that the induction machine with auxiliary winding (Trias) provides higher operating performance in terms of signal distortion and harmonics, resistive losses, overheating, starting, and operating power factor. At full load, the Trias SCIG provides a power factor of almost 0.99. In addition, the machine shows a decrease in losses of approximately 27% and reduction of in-rush current, the fact that the machine avoids the problem of overheating.

TABLE 1: Experimental test results of a standard and trias induction machine.

Quantity	Standard	Trias
Voltage (V)	117	117
Current (A)	2.69	0.426
Power (W)	43.2	43.7
Power factor	−0.130	−0.870
Reactive power (VAR)	−311	−24.1

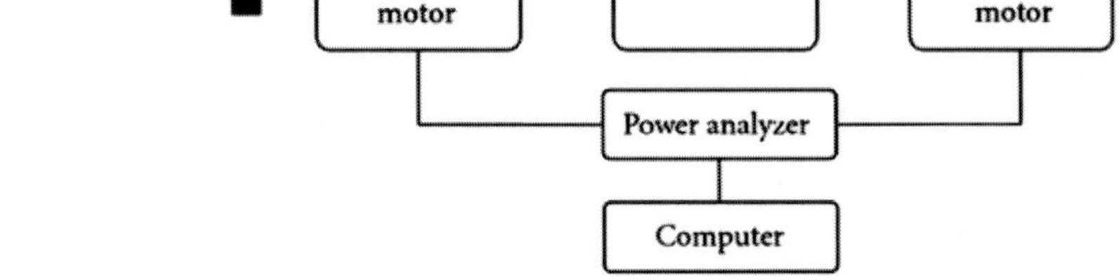

FIGURE 6: Typical measurement setup for an induction machine performance.

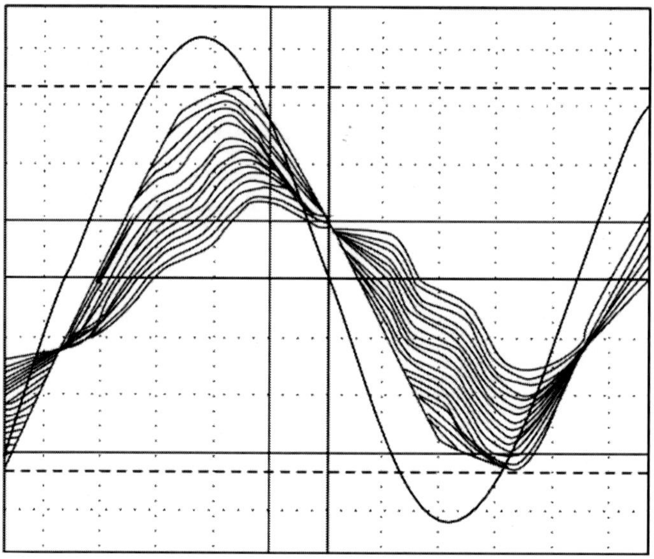

FIGURE 7: Signal acquired from an induction machine. (a) Standard. (b) With auxiliary winding.

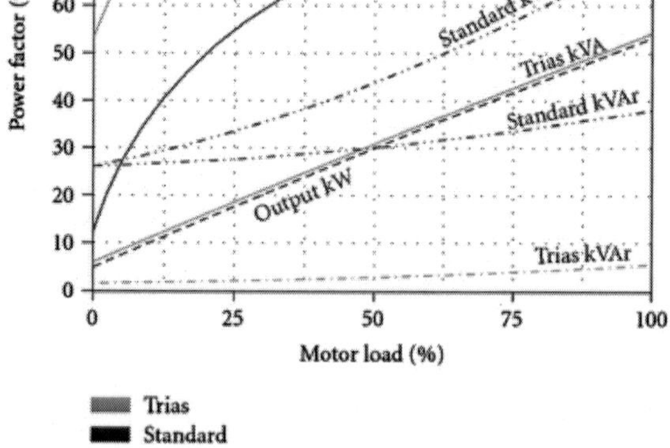

FIGURE 8: Power factor for an induction machine: standard and with auxiliary winding (Trias).

5.5 DISCUSSION AND CONCLUSION

The performance of an off-the-shelf three-phase induction machine can be enhanced for implementation as a generator in a SWEC to produce electricity to feed grid-connected or off-the-grid loads.

To facilitate the design of such machine, simulation and experimental procedures are presented to predict the steady-state performance of a three-phase induction generator with its stator windings connected under various loading conditions at any power factor. A passive auxiliary winding (LC excitation circuit) connected in wye configuration and magnetically coupled to the main winding of the induction machine has been successfully designed and implemented. The LC-excited induction machine uses capacitance and inductance to match or "tune" the natural occurring impedance in the inductive elements of a machine—allowing the machine to sustain itsown magnetic energyinternally, virtually independent of the power source. Also, the machine reduces load current up to 30%. Because the utility does not need to supply the magnetization current in the modified induction machine, the full load current is reduced. By reducing peak demand current up to 25%, the net inrush current is reduced. This creates a soft start, extending the life of the machine as well as the life of the SWEC.

The proposed technique involves mathematical modeling and simulation to calculate the values of capacitor and inductor. Experimental results obtained on the laboratory verify the validity of the technique.

REFERENCES

1. E. D. Bassett and F. M. Potter, "Capacitive excitation for induction generators," Electrical Engineering, vol. 35, pp. 540–545, 1935.
2. P. K. Shadhu Khan and J. K. Chatterjee, "Three-phase induction generators: a discussion on performance," Electric Machines and Power Systems, vol. 27, no. 8, pp. 813–832, 1999.
3. R. C. Bansal, D. P. Kothari, and T. S. Bhatti, "Induction generator for isolated hybrid power system applications: a review," in Proceedings of the 24th National Renewable Energy Convention, pp. 462–467, Bombay, India, December 2000.
4. C. Grantham, F. Rahman, and D. Seyoum, "A regulated self-excited induction generator for use in a remote area power supply," International Journal of Renewable Energy, vol. 2, no. 1, pp. 234–239, 2000.

5. R. C. Bansal, T. S. Bhatti, and D. P. Kothari, "Induction generator for isolated hybrid power system applications: a review," Journal of the Institution of Engineers, vol. 83, pp. 262–269, 2003.
6. B. Singh, R. B. Saxena, S. S. Murthy, and B. P. Singh, "A single-phase induction generator for lighting loads in remote areas," International Journal of Electrical Engineering Education, vol. 25, no. 3, pp. 269–275, 1988.
7. Y. H. A. Rahim, A. I. Alolah, and R. I. Al-Mudaiheem, "Performance of single phase induction generators," IEEE Transactions on Energy Conversion, vol. 8, no. 3, pp. 389–395, 1993.
8. O. Ojo and I. Bhat, "Analysis of single-phase self-excited induction generators: model development and steady-state calculations," IEEE Transactions on Energy Conversion, vol. 10, no. 2, pp. 254–260, 1995.
9. E. Muljadi, T. A. Lipo, and D. W. Novotny, "Power factor enhancement of induction machines by means of solid-state excitation," IEEE Transactions on Power Electronics, vol. 4, no. 4, pp. 409–418, 1989.
10. T. A. Lettenmaier, D. W. Novotny, and T. A. Lipo, "Single-phase induction motor with an electronically controlled capacitor," IEEE Transactions on Industry Applications, vol. 27, no. 1, pp. 38–43, 1991.
11. I. Tamrakar and O. P. Malik, "Power factor correction of induction motors using PWM inverter fed auxiliary stator winding," IEEE Transactions on Energy Conversion, vol. 14, no. 3, pp. 426–432, 1999.
12. C. Suciu, L. Dafinca, M. Kansara, and I. Margineanu, "Switched capacitor fuzzy control for power factor correction in inductive circuits," in Proceedings of the Power Electronics Specialists Conference, Galway, Irlanda, June 2000.
13. W. Hanguang, C. XIUMIN, L. Xianliang, and Y. Linjuan, "An investigation on three-phase capacitor induction motor," in Proceedings of Third Chinese International Conference on Electrical Machines, pp. 87–90, Xi'an, China, August 1999.
14. R. C. Bansal, "Three-phase self-excited induction generators: an overview," IEEE Transactions on Energy Conversion, vol. 20, no. 2, pp. 292–299, 2005.
15. J. M. Elder, J. T. Boys, and J. L. Woodward, "Self-excited induction machine as low cost generator," IEE Proceedings C, vol. 131, no. 2, pp. 33–41, 1984.
16. S. S. Murthy, "Novel self-excited self-regulated single phase induction generator," IEEE Transactions on Energy Conversion, vol. 8, no. 3, pp. 377–382, 1993.
17. T. Fukami, Y. Kaburaki, S. Kawahara, and T. Miyamoto, "Performance analysis of a self-regulated self-excited single-phase induction generator using a three-phase machine," IEEE Transactions on Energy Conversion, vol. 14, no. 3, pp. 622–627, 1999.
18. F. Parasiliti and M. Villani, "Design of high efficiency induction motors with die-casting copper rotors," in Energy Efficiency in Motor Driven Systems, F. Parasiliti and P. Bertoldi, Eds., pp. 144–151, Springer, 2003.
19. E. F. Brush, J. G. Cowie, D. T. Peters, and D. J. Van Son, "Die-cast copper motor rotors: motor test results, copper compared to aluminum," in Energy Efficiency In Motor Driven Systems, F. Parasiliti and P. Bertoldi, Eds., pp. 136–143, Springer, 2003.
20. R. C. Bansal, T. S. Bhatti, and D. P. Kothari, "Some aspects of grid connected wind electric energy conversion systems," Journal of the Institution of Engineers, vol. 82, pp. 25–28, 2001.
21. Nordisk Regelsamling (Nordic Grid Code), Nordel, 2004.

22. T. S. Bhatti, R. C. Bansal, and D. P. Kothari, "Reactive power control of isolated hybrid power systems," in Proceedings of the International Conference on Computer Applications in Electrical Engineering Recent Advances, pp. 626–632, Roorkee, India, February 2002.
23. B. Singh, S. S. Murthy, and S. Gupta, "Analysis and design of STATCOM-based voltage regulator for self-excited induction generators," IEEE Transactions on Energy Conversion, vol. 19, no. 4, pp. 783–790, 2004.
24. J. M. Elder, J. T. Boys, and J. L. Woodward, "The process of self excitation in induction generators," IEE Proceedings B, vol. 130, no. 2, pp. 103–108, 1983.
25. S. N. Mahato, M. P. Sharma, and S. P. Singh, "Transient performance of a single-phase self-regulated self-excited induction generator using a three-phase machine," Electric Power Systems Research, vol. 77, no. 7, pp. 839–850, 2007.

CHAPTER 6

TIME DOMAIN MODELING AND ANALYSIS OF DYNAMIC GEAR CONTACT FORCE IN A WIND TURBINE GEARBOX WITH RESPECT TO FATIGUE ASSESSMENT

WENBIN DONG, YIHAN XING, AND TORGEIR MOAN

6.1 INTRODUCTION

With the growth of the share of wind energy in the energy market, the design and implementation of large scale wind turbines has become a common occurrence. However, since its inception the wind energy industry has experienced high gearbox failure rates [1]. In order to achieve their stated design life goals of 20 years, most systems require significant repairs or overhauls well before the intended life is reached [2–4]. Some firm conclusions about the nature of the failures have been made based on the work of Musial et al. [5]: (i) gearbox failures are not specific to a single gear manufacturer or turbine model, which are general; (ii) poor adherence to accepted gear industry practices, or otherwise poor workmanship, is not the primary source of failures; (iii) most gearbox failures do not begin as

This chapter was originally published under the Creative Commons Attribution License. Dong W, Xing Y, and Moan T. Time Domain Modeling and Analysis of Dynamic Gear Contact Force in a Wind Turbine Gearbox with Respect to Fatigue Assessment. Energies ***2012**,5 (2012). doi:10.3390/en5114350.*

gear failures or gear-tooth design deficiencies, and up to 10% of gearbox failures may be manufacturing anomalies and quality issues that are gear related; (iv) the majority of wind turbine gearbox failures appear to initiate in the bearings, and (v) it is believed that the gearbox failures observed in the earlier 500 kW to 1000 kW sizes 5 to 10 years ago may still occur in many of the larger 1 to 2 MW gearboxes being built today with the same architecture. With larger wind turbines, the cost of gearbox rebuilds, as well as the down time associated with these failures, has become a significant portion of the overall cost of wind energy [6]. Presently NREL is performing a long-term project to improve the accuracy of dynamic gearbox testing to assess gearbox and drivetrain options, problems, and solutions under simulated field conditions. In addition, in order to increase the long-term reliability of gearboxes and make their design more reasonable, there is increasing interest in utilizing time domain simulations and physical tests in the prediction of gearbox design loads, with the continual development of computer technology, simulation tools and measurement equipments. In several previous studies Klose et al. [7] performed an integrated analysis of wind turbine behavior and structural dynamics of a jacket support structure under combined wind and wave loads in the time domain. Seidel et al. [8] used the sequential coupling and the full coupling methods to simulate offshore loads on jacket wind turbines, and validated these methods using measurement data from the DOWNVInD project. Gao and Moan [9] performed long-term fatigue analysis of offshore fixed wind turbines using time domain simulations. Dong et al. [10] performed long-term fatigue analysis of multi-planar tubular joints for jacket-type offshore wind turbines using time domain simulations. Peeters et al. [11,12], Xing et al. [13] performed a detailed analysis of internal drive train dynamics in a wind turbine using multi-body simulations. However, there is, at present, limited literature concerning long-term time-domain based analysis of mechanical components, e.g., main shaft, gears and bearings, in the wind turbine drive train system under dynamic conditions. This is mainly due to the complexities involved in modeling and simulating the drivetrain with respect to the computation efforts and scale. Recently, Dong et al. [14] established and applied a long-term time domain based gear contact fatigue analysis of a wind turbine under dynamic conditions. In the present study, several practical problems of time domain based gear contact fatigue analysis encountered in [14] are described and discussed. These are: (1) the rotation reversal problem of gears under low wind speed conditions, (2) the statistical uncertainty effect due to the time domain simulation and (3) simplified long term contact fatigue analysis of gear teeth under dynamic conditions. Several useful suggestions to address these issues are proposed.

6.2 TIME-DOMAIN SIMULATION OF WIND TURBINES

In this study, a 750 kW land-based wind turbine from the Gearbox Reliability Collorative (GRC) project coordinated by the National Renewable Energy Laboratory (NREL) in Colorado, USA is used as the case study. This is a three-bladed upwind turbine. The nominal hub height is 55 m, the rotor diameter is 48.2 m; the rated generator speed is 22/15 rpm, which represents a two-speed generator [four-pole (4P) and six-pole (6P) generator] with rated power of 750 kW and 200 kW, respectively; the nominal cut-in wind speed is 3 m/s; the rated wind speed is 16 m/s; the cut-out wind speed is 25 m/s; stall-regulated control is applied; thc design wind class is

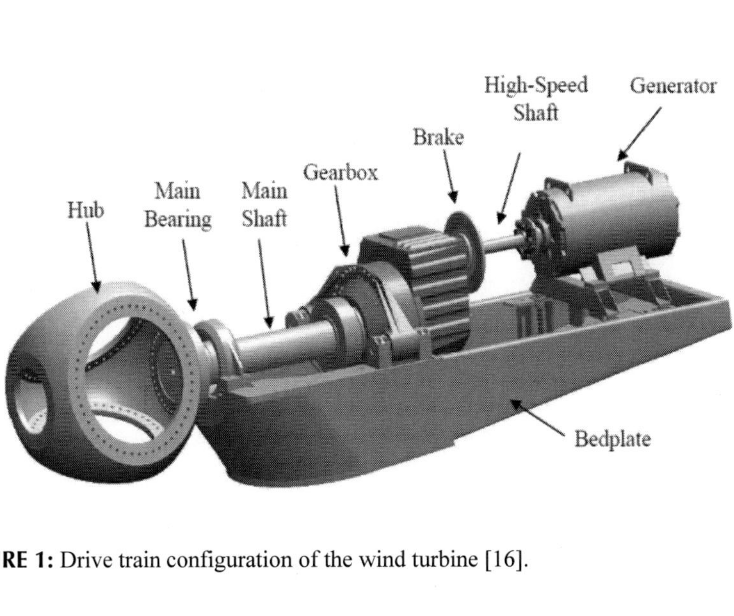

FIGURE 1: Drive train configuration of the wind turbine [16].

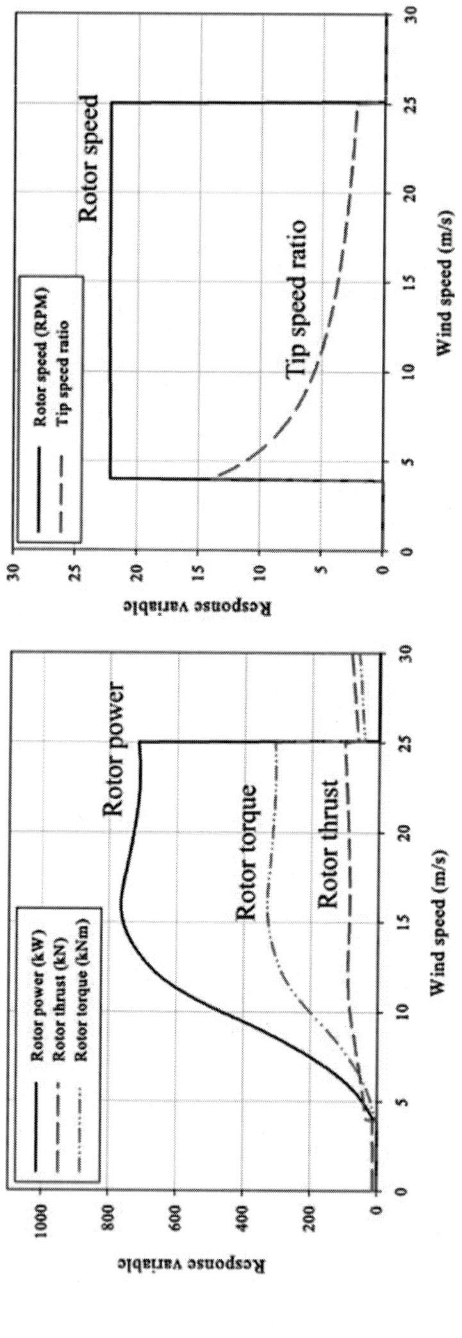

FIGURE 2: Drive train configuration of the wind turbine [17].

IEC Class II, and the design life is 20 years. The configuration of the drive train system of the wind turbine is as shown in Figure 1. The performance property of the wind turbine is as shown in Figure 2. More details about this wind turbine can be found in [15,16].

The analysis proceeds in two steps. First, global aero-elastic simulations are performed using the FAST code from NREL [18]. FAST is an aero-elastic code that computes the coupled wind turbine structural response under aerodynamic load effects. The time series of the main shaft torques are obtained and used as inputs in a multibody gearbox model in SIMPACK [19]. SIMPACK is a multi-purpose multibody code with special features available to model gearboxes. Figure 3 shows the gearbox internal components and Figure 4 shows the relative gearbox model in SIMPACK. Figure 5 shows an example of the calculation results of the torques in the mainshaft when using the 4P generator.

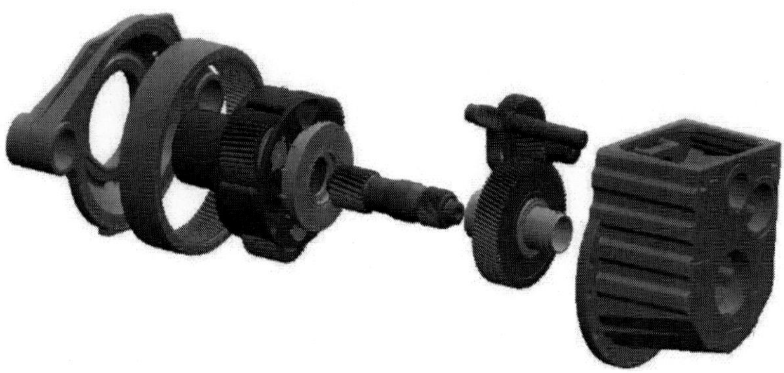

FIGURE 3: View of the gearbox internal components [16].

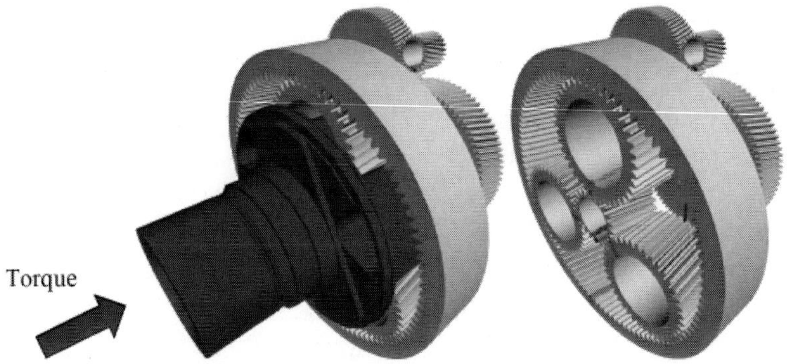

FIGURE 4: Gearbox model primitive in SIMPACK.

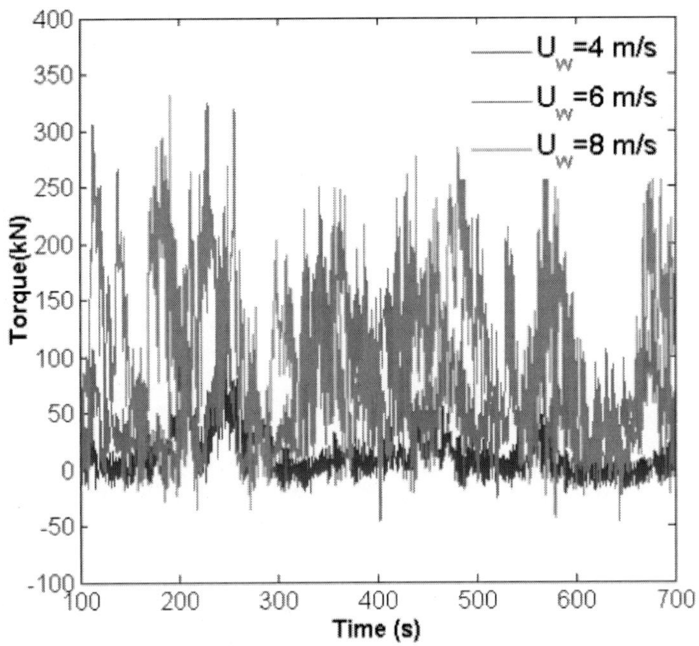

FIGURE 5: Time histories of main shaft torques when using the 4P generator.

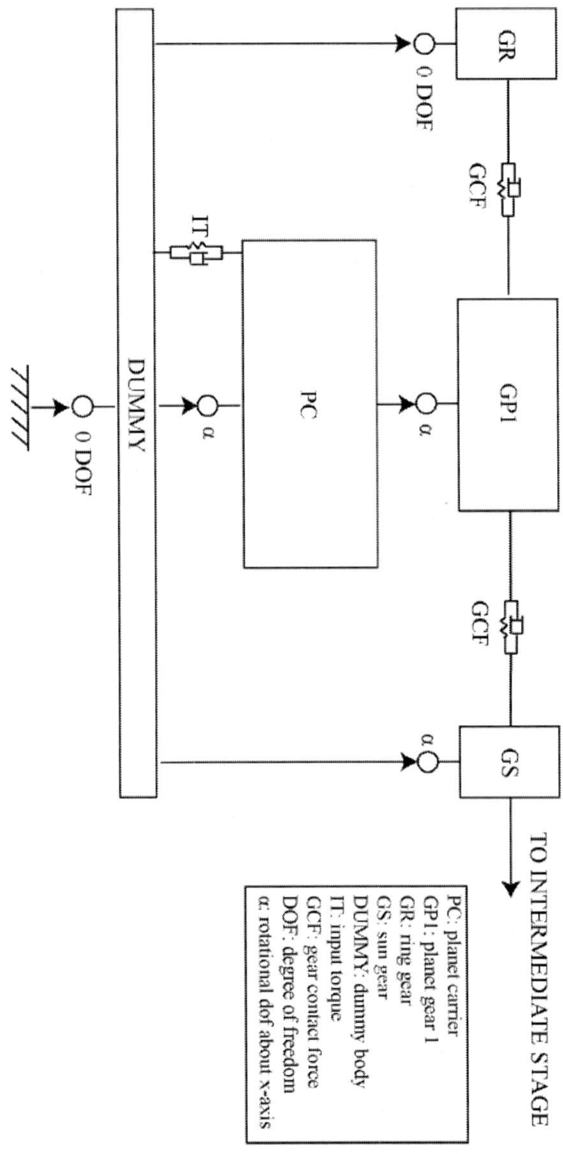

FIGURE 6: Topology diagram of gearbox model in SIMPACK.

In SIMPACK, each component of the gearbox is modeled as a rigid body and interconnected using joints and force elements. The topology diagram of the gearbox model is shown in Figure 6.

The gear pair force element in SIMPACK, FE 225, is used for modeling gear contact. FE225 models gear contact as a series of discrete springs and dampers. The gear stiffness is calculated in accordance with ISO 6336-1 [20]. This stiffness parameter depends on the location of the contact point and the gear geometry. The forces and torques acting on each individual gear are calculated as a function of the gear stiffness and the penetration depth at the gear teeth. FE225 also considers normal damping, coulomb friction, backlash and micro-geometry. The contact forces in meshing gears are obtained using the classical slicing method. Helical gears can be regarded as several very thin cylindrical gear wheels mounted on a mutual axis and individually rotated a small angle around their common axis [21]. In this way, a helical tooth is sliced into several independent cylindrical teeth. More details about the slicing method can be found in [22,23]. In this study, the time series of the gear contact forces at the contact point on a certain slice generated in the meshing gears for different wind speeds are used to perform the studies in Sections 3–5.

6.3 THE GEAR TORQUE REVERSAL PROBLEM

The two step analysis procedures as described in Section 2 are used. The time series of the wind turbine main shaft torques and the gear contact forces generated in meshing gears are obtained from FAST and SIMPACK simulations, respectively. In the analysis shown in Figure 5, the torques are negative for short time periods at low wind speeds, i.e., 4 m/s, 6 m/s and 8 m/s. This means that the gears do not mesh on a single side the entire time. Generally speaking, this phenomenon is bad for gearbox reliability. Figure 7 shows an example of the time series of the gear contact forces when using the 4P generator and a wind speed of 4 m/s. The notations, "tooth −1", "tooth 0" and "tooth +1", are also defined in Figure 8. They represent the different stages of gear meshings, which are engagement, middle and recess stage, respectively. In the analysis reported in Figure 7, the contact forces experienced by the gear teeth are not always positive, which is in consistent with the cases reported in Figure 5. This means that the gear contact is not merely on one side of the gear teeth, e.g., surface A. Contact occurs on surface B when the contact forces are negative, as shown in Figure 9(a). This is beneficial from a contact fatigue point of view. However, this is very bad from a tooth root bending fatigue point of view. Cracks could be initiated at the root location of gear tooth and propagate into the interior, which leads to failure. This is shown in Figure 9(a). Another important problem caused by this phenomenon is the postprocessing of the contact forces. In order to do the time domain based gear contact fatigue analysis, the time series of gear contact forces at a selected contact position on a certain gear tooth is required. However, the torque reversal problem makes the postprocessing difficult and inaccurate. A simplified method has to be applied, which is described in the following paragraph.

In this study, three different generator controllers are considered and compared at low wind speeds (4 m/s, 6 m/s and 8 m/s). These are the 4P controller, 6P controller and a simple variable speed controller (VS). The 4P controller and the 6P controller are obtained from NREL directly. The simple variable speed controller is designed in-house. The variable speed controller is designed based on the principle of maximizing the power

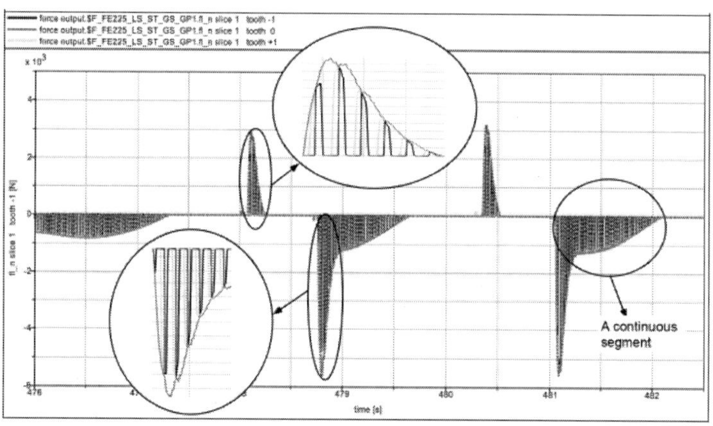

FIGURE 7: Time histories of gear contact force based on time domain simulation in SIMPACK ($U_w = 4$ m/s).

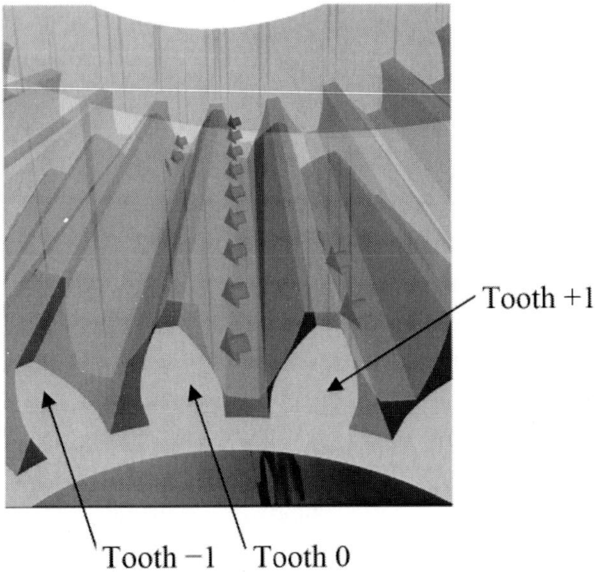

FIGURE 8: Scheme of meshing gears.

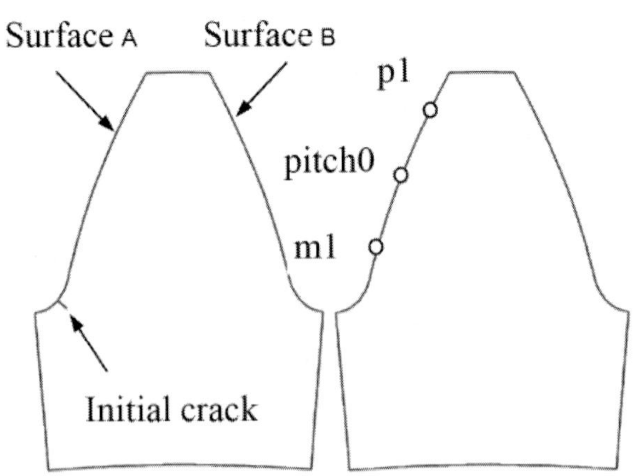

FIGURE 9: Scheme of a gear tooth.

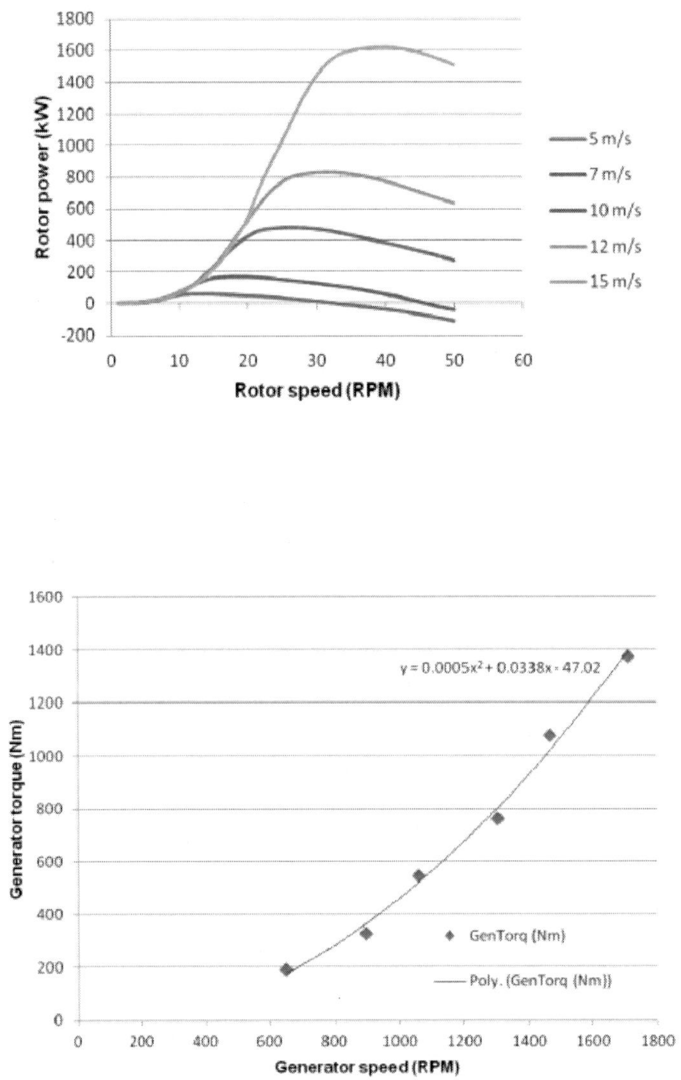

FIGURE 10: Design of a simple variable speed controller.

production at the low wind speeds. This means that the torque speed curve fit as shown on the right hand side of Figure 10 passes through maxima of the individual curves shown on the left hand side. Figure 11 shows the comparison of the torques for different generator controllers at $U_w = 4$ m/s. As observed in the figure, there are no negative torques. The 6P controller is better than the 4P controller, but there are still many negative torques. As the torque reversal problem is severe for the 4P and the 6P controllers at low wind speeds, a continuous segment taken from the entire time series of the contact forces for each wind speed is identified in terms of the maximum value of the mean contact forces, and is used to get the mean value and the standard deviation of the contact forces for each simulation sample from here on, which is a simplified method used in this study. It is noted that the segment lengths for different simulation samples are not uniform, which should be determined case by case.

Figure 12 shows the comparison of the power curves for different generator controllers with respect to three different wind speeds. In the analysis reported in this figure, there are no significant differences among the

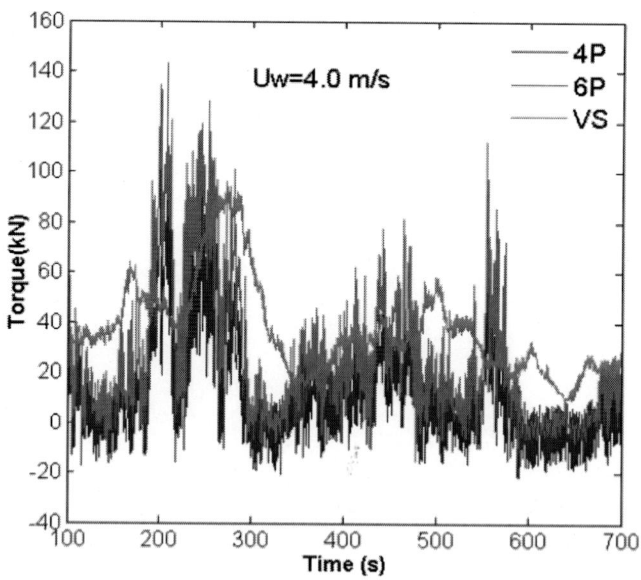

FIGURE 11: Time histories of main shaft torques using different generator controllers.

4P, the 6P and the VS controllers at $U_w = 4$ m/s and $U_w = 6$ m/s. The 4P and VS controllers produce more power than the 6P controller at $U_w = 8$ m/s. Furthermore, there are no negative values for the VS controller at all the wind speeds simulated.

Figure 13 (F_c represents the gear contact forces obtained from time domain simulations) shows the comparisons of the variation of mean contact forces with the increment of simulation samples at the three different contact points at different wind speeds and using different generators. As previously mentioned, p1 is the engagement point, pitch0 is the pitch point and m1 is the recess point. 20 simulations are performed for each wind speed. The simulation length is 700 s, with the first 100 s discarded. In the analysis reported in Figure 13, the variations of the mean contact forces at three different contact points are very similar. The mean contact force of the VS controller is smaller than those of the 4P and the 6P controllers. The simplified treatment of the time series of the contact forces for the 4P and

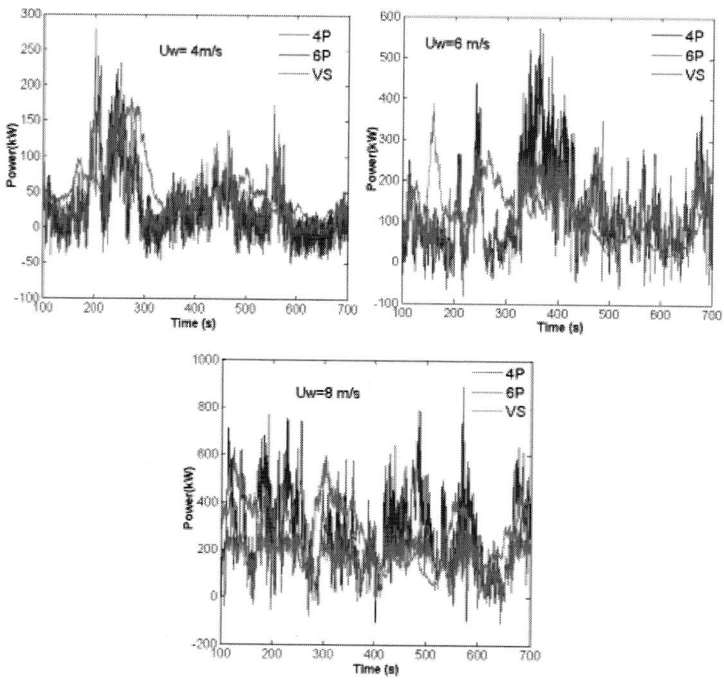

FIGURE 12. Power curves at different wind speeds using different generators.

the 6P controllers mentioned above could be conservative. The mean contact force for the 4P controller increases faster than the 6P and the VS controllers, with increasing wind speeds. Generally speaking, from a contact fatigue and bending fatigue point of view, the 6P and the VS controllers could be better than the 4P controller. From a power generation point of view, the 4P controller might be better than the 6P and the VS controllers, especially when the wind speeds are higher than 6 m/s.

6.4. STATISTICAL UNCERTAINTY EFFECT DUE TO TIME-DOMAIN SIMULATION

For wind turbines, their performances are subject to a number of uncertainties, which are caused by inherent physical randomness of the system or environment (named as aleatory undertainties, e.g., physical wind process) and lack of knowledge of the system or the environment (named as epistemic uncertainties, e.g., model uncertainty and statistical uncertainty). A rational treatment of these uncertainties in a quantitative manner associated with an engineering problem and its physical representation in an analysis are the essence of reliability analysis. In this section, the statistical uncertainty due to time domain simulation is considered, which is mainly due to that different sample data sets usually produce different statistical estimators such as the sample mean, std., etc.

For time domain simulation of wind turbines, one of the key components is the simulation of turbulent wind field. In this study, the turbulent wind field is simulated using the TurbSim code [24], which is a stochastic, full-field, turbulent-wind simulator. It uses a statistical model to numerically simulate time series of three-component wind-speed vectors at points in a two-dimensional vertical rectangular grid that is fixed in space. Figure 14 shows an example of a TurbSim wind field. In TurbSim, random phases (one per frequency per grid point per wind component) for the wind velocity time series are created using the random numbers generated by the pseudorandom number generator. For the same mean wind speed, if the random numbers are different, the wind velocity time series will be different. This will affect the calculations of aerodynamic forces applied on the blades and torques in the main shaft of wind turbine. Figure 15 shows an example of the torque time series obtained in FAST simulation for the same wind speed (Uw = 16 m/s) with respect to different random numbers. Generally speaking, the more simulation samples for the same mean wind speed, the better the simulation results. However, time domain simulations are usually very time consuming and the data size is very big, therefore it is necessary to identify a suitable sample size for a certain wind speed. This will cause the so-called statistical uncertainty. In this study the statistical uncertainty of the contact force calculation with respect to the number of simulations employed, at different wind speeds are estimated. The range of 1-h mean wind speed Uw is 4–24 m/s with an increment of 2 m/s. For each wind speed, 20 simulations are performed using different random seed numbers. For each simulation, a time history of the gear contact forces is obtained and used as a sample. Therefore, totally 20 samples for each wind speed are obtained.

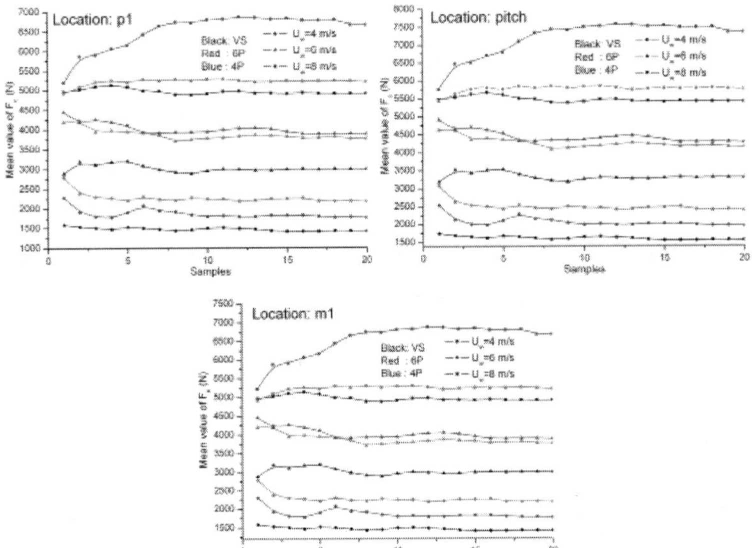

FIGURE 13: Variation of mean contact forces when using different generators at the different contact points, wind speeds and number of simulation samples.

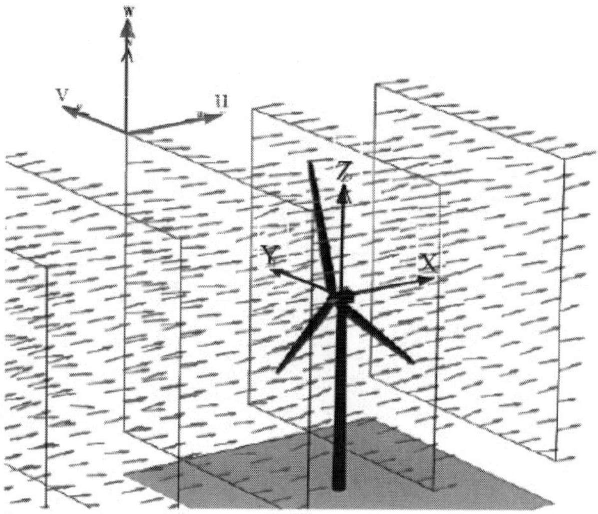

FIGURE 14: Example of wind field simulation in TurbSim [24].

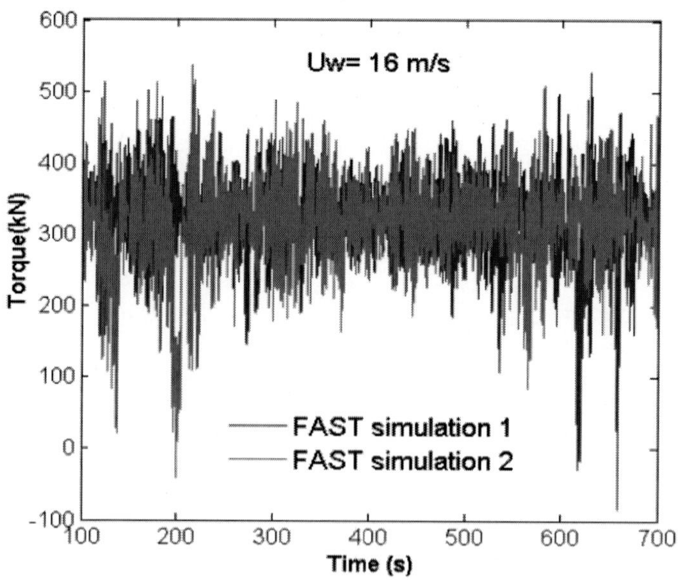

FIGURE 15: Time series of main shat torques in FAST simulation at the same wind speed with different simulations (random seeds are different).

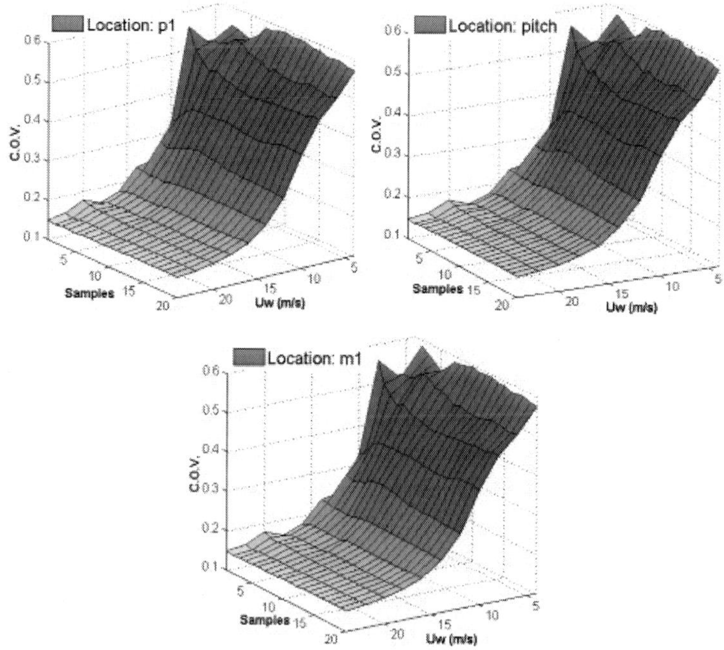

FIGURE 16: Variation of C.O.V. of the contact forces when using the 4P controller at different contact points, wind speeds and number of simulation samples.

Figure 16 shows the variation of the coefficient of variation (C.O.V.) of the gear contact forces at the three different contact points for different wind speeds and different simulation samples. The quantities (C.O.V.) in this figure are determined from the ensemble of x samples (x = 1, 2, 3, …, 20), which are the same as the quantities in Figures 17, 18. The 4P generator controller is used. The parameter C.O.V. is defined as follows:

$$C.O.V = \frac{\sigma_F}{\mu_F} \tag{1}$$

where μ_F represents the mean value of the contact forces; σF represents the standard deviation of the contact forces.

Figure 17 shows the variation of the parameter ζ at the three different contact points for different wind speeds and different simulation samples. The 4P generator controller is used. The parameter ζ is defined as follows:

$$\zeta = \frac{C.O.V._c^i - C.O.V._c^{20}}{C.O.V._c^{20}} \cdot 100\% \tag{2}$$

where $C.O.V._c^{\,i}$ represents the coefficient of variation of the contact forces based on i simulation samples (i = 1, 2, 3, …, 20).

In the analysis reported in Figure 16, the variations of the C.O.V. of the contact forces at three different contact points are very similar. At low wind speeds, the C.O.V. value can be up to 0.6. It is decreased significantly with the increment of wind speeds, which represents that the turbulence effect is decreased with the increment of wind speeds. In the analysis reported in Figure 17, the variations of the parameter ζ [Equation (2)] at three different contact points are very similar. The values of ζ at low wind speeds (UW < 12 m/s) are much higher than those at other wind speeds, especially when the simulation samples are less than 10. The maximum value of ζ can be up to 24%. The findings here suggest that there might be higher levels of uncertainty when using the simplified method discussed in the previous section. This is because the simplified method employs a portion of the original simulation length, i.e., shorter simulation length. It is, therefore, suggested that more samples be used when employing the simplified method. Based on the work in this study, at least 10 simulation samples might be used at low wind speeds, in order to keep the value of ζ within 5%.

In Figure 16, the 4P generator controller is used. In this study, when the 6P and the VS controllers are used, the C.O.V. values for U_W = 4 m/s, 6 m/s and 8 m/s are compared against the cases of the 4P controller, as shown in Figure 18. In the analysis reported in this figure, the variations of the C.O.V. values of the contact forces at three different contact points are similar for each controller. The C.O.V. values for the 6P and the VS controllers are less than that of the 4P controller. From an uncertainty level point of view, the benefits of the 6P and the VS controllers are increased with the increment of wind speeds. One reason is that the time series of the contact forces used for the 6P and the VS controllers are much longer than that of the 4P controller, especially for the VS controller. Figure 18 shows the comparison results at the pitch point. The cases at other points, e.g., the engagement point and the recess point, are similar to that of the pitch point, and not repeated herein. Based on the work in this study, if the

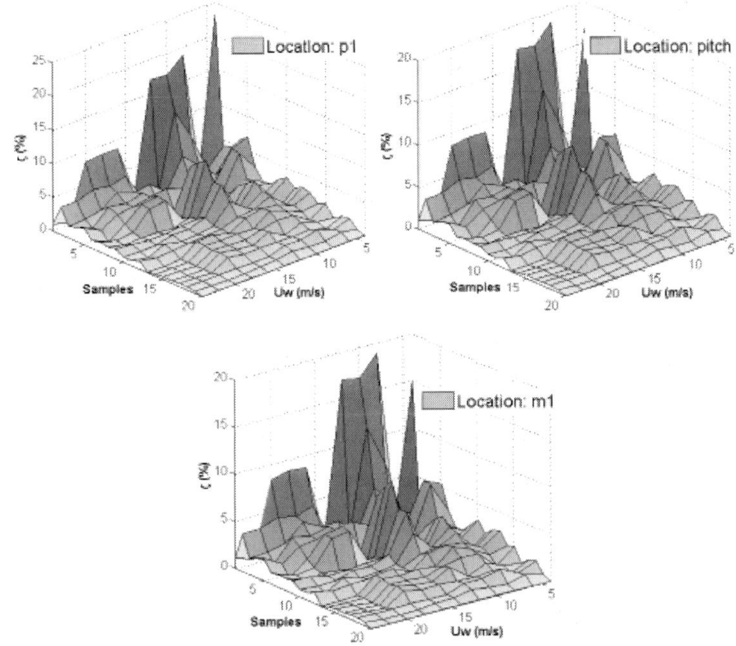

FIGURE 17: Variation of ζ [Equation (2)] when using the 4P controller at different contact points, wind speeds and number of simulation samples.

6P or the VS controller is applied, at least 6-8 simulation samples might be used at low wind speeds ($U_W < 12$ m/s) in order to obtain a relatively stable C.O.V. value of the contact forces.

In this section, the statistical uncertainty of the gear contact force calculation due to time domain simulation is investigated. It should be noted that a decoupled dynamic response analysis method and a simplified rigid gearbox model are applied as described in Section 2. These simplifications will cause the so-called model uncertainties, which can be reduced by using more refined method (e.g., fully coupled method) and more accurate model (e.g., gearbox model with flexible components). The availability of the decoupled analysis method used in this study is verified in [14]. The detailed analysis of model uncertainties is out of the scope in this paper and might be investigated in further work. In addition, the statistical uncertainty analysis in this study is mainly with respect to time domain based gear contact fatigue assessment in normal operations. It should be noted that the cases of wind turbine extreme loads analysis in normal operations are different. For extreme loads analysis, the peak values obtained from time histories of a certain variable should be used and the exceedance probability theory is applied. More details about wind turbine extreme loads analysis can be found in [25–28].

6.5 SIMPLIFIED GAR CONTACT FATIGUE ANALYSIS

Recently Dong, et al. [14] presented a simplified predictive pitting model for estimating gear service lives and verified its validity by comparing with the published experimental evidence. The model sets up a link between the global dynamic response analysis of wind turbine and the detailed contact fatigue analysis of gears in the drive train, which is given as follows:

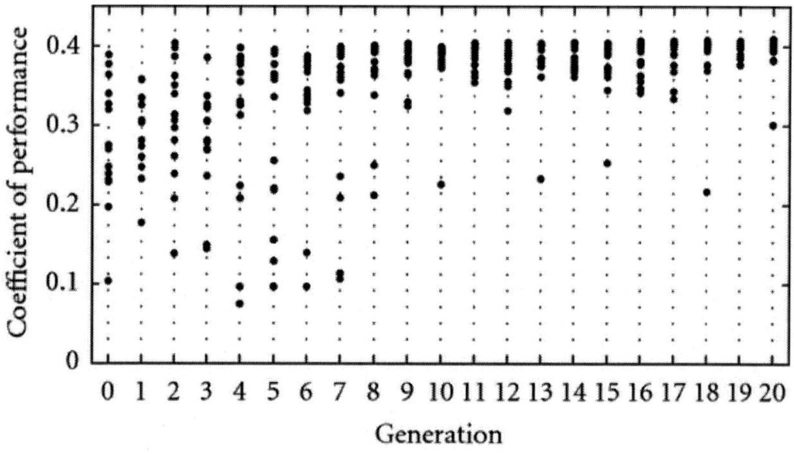

FIGURE 18: Variation of C.O.V. of the contact forces when using different controllers at the pitch contact point.

$$\zeta = \frac{C.O.V._c^{i} - C.O.V._c^{20}}{C.O.V._c^{20}} \cdot 100\% \tag{3}$$

where N_p represents the number of cycles for crack propatation. C and m represent the material constants. G_{2a} represents the geometry function. U is a factor related to crack closure. Δp_{max} represents the equivalent maximum contact pressure range, which is given as follows:

$$\Delta \bar{P}_{max} = \left(\int_0^{\infty} \Delta P_{max}^{m} \cdot f_{\Delta p_{max}}(\Delta p_{max}) d\Delta p_{max} \right)^{1/m} \tag{4}$$

where Δp_{max} represents the maximum contact pressure range, which can be calculated from time domain simulations or field tests. $f_{\Delta pmax}$ represents the probability density distribution of $\Delta_{pmax.}$

In order to obtain Δp_{max}, accurate postprocessing of the tooth contact loads is important. Figure 19 shows the sun gear with the gear teeth numbered. In order to perform time-domain based gear contact fatigue analysis, the time series of the contact forces for each gear tooth should be obtained by postprocessing the MBS simulation results. In reality, this procedure is very time consuming and inconvenient, especially for low wind speeds where the torque reversal problem is severe. A simplified approach is, therefore, desired. In this study the mean values and the standard deviations of the contact forces at three different locations on a representative tooth surface of the sun gear using three different methods are calculated. The three locations are as shown in Figure 9(b). The three different methods are described as follows:

- Maximum damage method: for each wind speed, a most dangerous gear tooth is identified in terms of the maximum mean contact force. A dummy gear tooth is then defined. It is further assumed that the time series of the contact forces of the most dangerous gear tooth for each wind speed are all applied on this dummy gear tooth, which is taken as the representative of all 21 gear teeth.

- Minimum damage method: this method is similar to the first one, for each wind speed, a safest gear tooth with the minimum mean gear tooth contact force is identified. A dummy gear tooth is then also defined. It is also further assumed that the time series of contact forces of the most safe gear tooth for each wind speed are all applied on this dummy gear tooth, which is also taken as the representative of all 21 gear teeth.
- Simple average method: the time series of the gear contact forces from SIMPACK simulations are used directly. It is assumed that the time series of the contact forces at the same contact position on each tooth surface of the sun gear are the same.

Figure 20 shows the comparisons of the mean contact forces using the three different methods at the three different contact points at different wind speeds.

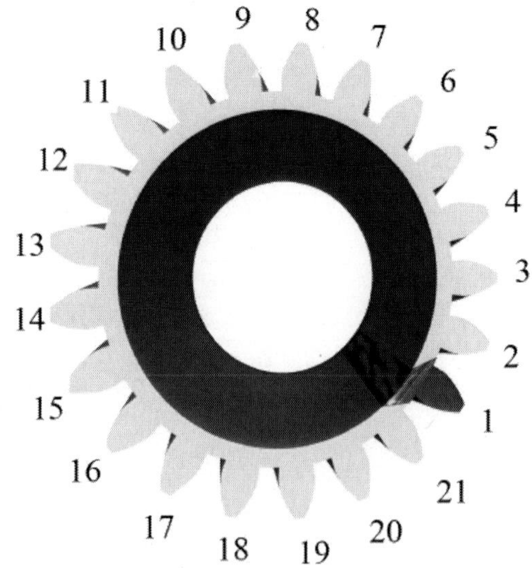

FIGURE 19: Front view of the sun gear in the SIMPACK model.

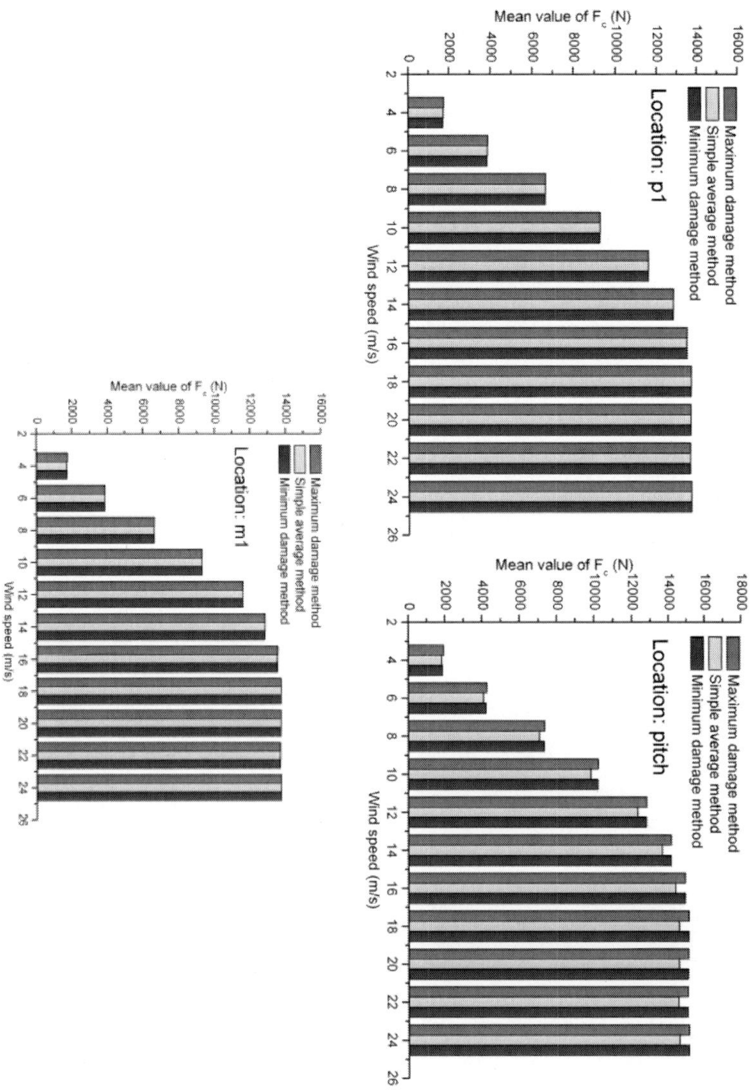

FIGURE 20: Comparison of mean contact forces when using different methods at different contact points and wind speeds (4P generator).

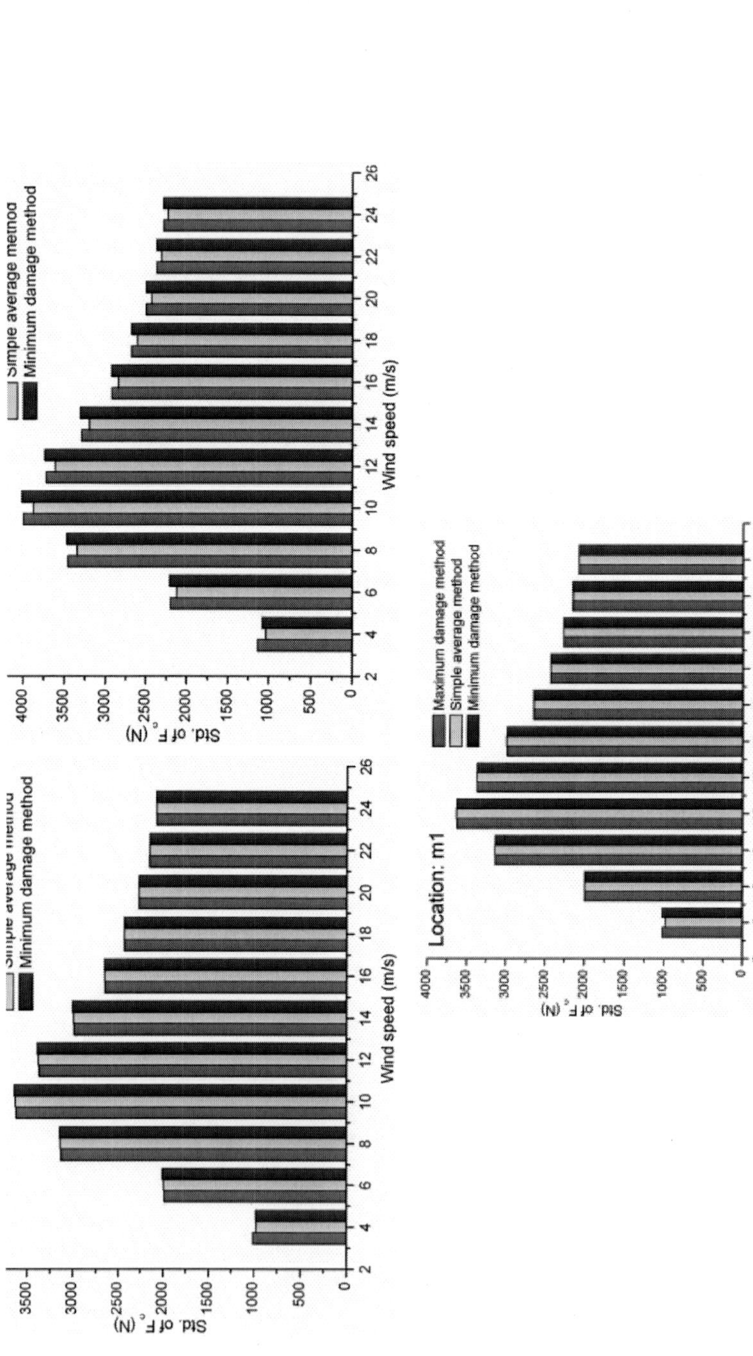

FIGURE 21: Comparison of standard deviations of contact forces when using different methods at different contact points and wind speeds (4P generator).

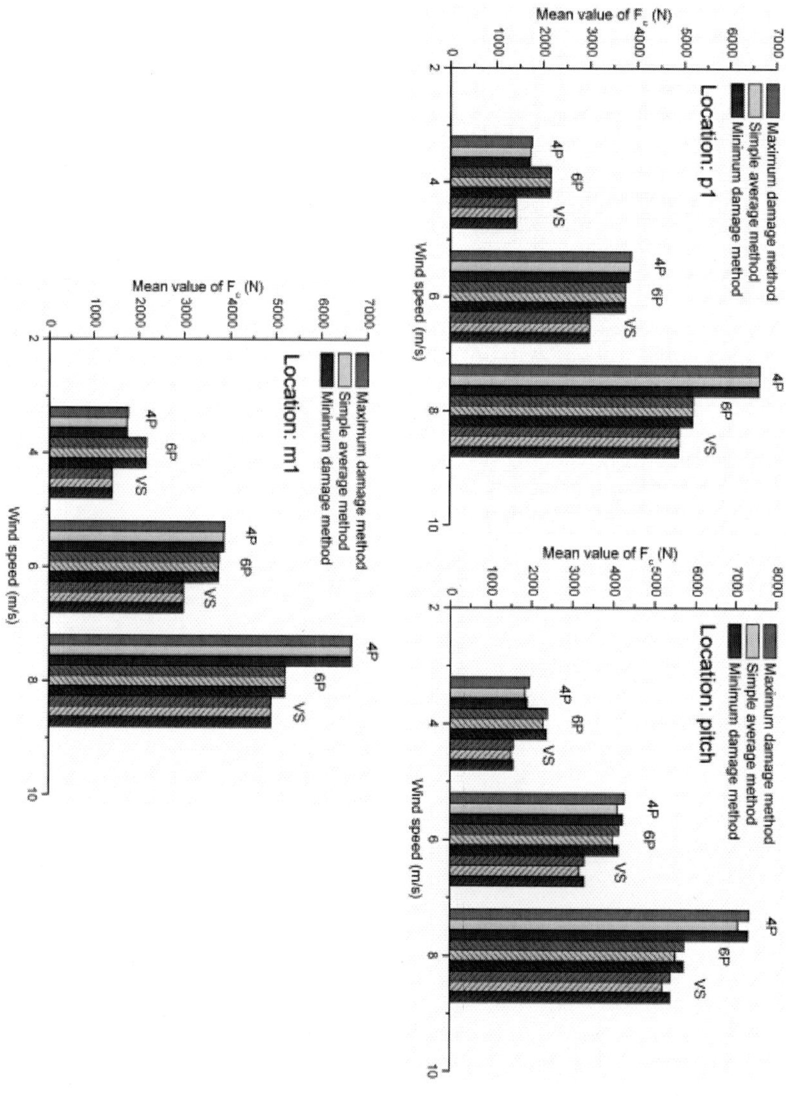

FIGURE 22: Comparison of mean contact forces when using different methods at different contact points, generators and wind speeds.

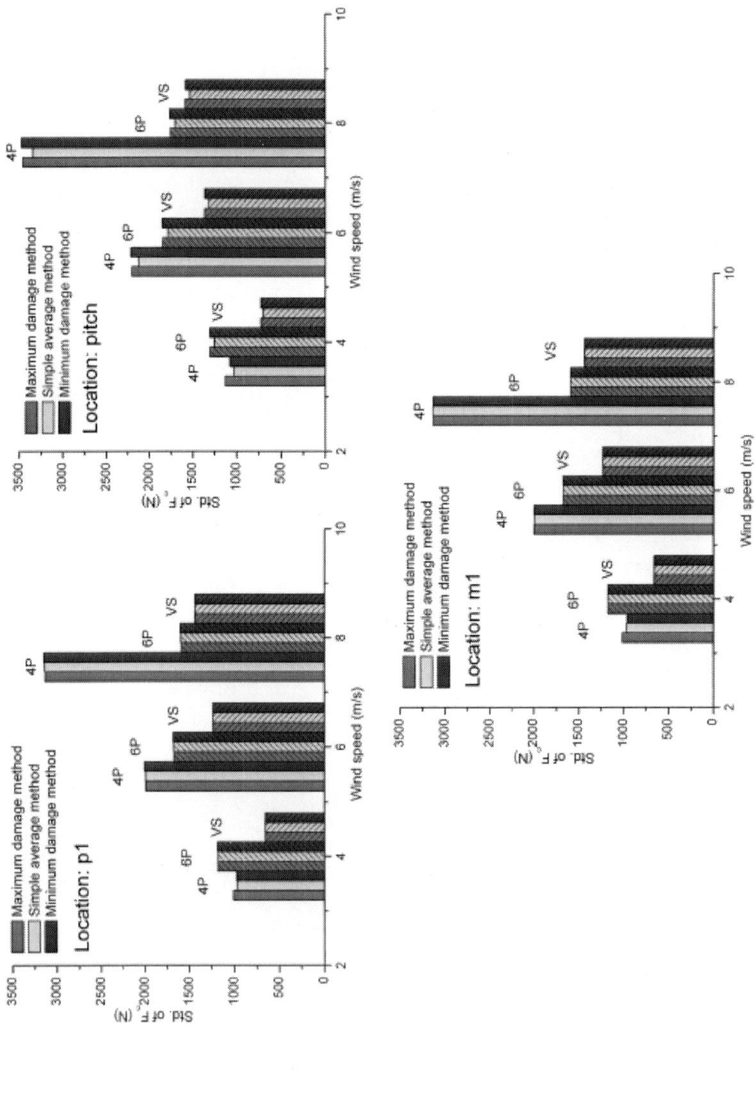

FIGURE 23: Comparison of standard deviations of contact forces when using different methods at different contact points, generators and wind speeds.

Figure 21 shows the comparisons of the standard deviations of the contact forces. The 4P controller is applied here. In the analysis reported in these figures, at the contact points p1 and m1, the mean contact forces and the standard deviations for different wind speeds are almost the same with respect to the three different methods mentioned above. At the contact point pitch0, the mean contact forces and the standard deviations for different wind speeds using the simple average method are a little smaller than those using the maximum damage method and minimum damage method, which is slightly not conservative. In addition, the cases of the 6P and the VS controllers are also considered in this study, and compared with the results of the 4P controller, as shown in Figures 22–23. In the analysis reported in these figures, the cases of the 6P and the VS controllers are very similar to the case of the 4P controller. Figures 20–23 show the validity of the simple average method with respect to different wind speeds and different generator controllers.

6.6 CONCLUSIONS

In this paper, three practical problems encountered in time domain based gear contact fatigue analyses are discussed. The main conclusions are presented below:

1. The reverse rotation problem is severe at low wind speeds (e.g., 4 m/s–8 m/s) for the 4P and the 6P generator controllers. In order to avoid it, the VS generator controller could be used. At low wind speeds, a continuous segment taken from the entire time series of the gear contact forces with respect to the 4P and the 6P generator controllers, which has the maximum mean contact force, might be used to do the time-domain based gear contact fatigue analysis, and the results could be on the conservative side.
2. The variations of the C.O.V. values at different contact points are similar. In order to keep the value of ζ [Equation (2)] within 5%, at least 10 simulation samples might be used at low wind speeds (U_w < 12 m/s) for the 4P generator controller if the simplified method mentioned in Section 3 is employed, and at least 6–8 simulation

samples might be used for the 6P and the VS generator controllers. For high wind speeds (U_w > 12 m/s), 5–6 simulation samples might be ok for the 4P, the 6P and VS generator controllers.

3. The simple average method is equally accurate for different wind speeds and different generator controllers, and is more efficient than the maximum damage method and the minimum damage method.

In this study, only the main shaft torque loads are considered. The effects of non-torque loads could be investigated in future work. In addition, a simple rigid body gearbox model is used in this paper, more refined gearbox models, e.g., with flexible components modeled, could be applied in future work. Furthermore, time-domain simulations of larger megawatt wind turbines (onshore and offshore) could be also performed in future work.

REFERENCES

1. McNiff, B.; Musial, W.D.; Errichello, R. Variations in Gear Fatigue Life for Different Wind Turbine Braking Strategies; Solar Energy Research Institute: Golden, CO, USA, 1990.
2. Facing up to the gearbox challenge: A survey of gearbox failure and collected industry knowledge. Windpower Monthly, November 2005, Volume 21, No. 11.
3. Rasmussen, F.; Thomsen, K.; Larsen, T.J. The Gearbox Problem Revisited; Riso Fact Sheet AED-RB-17(EN); Riso National Laboratory: Roskilde, Denmark, 2004.
4. Tavner, P.J.; Xiang, J.; Spinato, F. Reliability analysis for wind turbines. Wind Energy 2006, 10, 1–18.
5. Musial, W.; Butterfield, S.; McNiff, B. Improving Wind Turbine Gearbox Reliability. In Proceedings of European Wind Energy Conference, Milan, Italy, 7–10 May 2007.
6. Oyague, F.; Gorman, D.; Sheng, S. NREL Gearbox Reliability Collaborative Experimental Data Overview and Analysis. In Proceedings of Windpower 2010 Conference and Exhibition, Dallas, TX, USA, 23–26 May 2010.
7. Klose, M.; Dalhoff, P.; Argyriadis, K. Integrated Load and Strength Analysis for Offshore Wind Turbines with Jacket Structures. In Proceedings of the 17th International Offshore (Ocean) and Polar Engineering Conference (ISOPE 2007), Lisbon, Portugal, 1–6 July 2007.
8. Seidel, M.; Ostermann, F.; Curvers, A.P.W.M.; Kuhn, M.; Kaufer, D.; Boker, C. Validation of offshore load simulations using measurement data from the DOWNVInD

project. In Proceedings of European Offshore Wind Conference, Stockholm, Sweden, 14–16 September 2009.
9. Gao, Z.; Moan, T. Long-term fatigue analysis of offshore fixed wind turbines based on time-domain simulations. In Proceedings of the International Symposium on Practical Design of Ships and Other Floating Structures (PRADS), Rio de Janeiro, Brazil, 19–24 September 2010.
10. Dong, W.B.; Gao, Z.; Moan, T. Fatigue reliability analysis of jacket-type offshore wind turbine considering inspection and repair. In Proceedings of European Wind Energy Conference, Warsaw, Poland, 19–23 April 2010.
11. Peeters, J.; Vandepitte, D.; Sas, P. Analysis of internal drive train dynamics in a wind turbine. Wind Energy 2006, 9, 141–161.
12. Peeters, J. Simulation of Dynamic Drive Train Loads in a Wind Turbine. Ph.D. Thesis, Department of Mechanical Engineering, Division of Production Engineering, Machine Design and Automation (PMA), Katholieke Universiteit Leuven, Leuven, Belgium, 2006.
13. Xing, Y.H.; Moan, T. Wind turbine gearbox planet carrier modeling and analysis in a multibody setting. Wind Energy 2012, submitted.
14. Dong, W.B.; Xing, Y.H.; Moan, T.; Gao, Z. Time domain based gear contact fatigue analysis of a wind turbine drivetrain under dynamic conditions. Int. J. Fatigue 2012, in press.
15. Bir, G.S.; Oyague, F. Estimation of Blade and Tower Properties for the Gearbox Research Collaborative Wind Turbine; Technical Report NREL/EL-500-42250; National Renewable Energy Laboratory (NREL): Golden, CO, USA, 2007.
16. Oyague, F. GRC Drive Train Round Robin GRC 750/48.2 Loading Document (IEC 61400-1 Class IIB); National Renewable Energy Laboratory: Golden, CO, USA, 2009.
17. Xing, Y.H.; Karimirad, M.; Moan, T. Modeling and analysis of floating wind turbine drivetrain, Wind Energy 2012, submitted.
18. Jonkman, J.M.; Buhl, M.L., Jr. FAST User's Guide; Technical Report NREL/EL-500-38230; National Renewable Energy Laboratory (NREL): Golden, CO, USA, 2005.
19. SIMPACK Reference Guide, SIMPACK Release 8.9. September 1, 2010/SIMDOC v8.904; SIMPACK AS: Munich, Germany, 2010.
20. ISO 6336–1. Calculation of Load Capacity of Spur and Helical Gears—Part 1: Basic Principles, Introduction and General Influence Factors, 2nd ed.; The International Organization for Standardization: Geneva, Switzerland, 2006.
21. Flodin, A.; Andersson, S. A simplified model for wear prediction in helical gears. Wear 2001, 241, 285–292.
22. Haines, D.J.; Ollerton, E. Contact stress distributions on elliptical contact surfaces subjected to radial and tangential forces. Proc. Inst. Mech. Eng. 1963, 177, 95–114.
23. Kaller, J.J. Three-Dimensional Elastic Bodies in Rolling Contact; Kluwer Academic Publishing: Dordrecht, The Netherlands, 1990.
24. Jonkman, B.J. TurbSim User's Guide, version 1.50; Technical Report NREL/TP-500–46198; National Renewable Energy Laboratory (NREL): Golden, CO, USA, 2009.

25. Cheng, P.W.; van Bussel, G.J.W.; van Kuik, G.A.M.; Vugts, J.H. Reliability-based design methods to determine the extreme response distribution of offshore wind turbines. Wind Energy 2003, 6, 1–22.
26. Agarwal, P.; Manuel, L. Extreme loads for an offshore wind turbine using statistical extrapolation from limited field data. Wind Energy 2008, 11, 673–684.
27. Fogle, J.; Agarwal, P.; Manuel, L. Towards an improved understanding of statistical extrapolation for wind turbine extreme loads. Wind Energy 2008, 11, 613–635.
28. Nilanjan, S.; Gao, Z.; Moan, T.; Næss, A. Short term extreme response analysis of a jacket supporting an offshore wind turbine. Wind Energy 2012, in press.

PART III

TOWER AND FOUNDATION

CHAPTER 7

WIND TURBINE TOWER VIBRATION MODELING AND MONITORING BY THE NONLINEAR STATE ESTIMATION TECHNIQUE (NSET)

PENG GUO AND DAVID INFIELD

7.1 INTRODUCTION

Vibration can be a good indicator of the operating conditions of a range of mechanical components and structures and thus can support condition monitoring of important wind turbine components such as the rotor, drive train and tower [1,2]. Analysis of vibration signals in both the time and frequency domain can be used to identify incipient failure of these components, but the vibration sensor and analysis methods for tower and drive train are different. For the tower, because the vibration frequency is quite low, a low frequency sensor (0–200 Hz) and an appropriate model based analysis method are used, while for the drive train bearing and gearbox, a high frequency acceleration sensor (3–20 kHz) and fast Fourier transform (FFT), Cepstrum methods are used [3]. However, there are two difficulties in the application of vibration analysis to wind turbines. First, large-scale wind turbines operate these days in a variable speed mode to optimize performance in relation to time changing wind speed and so the rotational speed of the rotor, gearbox and generator are changing significantly in time. Because the rotation speed of the gearbox is changing, the width of the vibration sidebands is not fixed, and this creates difficulties in locating the exact locations of gear or bearing faults. It is conventional as in [4] to use order analysis to deal with this problem, or equivalently azimuthal data sampling (rather than fixed time interval sampling) in which the rotor vibration is analyzed based on samples recorded at equidistant rotational angles instead of time equidistant samples. Second, there is strong aerodynamic and vibrational coupling between different turbine components and thus many interconnected factors may influence the vibration signatures. Rotor dynamics and control can for example, significantly influence tower vibration (TV). When the wind speed is above the rated one, the blade angle will normally be adjusted to maintain the rated power. This will result in changes to the aerodynamic forces acting on the rotor, and thus can lead directly to changes in tower vibration (both frequencies and amplitudes). It therefore makes sense to analyze vibration in wider context.

In recent years, wind turbine condition monitoring using supervisory control and data acquisition system (SCADA) data analysis is increasingly common. The SCADA system for a wind turbine records hundreds of important variables that can give a more comprehensive indication of the wind turbine health condition. The work reported in [5] starts from basic laws of physics applied to the gearbox to derive robust relationships between temperature, efficiency, rotational speed and power output. With this relationship, an abnormal rise in the gearbox oil temperature as represented in the SCADA data can be used to predict gearbox failure. In [6], the authors use SCADA data and data mining algorithms to predict possible wind turbine faults. The study reported in [7] used a neural network to construct normal operating temperature models of the gearbox and generator based on SCADA data. When the residual between the model prediction and the measured value becomes very large, a potential fault is identified. In this paper we also use SCADA data for tower vibration modeling and monitoring. The vibration signals in the SCADA system are analyzed alongside other related variables to give an improved assessment of the tower and rotor condition.

This paper is arranged as follows: Section 2 gives a detailed description of the NSET modeling methodology. Section 3 introduces the SCADA data used and analyzes which factors or variables are most important with regard to their influence on tower vibration. The above and below rated operational regimes are dealt with separately. Section 4 uses the NSET technique to construct the two required sub-models for tower vibration. In Section 5, the TVM is used to detect the blade angle error/asymmetry. The paper finishes with a discussion and conclusions in Section 6.

7.2 TOWER VIBRATION MODELING METHOD: NONLINEAR STATE ESTIMATION TECHNIQUE (NSET)

NSET is a non-parametric model construction method first proposed by Singer [8]. It is now widely used in the nuclear power plant sensor calibration, electric product lifespan prediction and software aging research [9–11].

Assuming that there exist n variables or parameters of relevance for a particular process or device, then at time i , an observation of the variables can be written as an observation vector:

$$X(i) = [x_1 \ x_2 \ \cdots \ x_n]^T \tag{1}$$

Construction of a memory matrix D is the first step of NSET modeling approach. During a period of normal operation of the process or device, m historical observation vectors are collected covering the range of different operating conditions (such as high or low load, start up, before shut down, etc.) that the process or device is subject to, so as to construct the memory matrix D as:

$$D = [X(1)\, X(2) \ \cdots \ X(m)]$$
$$= \begin{bmatrix} x_1(1) & x_1(2) & \cdots & x_1(m) \\ x_2(1) & x_2(2) & \cdots & x_2(m) \\ \vdots & \vdots & & \vdots \\ x_n(1) & x_n(2) & \cdots & x_n(m) \end{bmatrix}_{nxm} = \begin{bmatrix} D_{11} & D_{12} & \cdots & D_{1m} \\ D_{21} & D_{22} & \cdots & D_{2m} \\ \vdots & \vdots & \cdots & \vdots \\ D_{n1} & D_{n2} & & D_{nm} \end{bmatrix}_{nxm} \tag{2}$$

Each observation vector in the memory matrix represents an operating state of the process or device. With proper selection of the m historical observation vectors, the subset space spanned by the memory matrix D can represent the whole normal working space of the process or device. The construction of memory matrix D is actually the procedure of learning and memorizing the normal behavior of the process or device.

The work reported in [12] provides a systematic approach to data vector selection and memory matrix construction. The input to NSET is a new observation vector X_{obs} obtained at some time and the output from NSET is a prediction X_{est} for this input vector for the same moment in time. For each input vector X_{obs}, NSET will produce a m dimensional weighting vector W :

$$W = [w_1\ w_2\ \cdots\ w_m]^T \tag{3}$$

with:

$$X_{est} = D \cdot W = w_1 \cdot X(1) + w_2 \cdot X(2) + \cdots + w_m \cdot X(m) \tag{4}$$

Equation (4) means that estimation in NSET is the result of a linear combination of the m historical observation vectors in the memory matrix D . The residual between the NSET estimation and the input is:

$$\varepsilon = X_{obs} - X_{est} \tag{5}$$

The residual sum of squares for ε is:

$$S(w) = \sum_{i=1}^{n} \varepsilon_i^2 = \varepsilon^T \varepsilon$$

$$= (X_{obs} - X_{est})^T (X_{obs} - X_{est})$$

$$(X_{obs} - DW)^T (X_{obs} - DW) = \sum_{i=1}^{n} \left(X_{obs}(i) - \sum_{j=1}^{m} w_j D_{ij} \right)^2 \tag{6}$$

In order to obtain the weighting vector W , we need to minimize the residual sum of square and let the partial derivatives for w_1, w_2, ... , w_m to be zero as follows:

$$\frac{\delta S(w)}{\delta w_k} = -2\sum_{i=1}^{n}\left(X_{obs}(i) - \sum_{j=1}^{m} w_j D_{ij}\right) D_{ik} = 0 \tag{7}$$

Equation (7) can be written as:

$$\sum_{i=1}^{n} X_{obs}(i) D_{ik} = \sum_{i=1}^{n}\sum_{j=1}^{m} w_j D_{ij} D_{ik} = \sum_{j=1}^{m}\left(\sum_{i=1}^{n} D_{ij} D_{ik}\right) w_j, k = 1,2,\cdots,m \tag{8}$$

If Equation (8) is written in matrix form:

$$D^T \cdot D \cdot W = D^T \cdot X_{obs} \tag{9}$$

From Equation (9), we can obtain the weighting vector as:

$$W = (D^T \cdot D)^{-1} \cdot (D^T \cdot X_{obs}) \tag{10}$$

Substitution of Equation (10) into Equation (4) gives the model predicted vector as:

$$X_{est} = D \cdot W = D \cdot (D^T \cdot D)^{-1} \cdot (D^T \cdot X_{obs}) \tag{11}$$

From Equation (11), we can clearly see that the predicted vector is the linear combination of the historical observation vectors in the memory matrix, as mentioned above. In Equation (11), $D^T \cdot D$ denotes the dot product between every two vectors in the memory matrix, and $D^T \cdot X_{obs}$ the dot product between the new input vector and each vector in the memory matrix. Euclidean distance is the simplest way to identify the relationship (distance) between any two vectors, and within NSET is used an intuitive measure of the similarity between vectors and so, in order to give NSET a more direct physical interpretation, this norm is used as nonlinear operator and replaces the dot product in $D^T \cdot D$ and $D^T \cdot X_{obs}$ in Equation (11).

The nonlinear operator for Euclidean distance in n-space is simply:

$$\otimes(X,Y) = \sqrt{\sum_{i=1}^{n}(x_i - y_i)^2} \tag{12}$$

When Equation (12) is used to replace the dot product in Equation (11), the result is:

$$\tilde{X}_{est} = D \cdot (D^T \otimes D)^{-1} \cdot (D^T \otimes X_{obs}) \tag{13}$$

In the construction of memory matrix D , the Euclidean distance between every two observation vectors of the m vectors should be big enough to ensure that the condition number is not excessive. Otherwise, it will be very difficult to calculate the inverse matrix and the NSET model may become ill conditioned.

If we are only interested in predicting one parameter such as x_n in the observation vector, then Equation (13) could be simplified as follows:

$$\begin{aligned} x_{nest} &= [x_n(1)\ x_n(2)\ \cdots\ x_n(m)] \cdot W \\ &= [x_n(1)\ x_n(2)\ \cdots\ x_n(m)] \cdot (D^T \otimes D)^{-1} \cdot (D^T \otimes X_{obs}) \end{aligned} \tag{14}$$

In this case, the prediction for x_n is simply a linear combination of the m historic observation values of x_n . The Euclidean norm is used to calculate the similarity between the new input vector X_{obs} and the m vectors of the memory matrix. Assuming that the new input measurement is most similar (in the Euclidian sense) to the vector X(i) in memory matrix, then, the Euclidean distance between them is the smallest of all m possible distances and the weight w_i corresponding to X(i) is the largest within W . In summary, the vector in memory matrix that has the best similarity with the new input will contribute the most to the prediction for x_n.

When the process or device works normally, the input observation vector of NSET should be located in the normal working space that is represented by the memory matrix D , and it is thus similar to some of the historical vectors in the memory matrix. In the case, the NSET estimation should be highly accurate. When problems or faults arise with the process or device, its dynamic characteristics will change, and the new observation vector will deviate from the normal working space. In this case the linear combination of the historical vectors in the memory matrix will not provide an accurate estimate of the input and the residual will increase in magnitude, sometimes very significantly.

NSET is quite different from the Artificial Neural Network (ANN), a very common data driven modeling method, in following two respects:

1. An ANN uses historical data to train the network. During the training, the network absorbs the information from the training data into the weights. After training the data is discarded. For each new input vector, the weights of the network remain constant and the prediction is the nonlinear combination of the variables in the input vector. And the weight for the network has no clear meanings. In contrast, with NSET modeling, for each new observation vector, the weights W are individually generated by (14). Prediction with an NSET model is the linear combination of the historical observation data. The weights for NSET model show the similarity between the new input vector and vectors already in the memory matrix.
2. It is difficult to determine the structure for an ANN. In practice, it heavily depends on the user's experience to choose the number of neurons and the number of hidden layers. ANNs with a simple structure generally don't have enough modeling ability, while those having a complex structure will often over-fit the problem.

> NSET is a non-parametric modeling method and does not need a pre-determined structure. Good construction of the memory matrix alone will ensure satisfactory modeling accuracy. The modeling abilities for these two contrasting methods have been compared for a particular application [12], and confirm the comments above.

When NSET is used for wind turbine condition monitoring, the operational time span covered by NSET model (i.e., from which the memory matrix is selected) should be carefully considered. The ambient temperature and wind speed distribution can be quite different according to the time of year, and this is certainly true of wind turbine studied here, which is located in Zhangjiakou, north of Beijing where there are pronounced seasonal variations. Such meteorological parameters have a significant influence on the operation of wind turbine components. In order to achieve satisfactory model accuracy, the time span covered by the NSET model should not be too long, and ideally should be constrained to be within a particular season. This does mean that an NSET model would have to be constructed for each season, and although this adds to the effort required, the task should not be onerous once the procedures for model construction are in place. A related issue is whether the memory matrix should be renewed to reflect new operation conditions for wind turbine. It is attractive to add to the memory matrix new vectors representing more extreme external conditions than might have been available when the matrix was first formed, but care must be taken to ensure that the wind turbine is still operating normally. The danger is that faulted operation is incorporated into the matrix, making it then less likely to identify future faults as anomalies. These difficulties concerning renewal or amendment of the memory matrix relate to whether we can distinguish an observation vector representing a normal operating condition from one associated with a fault. The former could be added to the memory matrix while the later should be rejected. Principal Components Analysis (PCA) could perhaps be used to distinguish these two categories of observation vectors.

7.3 WIND TURBINE SCADA DATA PREPARATIONS AND TOWER VIBRATION ANALYSIS

The machine studied in this paper is a GE model 1.5S LE 1.5 MW-rated variable pitch, variable speed wind turbine, located in Zhangjiakou, northwest of Beijing. The cut-in and rated wind speeds for wind turbine are 3 m/s and 12 m/s, respectively. The SCADA system records all wind turbine parameters every 10 min. This 10-minute resolution data is a time-averaged value. Each record includes a time stamp, power, wind speed, blade angle, tower and drive train vibration amongst many others. The accelerometer for measuring tower vibration is mounted at the top of tower, where it meets the nacelle. The accelerometer for drive train vibration (DTV) is mounted on the high-speed shaft bearing. 10-minute SCADA data from the wind turbine from March to April 2006 was used, and there were 8784 10-minute records, covering a period of 61 days. Data quality was good and there were no missing records during this period.

For a large-scale wind turbine, there are several different operational regimes reflecting different wind speed ranges. When the wind speed is between cut-in and rated ones, the wind turbine runs in a Maximum Power Point Tracking (MPPT) regime. In this regime, the blade angle is usually fixed (at around two degrees depending on the blade design) and the rotational speed for rotor is controlled to be proportional to wind speed in order to maintain operation at C_{pmax} and thus maximize energy capture. When the wind speed is above the rated wind speed, the wind turbine is controlled to operate at a fixed (rated) power output regime. In this control regime, the power is limited electronically through the variable speed drive converter to rated power, while at the same time the wind turbine's aerodynamic power is kept constant on average by adjusting the blade angle to limit the rotor speed within an acceptable range. In these two operating regimes, the tower vibration signals recorded by the SCADA are of course quite different. Figure 1 shows trends of tower vibration and related variables from 25/03/2006 to 29/03/2006. Figure 2 shows trends from 17/04/2006 to 22/04/2006. The physical units used for tower vibration and related variables are shown in Table 1.

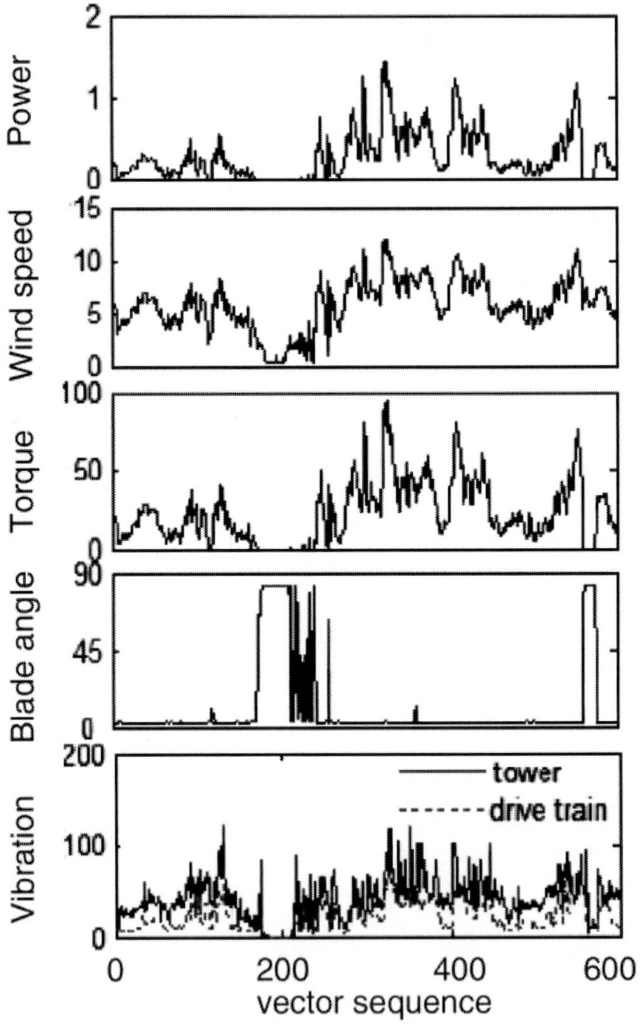

FIGURE 1: Trends for tower vibration and related variables with below rated wind speed.

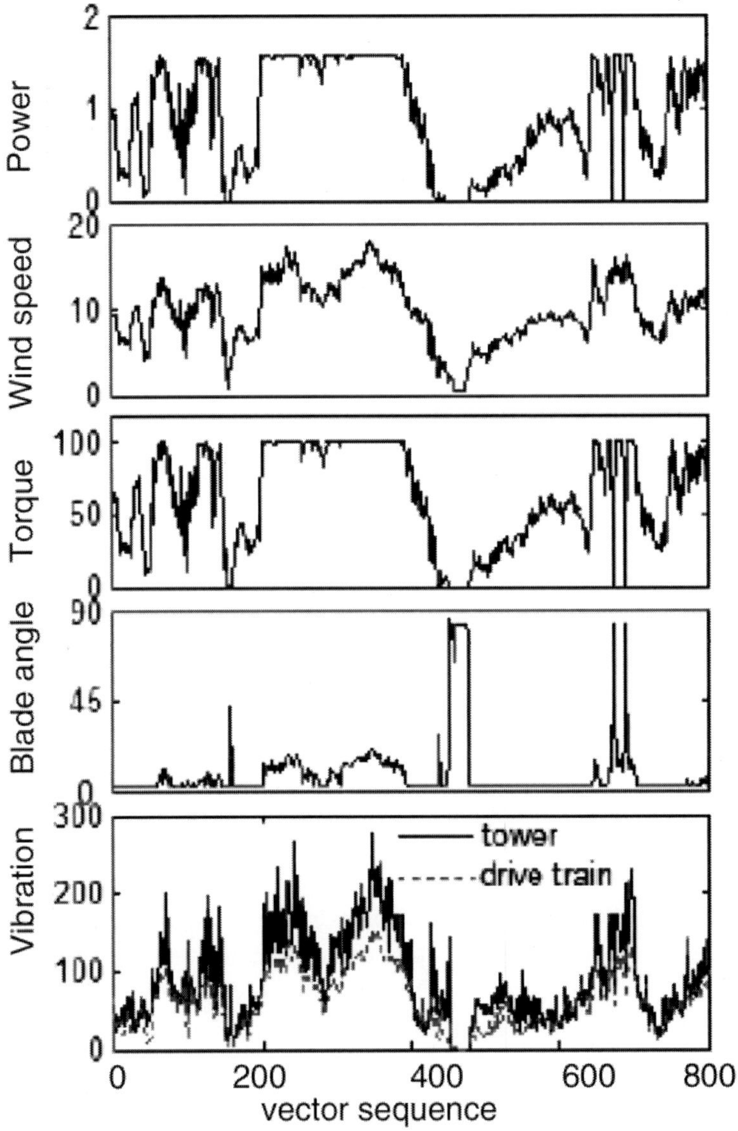

FIGURE 2. Trends for tower vibration and related variables with some operations above the rated values.

TABLE 1: Physical units for SCADA variables.

Variable name	Physical unit	Notice
Tower vibration	mm/s^2	Bandwidth: 0–200 Hz
Drive train vibration	mm/s^2	Bandwidth: 3–20 kHz
Power	MW	Rated: 1.5 MW
Wind speed	m/s	Rated: 12 m/s
Torque	%	Rated: 880 kNm
Blade angle	degree	Below rated: 2

7.3.1 TOWER VIBRATION ANALYSIS BELOW THE RATED WIND SPEED

Below rated wind speed, the pitch angle of this GE turbine is fixed at 2 degrees. From Figure 1, we can find that the following variables have a great influence on tower vibration magnitude.

1. Wind speed. Wind speed is stochastic and produces time varying forces and loads on the rotor. Most relevant to this analysis are the torque and thrust, both approximately proportional to wind speed squared below rated. Even below rated, the higher the wind speed the larger magnitude tower vibration, as shown in Figure 1. This is because the amplitude of thrust variation increases with wind speed, and wind speed standard deviation also increases with wind speed, assuming roughly constant turbulence intensity.
2. Torque and power. At Cpmax regime, torque will increase approximately with wind speed squared as indicated above, output power with wind speed cubed. Torque and power reflect how hard the wind turbine works. The higher torque and power is, the higher the rotating speeds for rotor and drive train become that will lead to increased tower vibration.
3. Drive train vibration. Drive train for wind turbine includes main bearing, gearbox, and generator bearing. Because the drive train is located in the nacelle, vibration of the drive train will be transmitted to the supporting structure, in this case through the yaw bearing to the tower and will directly influence tower vibration.

In Figure 1, at point 175 (27/03/2006 02:14:05 AM), the wind turbine went through an emergency shut down and the blade pitched from 2 degrees to 90 degrees to provide aerodynamic braking of the rotor as is normal for such an emergency stop (in this case, a remote manual stop). During such an event the aerodynamic forces on the rotor reverse over a very short period of time (typically less than 10 s) as it moves from turbine mode to propeller mode. This results in a large impulse force on the tower.

7.3.2 TOWER VIBRATION ANALYSIS ABOVE THE RATED WIND SPEED

Regarding Figure 2, we are interested in the period when the wind speed is above the rated value, that is, from points 199 to 400. During this period, the wind turbine is operating at constant power output regime. From Figure 2, we can see that the blade angle is regulating in accord with the wind speed. In this operating regime, the tower vibration is closely related to the following variables:

1. Blade angle. When the wind speed is above rated, the blade pitch for the GE model 1.5SLE is increased to regulate power. With an increase in blade pitch angle beyond the stall point, the aerodynamic lift coefficient blade decreases and the drag force coefficient increases rapidly. The Energies 2012, 5 5287 net effect is a significant increase in thrust and this result in increased tower deflection and vibration amplitudes.
2. Wind speed.
3. Drive train vibration.

The reasons for selecting wind speed and drive train vibration related to tower vibration are same as Section 3.1. In this operational regime, torque, output power, and rotational speed are approximately constant and thus have little influence on tower vibration.

A closer look at the magnitude of the difference between the tower vibration (TV) and drive train vibration (DTV) in Figure 2 reveals something interesting. This difference is relatively small when the blade angle is fixed, that is, when the wind turbine runs at Cpmax regime but the difference becomes considerable when the blade angle is changing, from data points 199 to 400, that is when the turbine is operating in the rated regime. The reason for this phenomenon lies with the main bearing characteristics. When the wind speed is low the thrust force on the rotor and tower is also small, and most of the load transmits to the drive train so that the vibration difference between them are small. In contrast, when the wind speed is high, the regulation of blade angle results in significant and rapid changes in thrust; this directly excites tower/rotor mode vibration. In this situation, the main bearing thrust ring structure, if suitably designed only a small part of the total load is transmitted to the drive train. As a result, the tower vibrates significantly while the drive train vibration remains similar to that approaching rated power.

From Figures 1 and 2, we can see that the variables that have greatest influence on tower vibration levels are quite different in the two distinct wind turbine operational regimes. And so the tower vibration model (TVM) should comprise two distinct sub-models corresponding to the two different turbine control regimes.

7.4 TOWER VIBRATION MODELING USING NONLINEAR STATE ESTIMATION TECHNIQUE (NSET)

The TVM is used to describe the complex relationship between tower vibration and the parameters that govern its behavior. In this paper, the TVM is constructed with use of the established Nonlinear State Estimation Technique (NSET) applied to SCADA data obtained when the wind turbine was working normally. This model can then be used as a reference to help detect incipient failure when contemporary data indicates a significant change in operational characteristics. NSET integrates the modeling variable (such as tower vibration) and its related variables (such as wind speed, power, toque, etc.) as a "related variable set". And at a sampling time, variables in the "related variable set" make an observation vector. After the TVM is constructed with NSET, by giving a new observation vector, the TVM NSET model can make a prediction for the tower vibration. The residual being the difference between the prediction and actual value for the tower vibration will reflect the deviation between the new input vector and the normal TVM. The magnitude and characteristics of the residual can be used to identify possible incipient failure for components such as the wind turbine rotor.

7.4.1 TOWER VIBRATION MODELING WITH NSET METHOD

Following the above section, the key steps for vibration modeling with NSET are in sequence: selection of the relevant variables to make up the observation vector and construct the memory matrix D using the SCADA data obtained from the wind turbine during periods of normal (healthy) operation. Historic data as shown in Figures 1 and 2 are used to validate the TVM. SCADA data from March to April but excluding these two sets used for validation, written as data set M , are used to model the tower vibration. As mentioned before, tower vibration has different influential variables in different operating regimes. Therefore, data set M is divided into to two subsets M_1 and M_2. M_1 includes the records which wind speed is between cut-in and rated wind speed, while records in M_2 are those which wind speed is between rated and cut out wind speed. M_1 and M_2 are used respectively to construct the sub-models for below and above the rated operation.

7.4.1.1 TVM FOR WIND SPEED BELOW THE RATED (SUB-MODEL A)

With the analysis in Section 3.1, the observation vector for regime below rated is made up from variables with the greatest influence on tower vibration, including the tower vibration parameter itself. It is perfectly acceptable in a NSET model to include the desired model output parameter such as tower vibration itself in the observation vector which is shown as Table 2.

TABLE 2: Observation vector below rated wind speed.

Working condition	Variables in the observation vector
below the rated (MPPT regime)	wind speed, torque, power, drive train vibration, tower vibration

For each record in subset M_1, the variables in Table 2 are selected to make up the historical observation vector. In total, the number of the historical observation vector available in M_1 is 5369. The second and critical step for NSET modeling is to selecting d1 (usually about several hundreds) representative historical observation vectors from the vectors available so as to form the memory matrix D_1. [12] has reported a systematic memory matrix construction method.

7.4.1.2 TVM FOR WIND SPEED ABOVE THE RATED (SUB-MODEL B)

Following the analysis in Section 3.2, observation vectors above rated take to include the following variables (Table 3).

TABLE 3: Observation vector above rated wind speed.

Working condition	Variables in the observation vector
above the rated (output leveling regime)	wind speed, blade angle, drive train vibration, tower vibration

One thousand forty seven (1047) historical observation vectors above the rated wind speed are available in M_2. With the same constructing method used before, d_2 historical observation vectors are selected to form the memory matrix D_2.

After the construction of memory matrices D1 and D2 , one or other of the two sub-models can be used to provide a prediction for any new input observation vector. In this paper, because we are only interested in the prediction for tower vibration alone, Equation (14) will be used to give the prediction result. Figure 3 shows how these two sub-models work together to give a prediction for tower vibration.

7.4.2 VALIDATION FOR THE NSET TOWER VIBRATION MODELS

Using the memory construction method as outlined in [12], the memory matrix D_1 is formed of 432 vectors, and D_2 has 261 vectors.

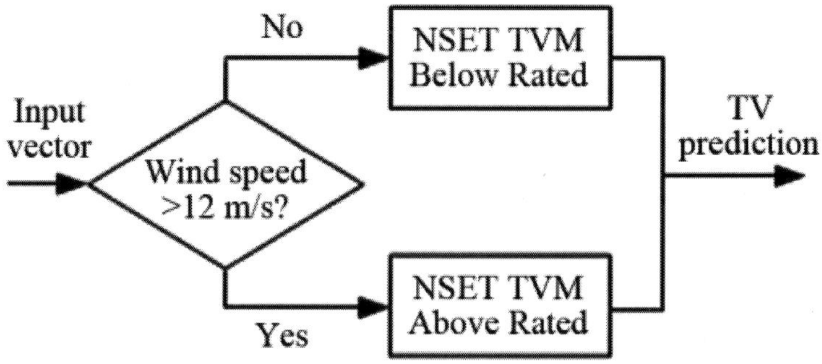

FIGURE 3. NSET modeling and prediction for tower vibration.

7.4.2.1 VALIDATION CASE 1:

The 600 records shown in Figure 1 are used to validate the TVM. During this period, wind speed is below the rated and only sub-model A is required for prediction of the tower vibration. Note that when the turbine is shuts down, the TVM cannot function and the prediction is thus zero. The validation result is shown in Figure 4. Note that in this figure, the pitch angle is shown in natural units (degrees) for ease of interpretation, rather than the scaled value between 0 and 1 for other parameters.

From Figure 4, we can see that when the wind turbine shuts down or starts up, the blade angle will pitch to the 90 or 2 degree setting (such as at points 175, 243, 260, 562, and 575). Because the blade pitches very quickly, the corresponding large change in aerodynamic loads result in abnormally large vibration magnitudes and large NSET model residuals. After removing these above points, sub-model A has a good prediction for tower vibration.

7.4.2.2 VALIDATION CASE 2:

The 800 records shown in Figure 2 are used to validate the TVM for above rated operation. The records of this period cover wind speed both below and above the rated. Sub-models A and B work together to give the prediction for tower vibration according to the logic of Figure 3. Validation is shown

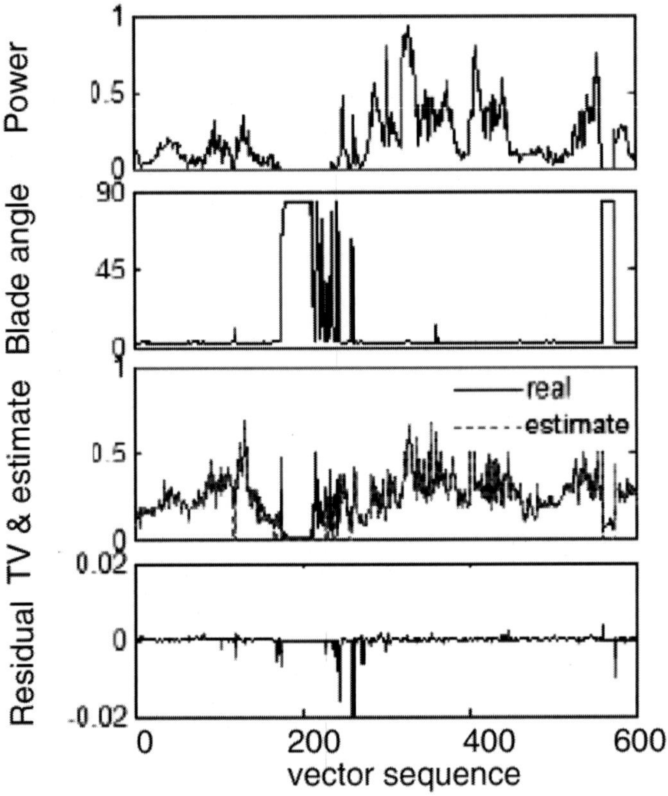

FIGURE 4: Validation for sub-model A.

in Figure 5. After removing the isolated large residuals caused by wind turbine shut downs and starts ups (such as at points 427, 674 and 688), the combination of these two sub-models demonstrates satisfactory modeling accuracy.

7.5 TVM USED FOR ROTOR CONDITION MONITORING

The analysis of Section 3 above shows that the rotor aerodynamic characteristics have a significant impact on tower vibration. Incipient rotor failure might be expected to lead to abnormal rotor aerodynamics and these

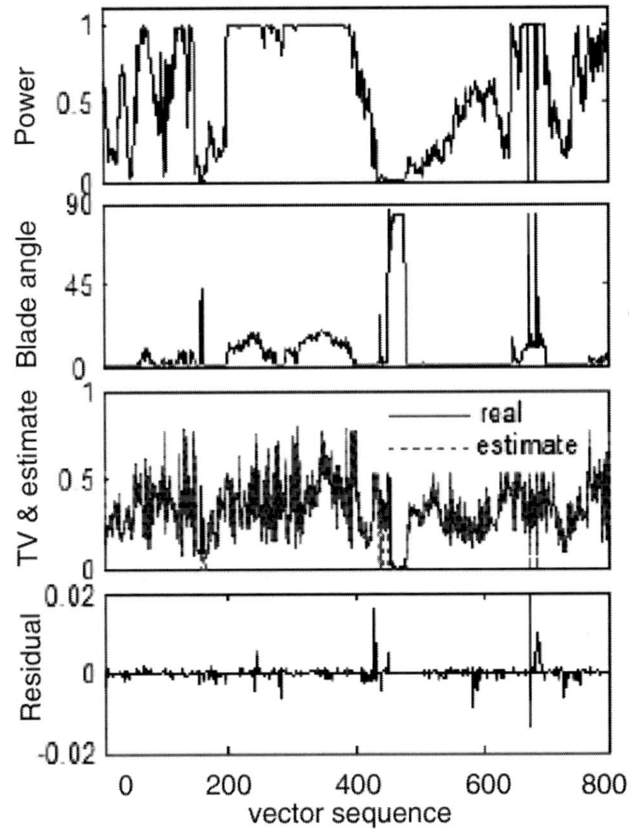

FIGURE 5: Validation for sub-model B.

changes could be detected through close monitoring and analysis of tower vibration. The TVM captures essential aspects of the relationship between the tower vibration and the key turbine parameters during normal healthy operation. When changes indicative of incipient failure of rotor occur, this normal relationship between the variables in the observation vector will change and deviate from the TVM. As a result, the TVM will no longer give an accurate prediction of tower vibration; the residual between the NSET model prediction and the measured values will become significant. Standard hypothesis testing [13], can be used to determine whether the differences are statically significant.

Blade angle asymmetry is a common kind of rotor fault and can lead to unacceptable fatigue damage. When this fault occurs, the blade angles for the three blades become different from each other leading to asymmetry of aerodynamic loading. If wind turbine runs in this way for extended periods, the unwanted asymmetric loads can cause serious damage to the drive train and even the supporting structure. Blade angle asymmetry could be detectable using the TVM developed in Section 4.

7.5.1 BLADE ANGLE ASYMMETRY DETECTION

For the wind turbine studied here, at 10:51 on 01/04/2006, the turbine underwent an emergency shut down due to excessive blade angle asymmetry. Information regarding this shutdown was recorded by the SCADA system and is shown in Table 4.

TABLE 4: Failure data.

Wind turbine ID	Date	Time	Failure code	Failure Text
15401801	01/04/2006	10:51:57	144	Blade angle asymmetry
15401801	01/04/2006	10:51:57	184	Shut down

We select 400 records around this failure as input vectors for the TVM constructed in Section 4 (starting 316 data points prior to shutdown). The trend for tower vibration residuals and trends for other related variables are shown in Figure 6.

The failure mentioned above occurred at point 316, and the blade angle pitched to 90 degrees as part of the emergency stop. In the trends for tower vibration and drive train vibration, the difference between these two are small before point 275. But after point 275, the tower vibration was much higher than before and the difference between the two was sharply increased. This abnormal change in the relationship between these variables is detected in a timely manner by the TVM and the residuals change in a statistically way after this point. With proper setting of the alarm threshold

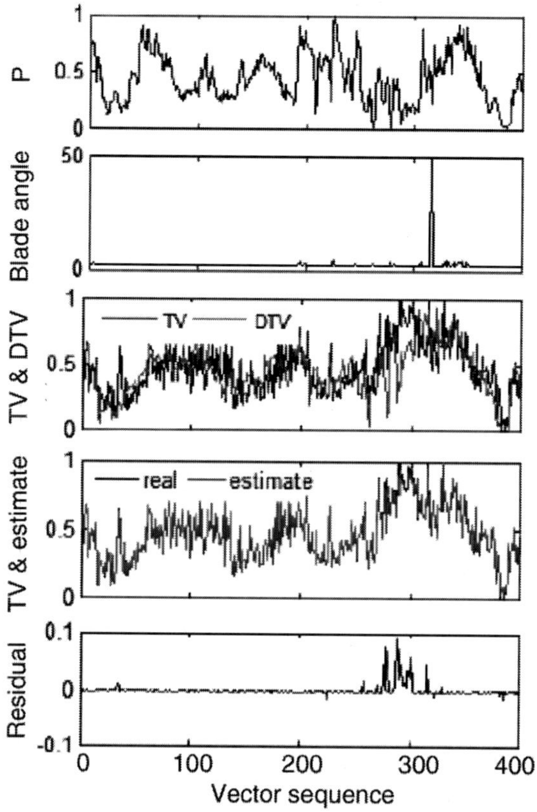

FIGURE 6: Trends for blade angle asymmetry

value or using moving window method as in [12], the rotor failure such as blade angle asymmetry can be robustly detected before serious damage is caused to the wind turbine. How to set the threshold for failure detection is not the purpose for this paper and readers can refer to papers [12,13] for more details on threshold determination. Using the moving window method, this blade angle asymmetry was detected at point 279, well ahead the wind turbine shut down at 316.

7.6 DISCUSSION AND CONCLUSIONS

This paper has characterized wind turbine tower vibration, both below and above the rated wind speed. The NSET method has been used to model the dependence of the tower vibration on the most influential parameters under normal operational conditions. The derived tower vibration model has been used to detect one specific kind of rotor fault: blade angle asymmetry. The following conclusions can be drawn:

1. For wind turbine condition monitoring, it can be misleading to analyze the vibration signal alone. Because of the strong impact of wind on a turbine and the coupling amongst the different wind turbine components and vibrational modes, vibration analysis must take other related factors into account to give a more accurate representation of the turbine so as to be useful for condition monitoring and diagnostics. For example, it is essential when analyzing a wind turbine rotor, to take both wind speed and rotational speed into account.
2. The results presented have demonstrated that tower vibration must be analyzed in the context of the rotor and its different operational regimes. Since the aerodynamic forces acting on the rotor are very sensitive to the blade angle, blade angle asymmetries will lead to significant differences in the thrust on individual blades. The unbalanced thrust force on the rotor will excite the supporting tower structure and cause the tower's behavior and vibration to deviate from the normal operational condition. Therefore, monitoring the tower vibration provides a useful method for detecting rotor aerodynamic asymmetries caused for example by poor blade pitch adjustment or blade pitch control faults. NSET has been shown to be an effective technique to model the relationship between tower and rotor dynamics. The NSET tower vibration model (TVM) is able to accurately represent the relationship between rotor loads and tower vibration and thus to detect incipient rotor faults (in this case blade asymmetry) in a timely manner. Admittedly only one example of successful fault identification has been presented in this study, and

this cannot prove that all such faults would be identified in a timely and thus useful manner. Access to much larger data sets is required in order to provide a statically significant sample of faults for detection, and this is work in progress. Nevertheless, the methodology presented here is underpinned by an engineering knowledge of the turbine and how it is operated, and this together with the successful fault identification allows the conclusion that the technique has promise and merits further development. It is also worth noting that blade pitch asymmetry is not the only means by which off axis aerodynamic loads could be generated that could be seen as abnormal, in contract to wind shear which is of course to be expected. Other conditions that would create abnormal off axis loads could include poor yaw control, damage to individual blades, and blade icing. All of these faults should in principal be detectable using the methodology presented here, and will be the subject of future research.

REFERENCES

1. Hameed, Z.; Hong, Y.S.; Cho, Y.M.; Ahn, S.H.; Song, C.K. Condition monitoring and fault detection of wind turbines and related algorithms: A review. Renew. Sustain. Energy Rev. 2009, 1, 1–39.
2. García Márquez, F.P.; Tobias, A.M.; Pinar Pérez, J.M.; Papaelias, M. Condition monitoring of wind turbines: Techniques and methods. Renew. Energy 2012, 46, 169–178.
3. Zhang, Z.; Verma, A.; Kusiak, A. Fault analysis and fault condition monitoring of the wind turbine gearbox. IEEE Trans. Energy Convers. 2012, 2, 526–535.
4. Caselitz, P.; Giebhardt, J. Rotor condition monitoring for improved operational safety of offshore wind energy converters. J. Solar Energy Eng. 2005, 5, 253–261.
5. Feng, Y.; Qiu, Y.; Crabtree, C.J.; Long, H.; Tavner, P.J. Monitoring wind turbine gearboxes. Wind Energy 2012, in press, doi:10.1002/we.1521.
6. Kusiak, A.; Li, W. The prediction and diagnosis of wind turbine fault. Renew. Energy 2011, 36, 16–23.
7. Zaher, A.; McArther, S.D.J.; Infield, D.G.; Patel, Y. Online wind turbine fault detection through automated SCADA data analysis. Wind Energy 2009, 6, 574–593.
8. Gross, K.C.; Singer, R.M.; Wegerich, S.W.; Herzog, J.P. Application of a model-based fault detection system to nuclear plant signals. In Proceedings of 9th International Conference on Intelligent Systems Application to Power System, Seoul, Korea, 6–10 July 1997; pp. 212–218.

9. Bockhorst, F.K.; Gross, K.C.; Herzog, J.P.; Wegerich, S.W. MSET modeling of Crystal River-3 venturi flow meters. In Proceedings of International Conference on Nuclear Engineering, San Diego, CA, USA, 10–15 May 1998; pp. 425–429.
10. Cheng, S.F.; Pecht, M. Multivariate state estimation technique for remaining useful life prediction of electronic products. In Proceedings of AAAI Fall Symposium on Artificial Intelligence for Prognostics, Arlington, VA, USA, 9–11 November 2007; pp. 26–32.
11. Cassidy, K.J.; Gross, K.C.; Malekpour, A. Advanced pattern recognition for detection of complex software aging phenomena in online transaction processing servers. In Proceedings of International Conference on Dependable Systems and Networks (DSN) 2002, Washington, DC, USA, 23–26 June 2002; pp. 478–482.
12. Guo, P.; Infield, D.; Yang, Y. Wind turbine generator condition monitoring using temperature trend analysis. IEEE Trans. Sustain. Energy 2012, 1, 124–133.
13. Wang, Y.; Infield, D. SCADA data based nonlinear state estimation technique for wind turbine gearbox condition monitoring. In Proceedings of European Wind Energy Association Conference 2012, Copenhagen, Denmark, 16–19 April 2012; pp. 621–629.

PART IV

CONTROL SYSTEMS

CHAPTER 8

TWO LQRI BASED BLADE PITCH CONTROLS FOR WIND TURBINES

SUNGSU PARK AND YOONSU NAM

8.1 INTRODUCTION

The main objective of wind turbine control is to make wind power production economically more efficient. This objective is often achieved in two distinct regions, i.e., the below rated wind speed and the above rated wind speed regions. In the below rated wind speed region, generator torque control is used primarily to control rotor speed to track the maximum power coefficient in order to maximize energy capture. In the above rated wind speed region, the blade pitch control is used primarily to regulate the rotor speed in order to regulate the aerodynamic power within its design limit [1]. As the wind turbine sizes are increasing and their mechanical components are built lighter, the reduction of the structural loads becomes a very important task of wind turbine control because structural loads can reduce turbine reliability and lifespan and also may cause power fluctuations. In particular, the reduction of blade loads has received special interest. Wind speed variations across the turbine rotor during rotor rotation, which is caused by the large rotor blade size, the wind shear, turbulence and tower shadow effects, cause periodic oscillations in blade structural loads, and

This chapter was originally published under the Creative Commons Attribution License. Park S and Nam Y. Two LQRI based Blade Pitch Controls for Wind Turbines. Energies ***2012****,5 (2012). doi:10.3390/en5061998.*

this structural load is especially important in the above rated wind speed region because high structural loads arise from strong winds. Therefore the individual pitch control is sometimes considered since common collective pitch control cannot compensate for the periodic loads on the blades.

Individual pitch control has been investigated by a number of researchers and shown to be beneficial [2–18]. However, individual pitch control can reduce only the oscillation of blade bending moment, not its steady-state value. The collective pitch control can mitigate the magnitude of bending moments, but this is in conflict with the control objective of rotor speed regulation. A modern multi-input, multi-output (MIMO) control framework can be used to explicitly take into account the conflicted control objectives which are regulating rotor speed while reducing blade loads, and the so-called centralized pitch control can be designed where the collective and individual pitch commands are generated from the same controller [2–4]. The advantages of centralized pitch control include that it handles multiple control objectives. Although the design of centralized pitch control is desirable from the control point of view, the separate collective and individual pitch control system is still preferable to the majority of wind turbine industries since individual pitch control is considered as a secondary controller working as an on-off mechanism.

In this paper, we present a separate set of collective and individual pitch control algorithms. Both pitch control algorithms use the LQR control technique with integral action (LQRI), and utilize Kalman filters to estimate system states and wind speed [5–8,19]. Compared to previous works, our collective pitch controller can control the rotor speed and collective, i.e., the steady-state value of, blade bending moments together to improve the trade-off between rotor speed regulation and load reduction, while the individual pitch controller reduces the fluctuating loads on the blades. The individual pitch controller is designed separately as an additional loop around the system, and can be added on to the collective pitch controller. In this way, we utilize the advantages of both the central pitch control and the separate set of collective and individual pitch control systems. Our algorithm can compensate for the effect of wind disturbance and can reduce the blade loads significantly, while using the same blade bending moment measurements to those of previous works.

In the next section, the dynamics of the wind turbine is modeled as a time-varying system and is converted to two time-invariant systems for the collective and individual pitch controller designs respectively. In Section 3, the collective and individual pitch control algorithms are developed based on the LQRI and state estimation of the Kalman filter. The performance of control algorithms is evaluated in Section 4 using computer simulations, and conclusions follow in Section 5.

8.2 WIND TURBINE MODEL

A wind turbine is a highly nonlinear system and difficult to model. A very complex mathematical model containing several degrees of freedom is necessary to fully explore wind turbine system behavior. The wind turbine system under consideration in this paper is commercial 2 MW 3-bladed horizontal axis system. To model this wind turbine, the GH Bladed [20], commercial software, is used. The rotor blades are modeled with six modal frequencies in the flapwise direction and five modal frequencies in the edgewise direction. Tower motion is modeled with two modes both in fore-aft and side-side directions, respectively. The flexibility of the shaft connected to the rotor side is modeled by an equivalent spring constant and damping. The pitch actuator and generator torque dynamics are also modeled with second order and first order systems, respectively. This high fidelity model is used for simulations with the designed controller.

For the pitch controller design, a simple linear wind turbine model is required that sufficiently describes the dynamics of wind turbine. In this paper, the simple wind turbine model utilizes rigid rotor blades and drive-train, while tower is modeled by one mode of fore-aft motion and one mode of side-side motion [3,9,10]. Consider the blade coordinate system as shown in Figure 1(a), where the x-axis points in the direction along the main shaft, the z-axis points toward the blade tip, the y-axis forms right-handed rule, and its origin is at the blade root. Consider also the fixed hub coordinate system as shown in Figure 1(b), where the x-axis points in the direction along the main shaft and the z-axis is in an upward direction, and its origin is at the hub center.

Then, the moments on the hub can be expressed using blade root moments as follows:

$$M_x = \sum_{i=1}^{3} M_{x,i}^{b}$$

$$M_y = \sum_{i=1}^{3} \cos\Psi_i M_{y,i}^{b}$$

$$M_z = \sum_{i=1}^{3} \sin\Psi_i M_{y,i}^{b} \tag{1}$$

where Ψ_i is the blade azimuth angle defined as zero when the i-th blade is in the upward position, $M_{x,i}^{b}$ is the aerodynamic component of the i-th blade root moment in the x-axis, and $M_{y,i}^{b}$, is the measured i-th blade root moment in the y-axis of the blade coordinate system, and both are given as follows:

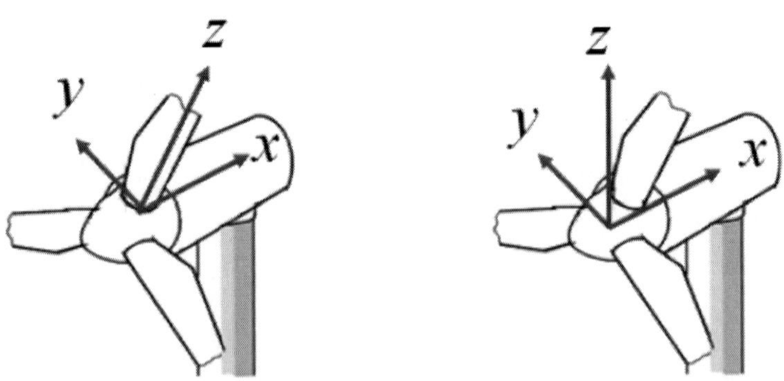

FIGURE 1: (a) Blade coordinate system; (b) Fixed hub coordinate system [21].

$$M^b_{x,i} = C_{M_x}(v_i, \Omega_r, \beta_i)\frac{1}{2}\rho\pi R_b^2 v_i^2$$

$$M^b_{y,i} = C_{M_y}(v_i, \Omega_r, \beta_i)\frac{1}{2}\rho\pi R_b^2 v_i^2 \tag{2}$$

where C_{Mx} and C_{My} are the moment coefficients, Ω_r is the rotor speed, β_i is the pitch angle of the i-th blade, ρ is the air density, R_b is the rotor radius, and v_i is the relative wind speed for the i-th blade, which is the sum of the blade effective wind speed $v_{0,i}$ and tower fore-aft motion as follows [9]:

$$v_i = v_{o,i} - \dot{x}_{fa} + \frac{3}{2H}\frac{3\dot{R}_b}{4}\dot{x}_{fa}\cos\Psi_\iota \tag{3}$$

where H is the tower height and x_{fa} is the tower fore-aft translation.

Similarly, the forces on the hub can be expressed as follows:

$$F_x = \sum_{i=1}^{3} F^b_{y,i}$$

$$F_y = \sum_{i=1}^{3} \cos\Psi_i F^b_{y,i} \tag{4}$$

where $F_{x,i}{}^b$, and $F_{y,i}{}^b$, are the aerodynamic components of the i-th blade forces in the x- and y-axis of blade coordinate system respectively, and are also given as follows:

$$F_{x,i}^{b} = C_{F_x}(v_i, \Omega_r, \beta_i)\frac{1}{2}\rho\pi R_b^2 v_i^2$$

$$F_{y,i}^{b} = C_{F_y}(v_i, \Omega_r, \beta_i)\frac{1}{2}\rho\pi R_b^2 v_i^2 \tag{5}$$

where C_{Fx} and C_{Fy} are the force coefficients.

Since the wind turbine model is highly nonlinear, it has to be linearized at some operating point for the controller design. The moments on the hub can be linearized as follows:

$$\delta M_x = \sum_{i=1}^{3}\left(\frac{\delta M_x^b}{\delta v}\delta v_{0,i} + \frac{\delta M_x^b}{\delta \beta}\delta\beta_i\right) + 3\frac{\delta M_x^b}{\delta\Omega_r}\delta\Omega_r - 3\frac{\delta M_x^b}{\delta v}\dot{x}_{fa}$$

$$\delta M_y = \sum_{i=1}^{3}\cos\Psi_i\left(\frac{\delta M_y^b}{\delta v}\delta v_{0,i} + \frac{\delta M_y^b}{\delta \beta}\delta\beta_i\right) - \frac{\delta M_y^b}{\delta v}\frac{27R_b}{16H}\dot{x}_{fa}$$

$$\delta M_z = \sum_{i=1}^{3}\sin\Psi_i\left(\frac{\delta M_y^b}{\delta v}\delta v_{0,i} + \frac{\delta M_y^b}{\delta \beta}\delta\beta_i\right) \tag{6}$$

where δ denotes the difference from equilibrium value. The forces on the hub can be linearized likewise as follows:

$$\delta F_x = \sum_{i=1}^{3}\left(\frac{\delta F_x^b}{\delta v}\delta v_{0,i} + \frac{\delta F_x^b}{\delta \beta}\delta\beta_i\right) + 3\frac{\delta F_x^b}{\delta\Omega_r}\delta\Omega_r - 3\frac{\delta F_x^b}{\delta v}\dot{x}_{fa}$$

$$\delta F_y = \sum_{i=1}^{3}\cos\Psi_i\left(\frac{\delta F_y^b}{\delta v}\delta v_{0,i} + \frac{\delta F_y^b}{\delta \beta}\delta\beta_i\right) - \frac{\delta F_y^b}{\delta v}\frac{27R_b}{16H}\dot{x}_{fa} \tag{7}$$

With the assumption of a rigid drive-train, the linearized rotor angular acceleration is described as:

$$J_e \delta \dot{\Omega}_r = \delta M_x - N_g \delta T_g \tag{8}$$

where J_e is the effective moment of inertia of rotor, generator and transmission, N_g is the gear ratio, and δT_g is the perturbed generator torque. The tower motion is approximated by one mode of fore-aft and one mode of side-side motion as follows:

$$M_t \ddot{x}_{fa} + d_t \dot{x}_{fa} + K_t x_{fa} = \delta F_x + \frac{3}{2H} \delta M_y$$

$$M_t \ddot{y}_{ss} + D_t \dot{y}_{ss} + K_t y_{ss} = \delta F_y + \frac{3N_g}{2H} \delta T_g \tag{9}$$

where M_t, D_t, K_t are tower modal mass, damping and stiffness, respectively, and y_{ss} is the tower side-side translation. The multiplier 3/(2H) is the ratio between displacement and rotation of the tower top, assumed that the tower is approximated with prismatic beam subjected to a bending force load [9].

Equations (6–9) describe wind turbine dynamic equations and show that the wind turbine has time-varying dynamics even under constant wind conditions. To make the control design problem time-invariant, the time-varying wind turbine model is transformed to a linear time-invariant model using the Coleman transform. The Coleman transform and its inversion are defined as [22]:

$$P = \begin{bmatrix} 1 & \cos\Psi_1 & \sin\Psi_1 \\ 1 & \cos\Psi_2 & \sin\Psi_2 \\ 1 & \cos\Psi_3 & \sin\Psi_3 \end{bmatrix}$$

$$P^{-1} = \begin{bmatrix} 1/3 & 1/3 & 1/3 \\ (2/3)\cos\Psi_1 & (2/3)\cos\Psi_2 & (2/3)\cos\Psi_3 \\ (2/3)\sin\Psi_1 & (2/3)\sin\Psi_2 & (2/3)\sin\Psi_3 \end{bmatrix} \tag{10}$$

where $\Psi_2 = \Psi_1 + 2\pi/3$ and $\Psi_3 = \Psi_1 + 4\pi/3$.

Transforming perturbed wind speed, pitch angles and blade moments in Equations (6) and (7) to the variables in the Coleman frame yields the following moment equations:

$$\begin{aligned}
\delta M_x &= 3\frac{\delta M_x^b}{\delta v}\left(\delta v_{o_c} - \dot{x}_{fa}\right) + 3\frac{\delta M_x^b}{\delta \beta}\delta\beta_c + 3\frac{\delta M_x^b}{\delta \Omega_r}\delta\Omega_r \\
\delta M_0 &= \frac{\delta M_y^b}{\delta v}\left(\delta v_{o_c} - \dot{x}_{fa}\right) + 3\frac{\delta M_y^b}{\delta \beta}\delta\beta_c + \frac{\delta M_y^b}{\delta \Omega_r}\delta\Omega_r \\
\delta M_d &= \frac{\delta M_y^b}{\delta v}\delta v_{o_d} + \frac{\delta M_y^b}{\delta \beta}\delta\beta_d - 3\frac{\delta M_y^b}{\delta v}\frac{9R_b}{8H}\dot{x}_{fa} \\
\delta M_q &= \frac{\delta M_y^b}{\delta v}\delta v_{o_q} + \frac{\delta M_y^b}{\delta \beta}\delta\beta_q
\end{aligned} \tag{11}$$

and force equations:

$$\begin{aligned}
\delta F_x &= 3\frac{\delta F_x^b}{\delta v}\left(\delta v_{o_c} - \dot{x}_{fa}\right) + 3\frac{\delta F_x^b}{\delta \Omega_r}\delta\Omega_r + 3\frac{\delta F_x^b}{\delta \beta}\delta\beta_c \\
\delta F_y &= \frac{3}{2}\frac{\delta F_y^b}{\delta v}\delta v_{o_d} + \frac{3}{2}\frac{\delta F_y^b}{\delta \beta}\delta\beta_d + \frac{\delta F_y^b}{\delta v}\frac{27R_b}{16H}\dot{x}_{fa}
\end{aligned} \tag{12}$$

where δv_{0c} and $\delta\beta_c$ are the perturbed collective wind speed and pitch angle respectively, δv_{0d} and δv_{0q} are the perturbed wind speed, $\delta\beta_d$ and $\delta\beta_q$ are the perturbed pitch angles, and δM_d and δM_q are the perturbed moments in the d-(tilt) and q-axis(yaw) of the Coleman frame, respectively, which are defined as follows:

$$\begin{bmatrix}\delta v_{0_c}\\ \delta v_{0_d}\\ \delta v_{0_q}\end{bmatrix} = P^{-1}\begin{bmatrix}\delta v_{0_1}\\ \delta v_{0_2}\\ \delta v_{0_3}\end{bmatrix}, \begin{bmatrix}\delta \beta_c\\ \delta \beta_d\\ \delta \beta_q\end{bmatrix} = P^{-1}\begin{bmatrix}\delta \beta_1\\ \delta \beta_2\\ \delta \beta_3\end{bmatrix}, \begin{bmatrix}\delta M_0\\ \delta M_d\\ \delta M_q\end{bmatrix} = P^{-1}\begin{bmatrix}\delta M_{y,1}^b\\ \delta M_{y,2}^b\\ \delta M_{y,3}^b\end{bmatrix} \tag{13}$$

The effective wind speed of each blade varies due to wind shear, turbulence and tower shadow effects, which results in periodic blade loading with the rotation of the rotor (so-called 1p, 2p, …, etc. loading). According to Equation (13), the 1p blade loading is transformed into constant loading in the Coleman frame, and the reduction of 1p blade loading can be achieved by reducing the constant values of the load in the Coleman frame. From Equation (11), these values can be controlled mainly by $\delta\beta_d$ and $\delta\beta_q$, and are almost decoupled from the collective pitch control $\delta\beta_c$, while the rotor speed and the collective blade moment can be controlled mainly by $\delta\beta_c$. This means that the collective and the individual pitch controls can be designed separately for their own control objectives.

8.3 PITCH CONTROLLER DESIGN

The time-invariant wind turbine dynamic Equations (8,9,11,12) can be written in state-space form as follows:

$$\begin{aligned}\dot{x} &= Ax + Bu + Gd\\ z &= Cx + Du + Fd\end{aligned} \tag{14}$$

where:

$$x = \begin{bmatrix}\delta\Omega_r & x_{fa} & \dot{x}_{fa} & y_{ss} & \dot{y}_{ss}\end{bmatrix}^T, u = \begin{bmatrix}\delta\beta_c & \delta\beta_d & \delta\beta_q & \delta T_g\end{bmatrix}^T$$
$$d = \begin{bmatrix}\delta v_{0_c} & \delta v_{0_d} & \delta v_{0_q}\end{bmatrix}^T, z = \begin{bmatrix}\delta\Omega_r & \delta M_0 & \delta M_d & \delta M_q\end{bmatrix}^T$$

The controller in this paper consists of three independent control loops: generator torque control, collective pitch control, and individual pitch control. The generator torque control is maintained constant at the above rated wind speed and the drive-train damper is included to damp the drive-train's torsional oscillation. The conventional PI-based collective pitch control is also designed for comparison purpose, which includes some low-pass filter and notch filter. However, the design of the conventional collective pitch controller is not within the scope of this paper. The collective and individual pitch controllers are designed in this paper.

As discussed in the previous section and from Equations (8) and (11), the collective wind speed and pitch angle mainly affect the rotor speed and the collective blade moments, while the d- and q-axis wind speeds and pitch angles mainly affect the d-and q-axis blade moments. Therefore, Equation (14) can be decomposed into two sets of equations. One equation based on the assumption that all d- and q-axis variables are zero in Equation (14) is given as follows:

$$\begin{aligned} \dot{x} &= Ax + B_1 u_1 + G_1 d_1 \\ z_1 &= C_1 x + D_1 u_1 + F_1 d_1 \end{aligned} \tag{15}$$

where:

$$u_1 = \delta\beta_c, d_1 = \delta v_{0_c}, z_1 = [\delta\Omega_r \ \ \delta M_0]^T$$

and the other equation based on the assumption that all collective variables are zero is given as follows:

$$\begin{aligned} \dot{x} &= Ax + B_2 u_2 + G_2 d_2 \\ z_2 &= C_2 x + D_2 u_2 + F_2 d_2 \end{aligned} \tag{16}$$

where:

$$u_2 = \left[\delta\beta_c \ \ \delta\beta_q\right]^T, d_2 = \left[\delta v_{0d} \ \ \delta v_{0q}\right]^T, z_2 = \left[\delta \mathrm{M}_d \ \ \delta M_q\right]^T$$

From Equations (14–16), it is clear that the system state variables x cannot be used directly as measurements for control feedback because the state variables in Equations (15) and (16) are different from those of Equation (14). The state variables in Equation (15) are influenced only by the collective wind speed and pitch angle, and those in Equation (16) by the d- and q-axis wind speeds and pitch angles, respectively, whereas the variables in Equation (14) are influenced by all of them. Therefore, instead of measuring the state variables, we should estimate those variables from measured rotor speed $\delta\Omega_r$ and moment δM_0 in the case of Equation (15), and measured moments δM_d and δM_q in the case of Equation (16).

8.3.1 COLLECTIVE PITCH CONTROLLER

The collective pitch controller is designed based on the dynamic Equation (15), where the inputs are the collective pitch angle $\delta\beta_c$ with the collective wind speed δv_{0c} , and the measured outputs are the rotor speed $\delta\Omega_r$ and moment δM_0. The collective wind speed is estimated here and used by the pitch controller. The wind speed d_1 in Equation (15) can be modeled as an unknown constant with the addition of white noise of power spectral density W_1 as follows:

$$\dot{d}_1 = w_1, w_1 \sim (0, W_1) \tag{17}$$

Now, the Kalman filter is designed to estimate system states and wind speed based on the following augmented system with the wind speed:

$$\begin{bmatrix} \dot{x} \\ \dot{d}_1 \end{bmatrix} = \begin{bmatrix} A & G_1 \\ 0 & 0 \end{bmatrix} \begin{bmatrix} x \\ d_1 \end{bmatrix} + \begin{bmatrix} B_1 \\ 0 \end{bmatrix} u_1 + \begin{bmatrix} 0 \\ 1 \end{bmatrix} w_1$$

$$z_1 = \begin{bmatrix} C_1 & F_1 \end{bmatrix} \begin{bmatrix} x \\ d_1 \end{bmatrix} + D_1 u_1 + v_1 \tag{18}$$

where v_1 is the measurement noise with the power spectral density of V_1.

Based on the state estimates, the LQR controller is designed, such that time domain performance criteria as minimal rotor speed variation and blade moment are directly included in the design. Since the standard LQR provides only proportional gains, Equation (15) is augmented with the integral of the rotor speed in order to cancel steady-state errors for step wind disturbances. Let $\delta\Omega_I$ be the integral of the rotor speed $\delta\Omega_r$, then the augmented system becomes:

$$\begin{bmatrix} \dot{x} \\ \delta\dot{\Omega}_I \end{bmatrix} = \begin{bmatrix} A & 0 \\ C_0 & 0 \end{bmatrix} \begin{bmatrix} x \\ \delta\Omega_I \end{bmatrix} + \begin{bmatrix} B_1 \\ 0 \end{bmatrix} u_1$$

$$y_1 = \begin{bmatrix} C_1 & 0 \\ 0 & 1 \end{bmatrix} \begin{bmatrix} x \\ \delta\Omega_I \end{bmatrix} + \begin{bmatrix} D_1 \\ 0 \end{bmatrix} u_1 \qquad (19)$$

where $C_0 = [1\ 0\ 0\ 0\ 0]$, and y_1 is the performance output. The LQRI based collective pitch control is determined such that it minimizes the cost function:

$$J = \int_0^\infty (y_1^T Q_1 y_1 + u_1^T R_1 u_1) dt \qquad (20)$$

where the trade-off between rotor speed regulation and blade load reduction can be explicitly considered in the weighting matrix Q_1.

The collective pitch control command is calculated in a straight forward manner as follows:

$$\delta\beta_c^{cmd} = K_{Xcol}\hat{x} + K_{Icol} \int_0^\infty \delta\Omega_r dt \qquad (21)$$

where $\hat{x}$ is the state estimate from the Kalman filter.

8.3.2 INDIVIDUAL PITCH CONTROLLER

The individual pitch controller is designed based on the dynamic Equation (16), where the inputs are the d- and q-axis pitch angles $\delta\beta_\delta$, $\delta\beta_q$ with the wind speeds δv_{0d}, δv_{0q}, and the measured outputs are d- and q-axis blade moments δM_d, δM_q.

Because the 1p variation of wind speed is transformed into a constant in the Coleman frame, the wind speeds 2 d in Equation (16) can be modeled as unknown constants with the addition of white noise of power spectral density 2 W as follows:

$$\dot{d}_2 = w_2, \qquad w_2 \sim (0, W_2) \tag{22}$$

The Kalman filter is designed based on the following augmented system with wind speeds:

$$\begin{bmatrix} \dot{x} \\ \dot{d}_2 \end{bmatrix} = \begin{bmatrix} A & G_2 \\ 0 & 0 \end{bmatrix} \begin{bmatrix} x \\ d_2 \end{bmatrix} + \begin{bmatrix} B_2 \\ 0 \end{bmatrix} u_1 + \begin{bmatrix} 0 \\ I_2 \end{bmatrix} w_2$$

$$z_2 = \begin{bmatrix} C_2 & F_2 \end{bmatrix} \begin{bmatrix} x \\ d_2 \end{bmatrix} + D_2 u_2 + v_2 \tag{23}$$

where I_2 denotes the identity matrix and v_2 is the measurement noise with the power spectral density of V_2.

Feedforward compensation can be utilized for rejecting the load caused by wind disturbance. Since the Kalman filter provides an estimate of the wind speed, we can design a feedforward controller on assumption that the wind and pitch angles dominate the blade moments in Equation (16) as follows:

$$u_{2\_ff} = -D_2^{-1} D_2 \hat{d}_2 \tag{24}$$

where $\hat{d}_2$ is wind speed estimate.

Again, since the standard LQR provides only proportional gains, Equation (16) is augmented with the integrals of the blade moments in order to cancel steady-state errors for step wind disturbances. Let z_I be the integrals of the blade moments z_2 , then the augmented system becomes:

$$\begin{bmatrix} \dot{x} \\ \dot{z}_I \end{bmatrix} = \begin{bmatrix} A & 0 \\ C_2 & 0 \end{bmatrix} \begin{bmatrix} x \\ z_I \end{bmatrix} + \begin{bmatrix} B_2 \\ D_2 \end{bmatrix} u_2$$

$$y_2 = \begin{bmatrix} C_2 & 0 \\ 0 & I_2 \end{bmatrix} \begin{bmatrix} x \\ z_I \end{bmatrix} + \begin{bmatrix} D_2 \\ 0 \end{bmatrix} u_2 \quad (25)$$

where y_2 is the performance output. The LQRI based individual pitch control is determined such that it minimizes the cost function:

$$J = \int_0^\infty (y_2^T Q_2 y_2 + u_2^T R_2 u_2)dt \quad (26)$$

The time domain performance criteria as minimal fluctuation of blade moments are directly included in weighting matrices Q_2 and R_2.

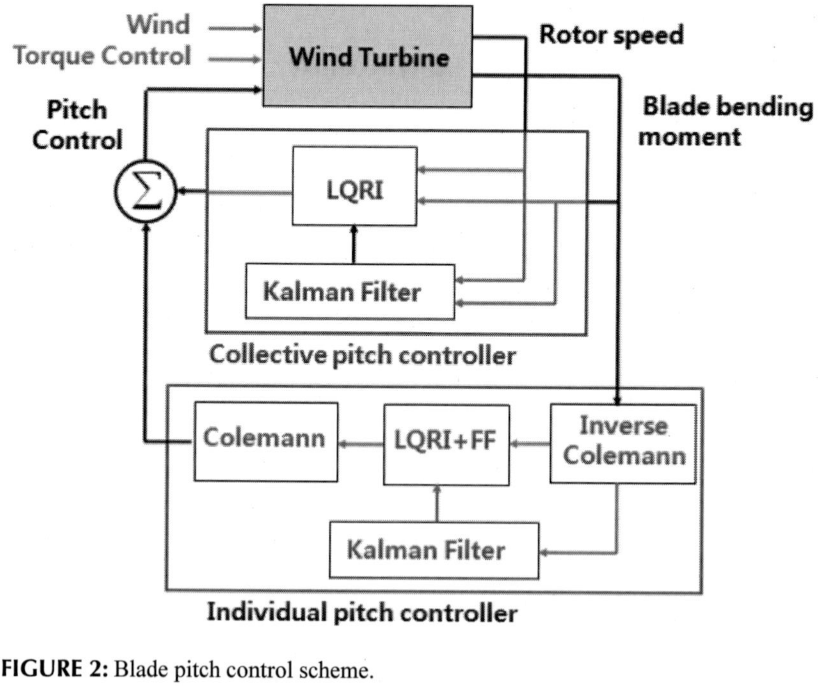

FIGURE 2: Blade pitch control scheme.

The feedback control law is calculated in a straight forward manner as follows:

$$u_{2\_fb} = K_{Xipc}\hat{x} + K_{Iipc}\int_{0}^{t} z_2 dt \quad (27)$$

where x is the state estimate from the Kalman filter. The individual pitch control commands, $\delta\beta_d^{cmd}$ and $\delta\beta_q^{cmd}$, calculated in the Coleman frame are obtained by summing the feedback control (27) and the feedforward control (24), and these control commands are transformed to the pitch command for each blade by the Coleman transform before adding it to the collective pitch command. The overall pitch control commands for each blade are given as follows:

$$\delta\beta_1^{cmd} = \delta\beta_c^{cmd} + \delta\beta_d^{cmd}\cos\Psi_1 + \delta\beta_q^{cmd}\sin\Psi_1$$

$$\delta\beta_2^{cmd} = \delta\beta_c^{cmd} + \delta\beta_d^{cmd}\cos\Psi_2 + \delta\beta_q^{cmd}\sin\Psi_2$$

$$\delta\beta_3^{cmd} = \delta\beta_c^{cmd} + \delta\beta_d^{cmd}\cos\Psi_3 + \delta\beta_q^{cmd}\sin\Psi_3 \quad (28)$$

The overall pitch control structure is shown schematically in Figure 2.

8.4 SIMULATIONS

The simplified linear model, which is used for the pitch controller design, is validated in Figures 3 and 4. In these figures, the first column shows the frequency responses of rotor speed of the high fidelity and simple turbine models to the three Coleman-transformed pitch angles and wind speeds. The second and the third columns are the frequency responses for the d- and q-axis blade moments, respectively. The frequency response plots of the high fidelity and simple turbine models show that the simple linear wind turbine model is an appropriate choice for the pitch controller design.

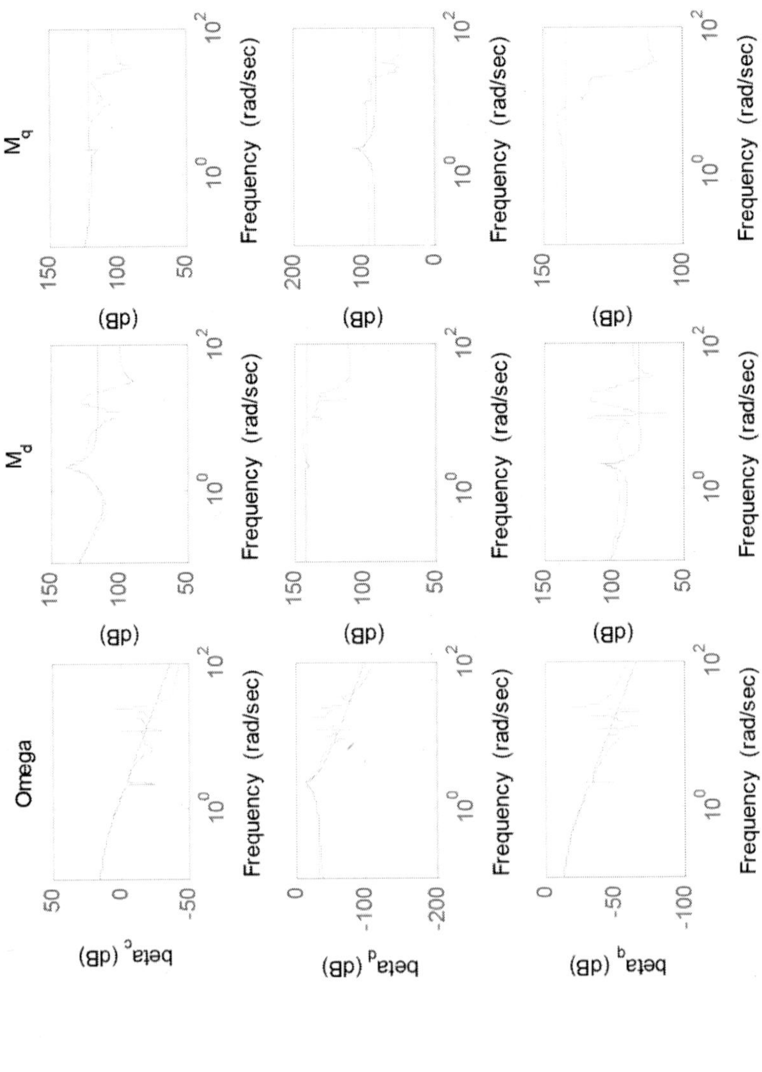

FIGURE 3: Frequency response from Coleman-transformed pitch angles to rotor speed, d- and q-axis blade moments, both for the high fidelity (red) and the simple models (blue).

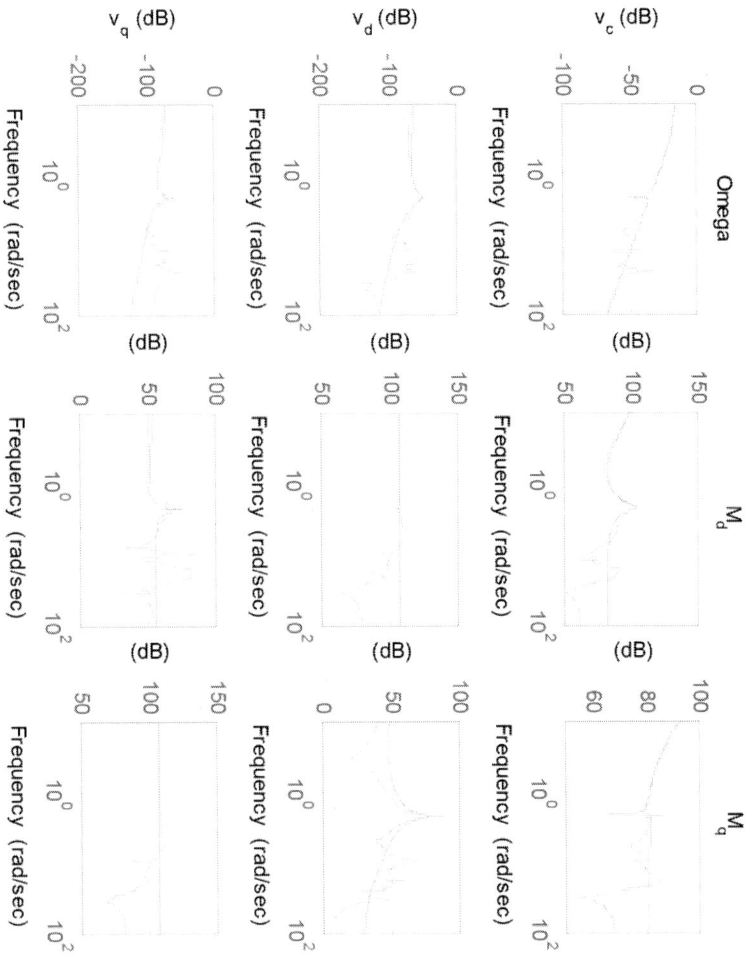

FIGURE 4: Frequency response from Coleman-transformed wind speeds to rotor speed, d- and q-axis blade moments, both for the high fidelity (red) and the simple models (blue).

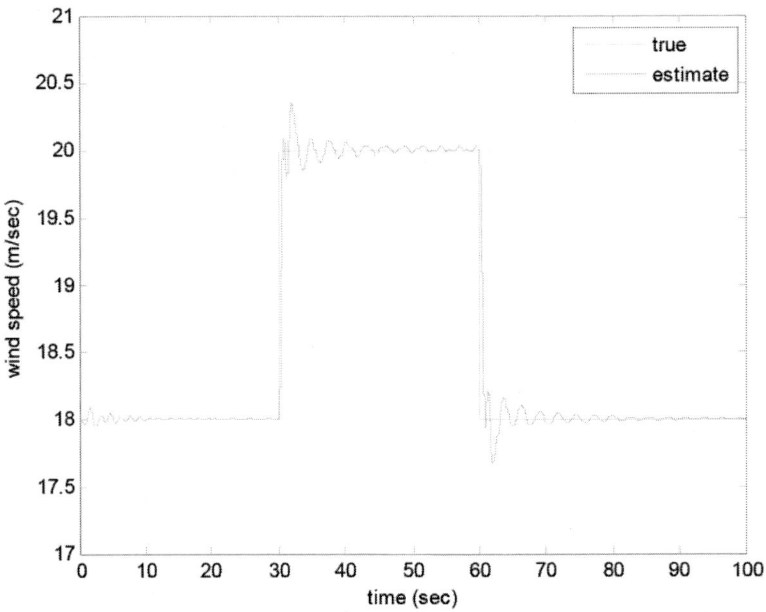

FIGURE 5: Wind speed profile.

Computer simulations are performed to evaluate the performance of the proposed collective and individual pitch controllers. The high fidelity wind turbine model described in Section 2 is used for simulations, and the drive-train damper is designed and implemented beforehand.

Two wind conditions are used in simulations. First, the steady wind with positive stepwise change shown in Figure 5 is considered and a wind shear is superimposed on the wind field. In Figure 5, the estimate of wind speed is also plotted. Although the wind speed profile in Figure 5 is unrealistic, it offers very clear view of the wind turbine dynamic behavior.

The trade-off between rotor speed regulation and blade load reduction is made and the results are shown in Figures 6–9. This trade-off is possible because the rotor speed regulation and blade load reduction are explicitly considered in the cost function. These figures also show the performance of individual pitch control compared to that of collective pitch control alone. From Figures 6 and 7, it can be seen that good regulation perfor-

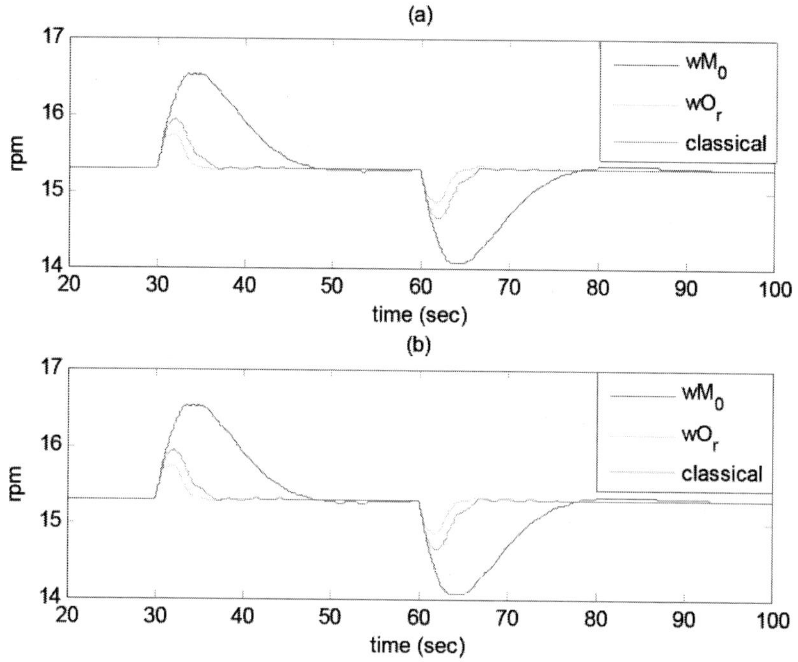

FIGURE 6: Responses of rotor speed (more weighting on blade moment(blue), more weighting on rotor speed(red), PI-based control(black)): (a) without IPC; (b) with IPC.

mance of rotor speed leads to significant overshoot in the blade loads. In other words, the rotor speed is well regulated and quickly compensated for the influences of wind speed changes, but it produces a large overshoot of collective blade bending moments when putting more weightings on the rotor speed regulation, however, the collective blade bending moments responds moderately at the cost of large overshoot and slow response of rotor speed when putting more weightings on the blade load reduction. For comparison purpose, the rotor speed and collective bending moment responses of the conventional PI-based collective pitch control are also plotted in Figures 6 and 7. Although conventional collective pitch control regulates rotor speed well, it produces a large overshoot of collective blade bending moments. Figures 6 and 7 also show that the individual pitch control does not significantly affect the rotor speed and bending moment responses, which explains the decoupling between the collective and individual pitch controls.

Figure 8 shows the responses of the blade bending moments. The individual pitch controllers achieve a significant reduction of blade bending moment oscillations compared to the collective pitch control.

Figure 9 shows the associated blade pitch control commands for the collective and individual pitch controllers, and that the load reduction is a consequence of increased pitch activity that constantly varies around the collective pitch angle to control the periodic blade bending moments.

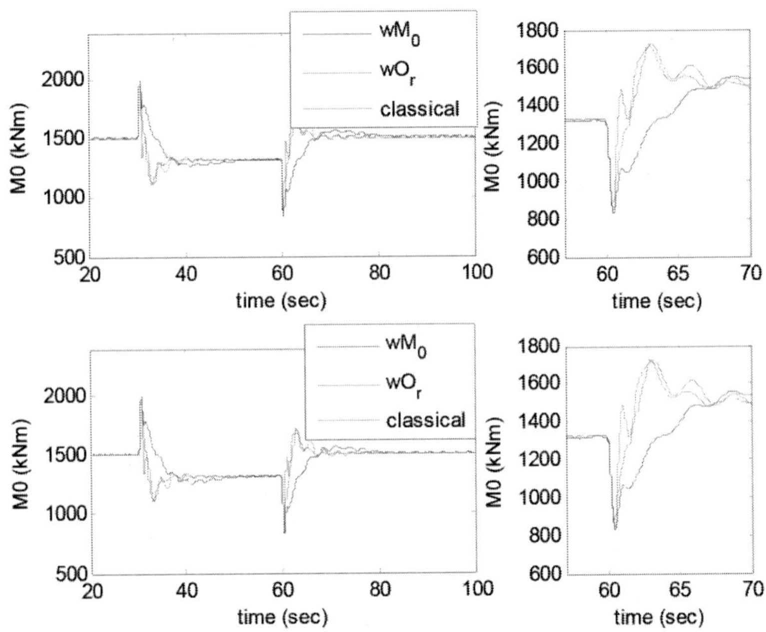

FIGURE 7: Responses of collective blade bending moments: (a) without IPC; (b) with IPC.

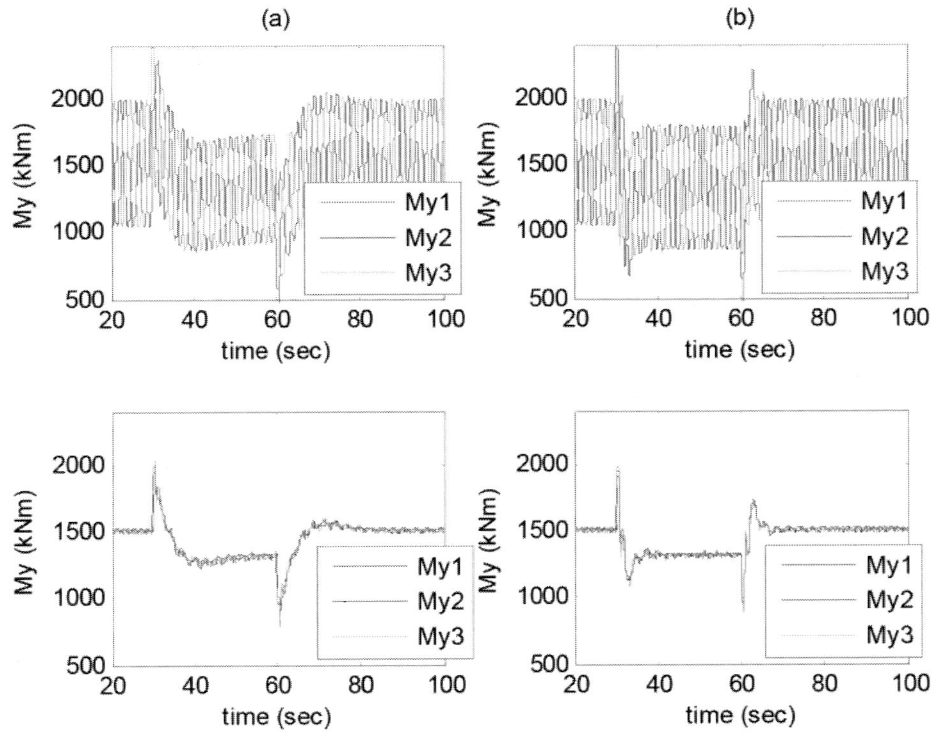

FIGURE 8: Responses of blade bending moments (without IPC (top) and with IPC (bottom)): (a) more weighting on blade moment; (b) more weighting on rotor speed.

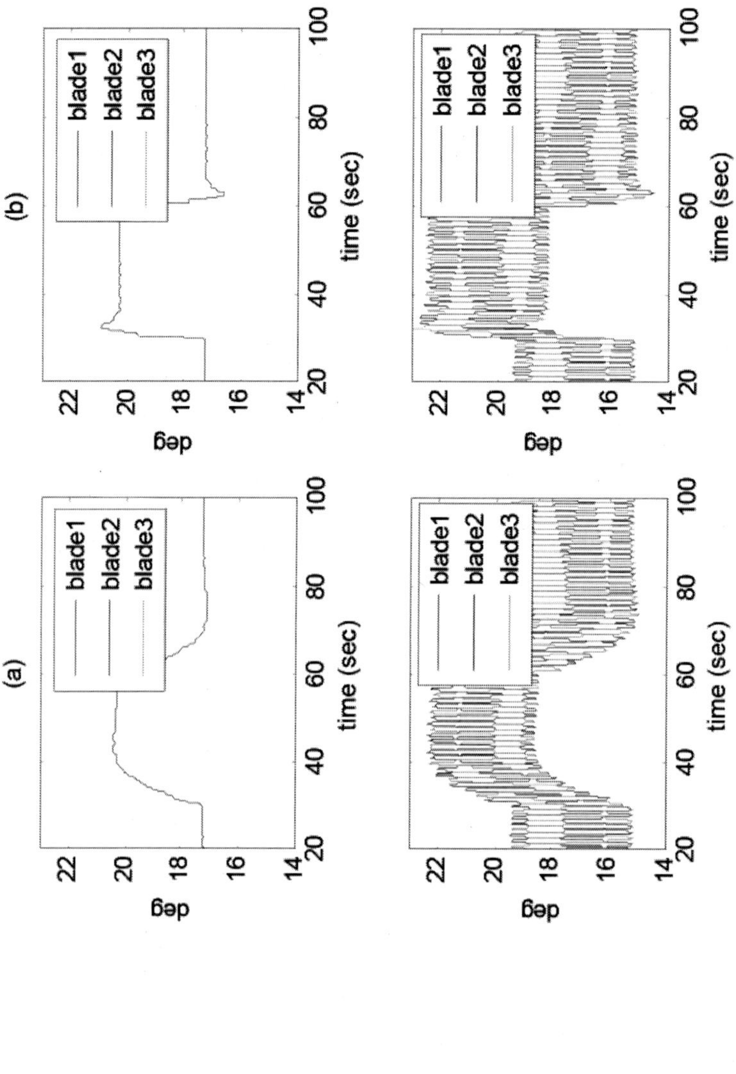

FIGURE 9: Responses of pitch commands (without IPC (top) and with IPC (bottom)): (a) more weighting on blade moment; (b) more weighting on rotor speed.

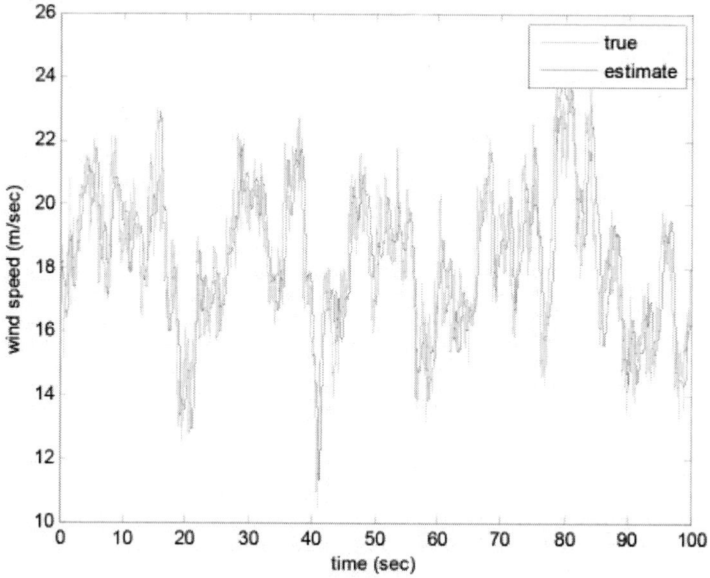

FIGURE 10: Turbulent wind speed profile.

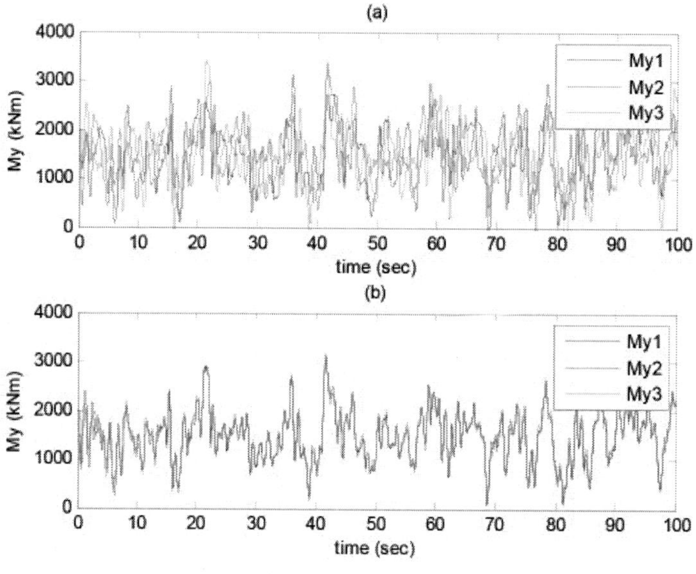

FIGURE 11: Responses of blade bending moments: (a) without IPC; (b) with IPC.

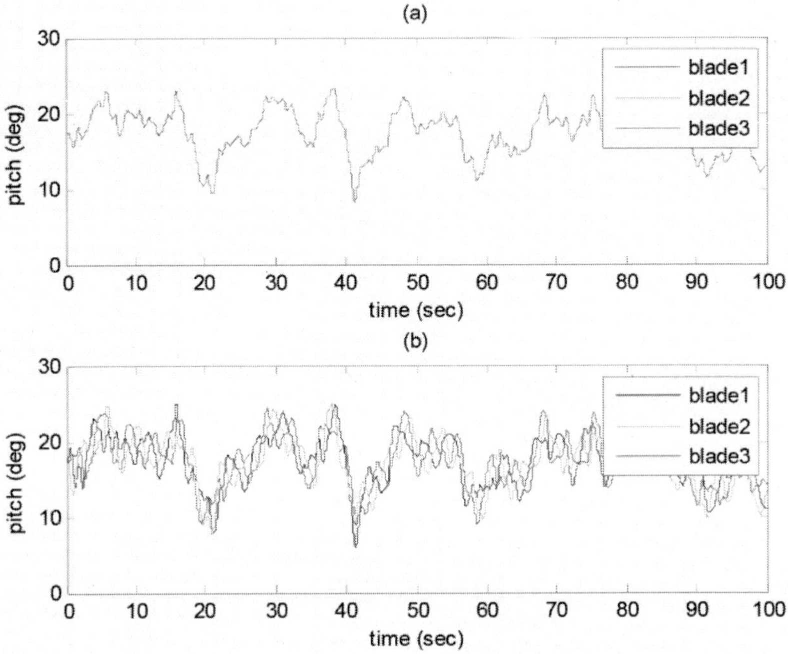

FIGURE 12: Responses of pitch commands: (a) without IPC; (b) with IPC.

A more realistic turbulent wind (TI = 18%) condition shown in Figure 10 is used for the second simulation runs with the same controllers, and the simulation results are shown in Figures 11–13, where the responses of the blade bending moments, the pitch commands, and the rotor speed are shown. Transforming the blade bending moments to the collective, and d-(tilt) and q-axis (yaw) moments in the Coleman frame, the effect of the individual controller becomes very apparent as shown in Figure 14. For comparison purpose, the rotor speed and collective bending moment responses of the conventional collective pitch control are also plotted in Figures 13 and 14. Slightly larger fluctuations than those of the proposed collective pitch control are observed.

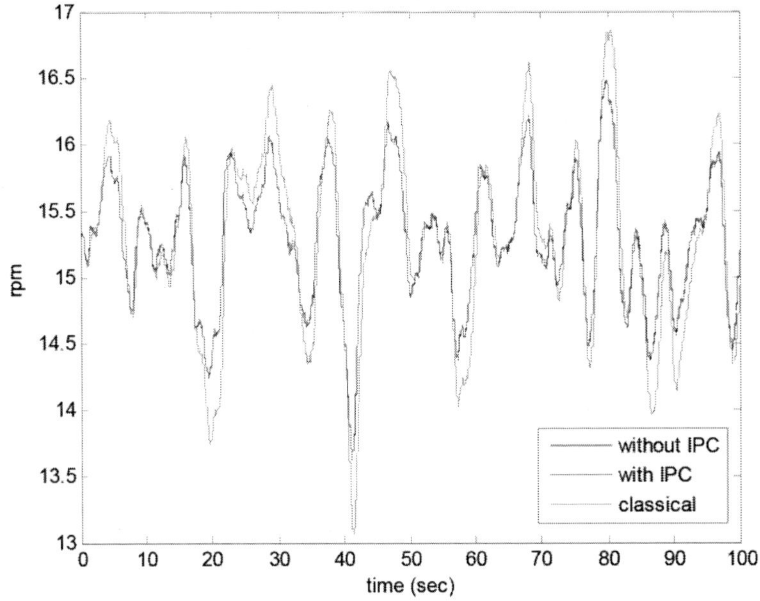

FIGURE 13: Responses of rotor speed.

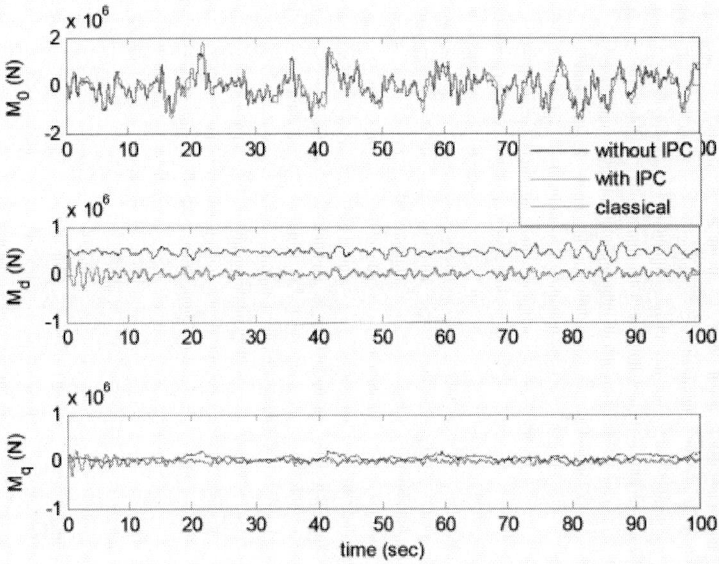

FIGURE 14: Responses of collective moment (top), tilt moment (middle) and yaw moment (bottom).

Considering all simulation cases, it can be seen that very good rotor speed regulation performance can be achieved, together with a significant reduction of blade bending moments by the proposed collective and individual pitch controllers.

8.5 CONCLUSIONS

In this paper, we presented separate sets of collective and individual pitch control algorithms for rotor speed regulation and blade load reduction for a wind turbine. The simple linear time-varying model was first derived by linearization, which is suitable for blade pitch controller design, but yet sufficiently describes the dynamics of wind turbine, and then converted into two time-invariant models by the Coleman transform for the collective and individual pitch controller designs.

With both the linear time-invariant models, the collective and individual pitch control algorithms were developed separately based on the LQRI and the state estimation of Kalman filter. Our algorithms take advantages of both central pitch control and the separate sets of collective and individual pitch control systems such that time domain performance criteria as rotor speed regulation and minimal bending moments can be directly included in the design and at the same time, both pitch control algorithms can be designed separately.

The states of both systems were estimated in the Coleman frame using Kalman filters, and these were used in the LQRI control. The collective pitch controller can control rotor speed and collective blade bending moments together to improve the trade-off between rotor speed regulation and load reduction, and the individual pitch controller can reduce the fluctuating loads on the blades. The collective pitch controller is a main controller, while the individual pitch control can be added to the collective pitch controller as an on-off mechanism.

Computer simulations were performed with a high fidelity model containing several degrees of freedom and steady and turbulent wind conditions. Simulation results showed that the proposed collective and individual pitch controllers achieved very good rotor speed regulation and significant reduction of blade bending moments.

REFERENCES

1. Laks, J.H.; Pao, L.Y.; Wright, A.D. Control of Wind Turbines: Past, Present, and Future. In Proceedings of the American Control Conference, St. Louis, MO, USA, 10–12 June 2009; pp. 2096–2103.
2. Stol, K.A.; Zhao, W.; Wright, A.D. Individual blade pitch control for the controls advanced research turbine (cart). J. Sol. Energy Eng. 2006, 128, 498–505.
3. Selvam, K.; Kanev, S.; van Wingerden, J.W.; van Engelen, T.; Vergaegen, M. Feedback-feedforward individual pitch control for wind turbine load reduction. Int. J. Robust Nonlinear Control 2008, 130, 72–91.
4. Thomsen, S.C.; Niemann, H.; Poulsen, N.K. Individual Pitch Control of Wind Turbines Using Local Inflow Measurements. In Proceedings of the 17th World Congress on the International Federation of Automatic Control, Seoul, Korea, 6–11 July 2008; pp. 5587–5592.
5. Munteanu, I.; Cutululisand, N.A.; Bratcu, A.I.; Ceanga, E. Optimization of variable speed wind power systems based on a LQG approach. Control Eng. Pract. 2005, 13, 903–912.
6. Lescher, F.; Camblong, H.; Briand, R.; Curea, O. Alleviation of Wind Turbines Loads with a LQG Controller Associated to Intelligent Micro Sensors. In Proceedings of the IEEE International Conference on Industrial Technology (ICIT 2006), Mumbai, India, 15–17 December 2006; pp. 654–659.
7. Nourdine, S.; Camblong, H.; Vechiu, I.; Tapia, G. Comparison of Wind Turbine LQG Controllers Designed to Alleviate Fatigue Loads. In Proceedings of the 8th IEEE International Conference on Control and Automation, Xiamen, China, 9–11 June 2010; pp. 1502–1507.
8. Selvam, K. Individual Pitch Control for Large Scale Wind Turbines; ECN-E-07-053; Energy Research Center of the Nertherlands: North Holland, The Nertherlands, 2007.
9. Petrovic, V.; Jelavic, M.; Peric, N. Identification of Wind Turbine Model for Individual Pitch Controller Design. In Proceedings of the 43rd International Universities Power Engineering Conference (UPEC 2008), Padova, Italy, 1–4 September 2008.
10. Jelavic, M.; Petrovic, V.; Peric, N. Estimation based individual pitch control of wind turbine. Automatika 2010, 51, 181–192.
11. Wilson, D.G.; Berg, D.E.; Resor, B.R.; Barone, M.F.; Berg, J.C. Combined Individual Pitch Control and Active Aerodynamic Load Controller Investigation for the 5 MW Up Wind Turbine. In Proceedings of the AWEA WINDPOWER 2009 Conference & Exhibition, Chicago, IL, USA, 4–7 May 2009.
12. Leithead, W.E.; Connor, B. Control of variable speed wind turbines: Design task. Int. J. Control 2000, 13, 1189–1212.
13. Balas, M.J.; Wright, A.; Hand, M.M.; Stol, K. Dynamics and Control of Horizontal Axis Wind Turbines. In Proceedings of the American Control Conference, Denver, CO, USA, 4–6 June 2003.
14. Wright, A.D. Modern Control Design for Flexible Wind Turbines; Technical Report NREL/TP-500-35816; National Renewable Energy Laboratory: Golden, CO, USA, 2004.

15. Ma, H.; Tang, G.; Zhao, Y. Feedforward and feedback optimal control for offshore structures subjected to irregular wave forces. Ocean Eng. 2006, 33, 1105–1117.
16. Bottasso, C.L.; Croce, A.; Savini, B. Performance comparison of control schemes for variable-speed wind turbines. J. Phys. Conf. Ser. 2007, 75, doi:10.1088/1742-6596/75/1/012079.
17. Wright, A.D.; Fingersh, L.J. Advanced Control Design for Wind Turbines; Technical Report NREL/TP-500-42437; National Renewable Energy Laboratory: Golden, CO, USA, 2008.
18. Van Engelen, T. Design Model and Load Reduction Assessment for Multi-rotational Mode Individual Pitch Control (Higher Harmonics Control); ECN-RX-06-068; Energy Research Centre of the Netherlands: North Holland, The Nertherlands, 2006.
19. Mateljak, P.; Petrovic, V.; Baotic, M. Dual Kalman Estimation of Wind Turbine States and Parameters. In Proceedings of the International Conference on Process Control, Tatranská Lomnica, Slovakia, 14–17 June 2011; pp. 85–91.
20. Bossanyi, E.A.; Quarton, D.C. GH Bladed—Theory Manual; Garrad Hassan & Partners Ltd.: Bristol, UK, 2008.
21. Lloyd, G. Rules and Guidelines IV: Industrial Services, Part I—Guideline for the Certification of Wind Turbines, 5th ed.; Germanischer Lloyd Windenergie: Hamburg, Germany, 2003.
22. Bir, G. Multiblade Coordinate Transformation and Its Application to Wind Turbine Analysis. In Proceedings of the 47th The American Institute of Aeronautics and Astronautics/Aerospace Sciences Meeting (AIAA/ASME), Orlando, FL, USA, 5–10 January 2009.

CHAPTER 9

POWER CONTROL DESIGN FOR VARIABLE-SPEEDWIND TURBINES

YOLANDA VIDAL, LEONARDO ACHO, NINGSU LUO, MAURICIO ZAPATEIRO, AND FRANCESC POZO

9.1 INTRODUCTION

Motivated by the high dependence that the global economy has on fossil fuels and environmental concerns, focus on alternative methods of electricity generation is increasing. In this trend towards the diversification of the energy market, wind power is the fastest growing sustainable energy resource [1].

Wind turbines with rudimentary control systems that aim to minimize cost and maintenance of the installation have predominated for a long time [1]. More recently, the increasing size of the turbines and the greater penetration of wind energy into the utility networks of leading countries have encouraged the use of electronic converters and mechanical actuators. These active devices incorporate extra degrees of freedom into the design, allowing for active control of the captured power. Static converters, used as an interface to the electric grid, enable variable-speed operation, at least up to rated speed. Due to external perturbations, such as random wind fluctuations, wind shear and tower shadows, variable speed control seems to be a good option for optimizing the operation of wind turbines [2]. Wind energy conversion systems are challenging from the control system viewpoint. Wind turbines inherently exhibit nonlinear dynamics and are exposed to large cyclic disturbances that may excite the poorly damped vibration modes of the drive-train and tower, see [1,3]. Additionally, it is difficult to obtain mathematical models that accurately describe the dynamic behavior of wind turbines because of the particular operating conditions. Moreover, this task is even more involved due to the current tendency towards larger and more flexible wind turbines. The lack of accurate models must be countered by robust control strategies capable of securing stability and certain performance features despite model uncertainties. The control problems are even more challenging when turbines are able to operate at variable speeds and pitch, see [4–6]. The best use of this type of turbine can only be achieved with several controllers, see [7,8].

A new control strategy for variable-speed, variable-pitch horizontal-axis wind turbines (HAWTs) is proposed in this paper. This control is obtained with a nonlinear dynamic chattering torque control strategy and a proportional integral (PI) control strategy for the blade pitch angle. This new control structure allows for a rapid transition of the wind turbine generated power between different desired values. This implies that it is possible to increase or decrease the WT power production with consideration of the power consumption on the network. This electrical power tracking is ensured with high-performance behaviors for all other state variables: including turbine and generator rotational speeds; and smooth and adequate evolution of the control variables.

This paper is organized as follows. In Section 2, the wind turbine modeling is presented. Section 3 briefly describes the National Renewable Energy Laboratory (NREL) wind turbine simulator FAST code [9]. The pitch and torque controllers are then presented in Section 4. Finally, in Section 5, the proposed controllers are validated with the FAST aeroelastic wind turbine simulator and their performance is compared to the controllers proposed in [10,11] to highlight the improvements of the provided method.

9.2 SYSTEM MODELING

The wind turbine consists of a rotor assembly, gear-box, and generator. The wind turbine rotor extracts the energy from the wind and converts it into mechanical power. A simplified model of the rotor was employed in [12–14]. This model assumes an algebraic relation between the wind speed and the extracted mechanical power, described with the following equation

$$P_m(u) = \frac{1}{2} C_p(\lambda, \beta) \rho \pi R^2 u^3$$

where ρ is the air density, R is the radius of the rotor, u is the wind speed, C_p is the power coefficient of the wind turbine, β is the pitch angle, and λ is the tip-speed ratio given by

$$\lambda = \frac{R\omega_r}{u}$$

where ω_r is the rotor speed. Thus, changes in the wind speed or rotor speed produce changes in the tip-speed ratio, leading to power coefficient variation; thus, the generated power is affected. The aerodynamic torque coefficient is related to the power coefficient as follows,

$$P_m = \omega_r T_a$$

the aerodynamic torque expression is described as

$$T_a = \frac{1}{2} C_q(\lambda, \beta) \rho \pi R^3 u^2$$

where

$$C_q(\lambda, \beta) = \frac{C_p(\lambda, \beta)}{\lambda}$$

For a perfectly rigid low-speed shaft, a single-mass model for a wind turbine can be considered [10,15–17],

$$J_{t\dot{\omega}r} = T_a - K_{t\omega r} - T_g$$

where J_t is the turbine total inertia (kg m^2), K_t is the turbine total external damping (Nm rad^{-1} s), T_a is the aerodynamic torque (Nm), and T_g is the generator torque (Nm). The scheme of the one-mass model is provided in Figure 1.

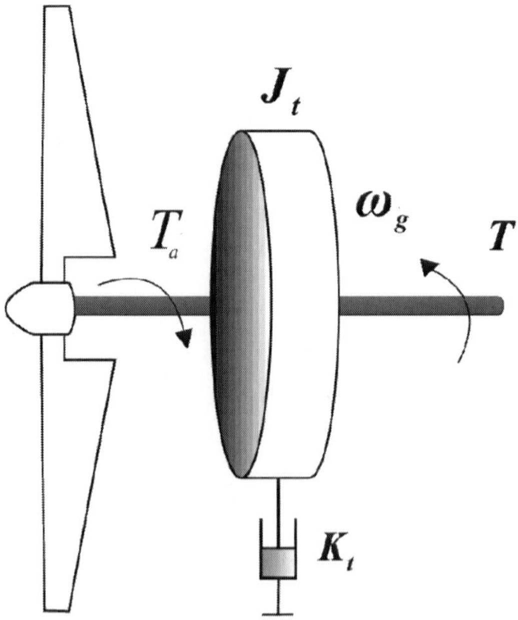

FIGURE 1: One-mass model of a wind turbine.

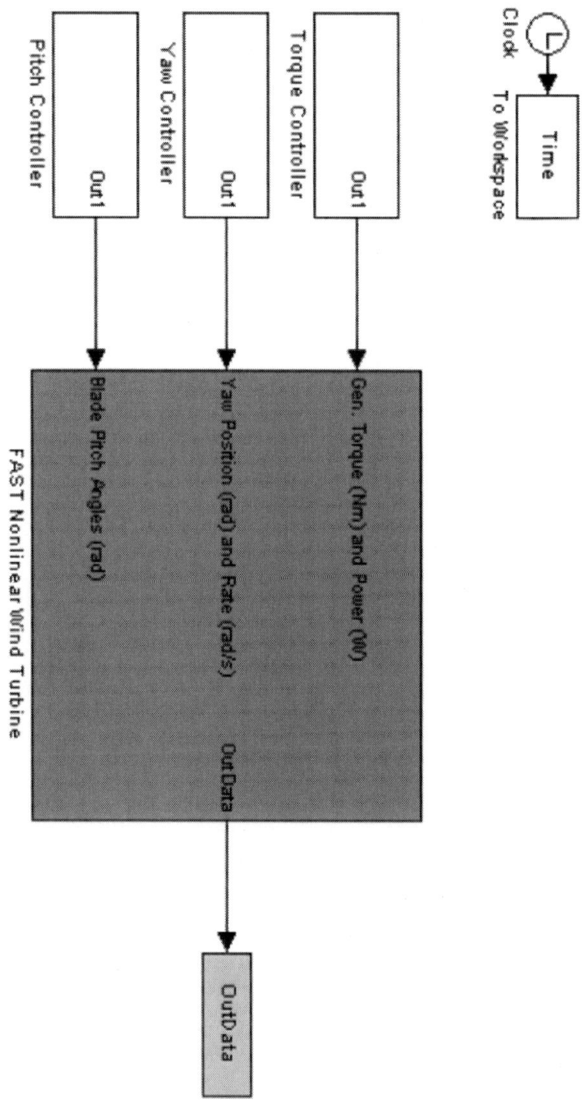

FIGURE 2: Simulink open-loop model.

9.3 BRIEF SIMULATOR DESCRIPTION (FAST)

The FAST code [9] is a comprehensive aeroelastic simulator capable of predicting the extreme and fatigue loads of two- and three-bladed HAWTs. This simulator was chosen for validation because, in 2005, it was evaluated by Germanischer Lloyd WindEnergie and found suitable for the calculation of onshore wind turbine loads for design and certification [18]. An interface between FAST and Simulink was also developed with MATLAB R®, enabling users to implement advanced turbine controls in Simulink R® a convenient block diagram form. The FAST subroutines are linked with a Matlab standard gateway subroutine so the FAST motion equations (in an S-function) can be incorporated in a Simulink model. This introduces tremendous flexibility for wind turbine control implementation during simulation. Generator torque, nacelle yaw, and pitch control modules can be designed in the Simulink environment and simulated while using the complete nonlinear aeroelastic wind turbine equations of motion, which are available in FAST. The wind turbine block contains the S-function block with the FAST motion equations and blocks that integrate the degree-of-freedom accelerations to obtain velocities and displacements. Thus, the equations of motion are formulated in the FAST S-function and solved using one of the Simulink solvers.

9.4 CONTROL STRATEGY

The developed MATLAB R® interface between FAST and Simulink has allowed us to implement the proposed torque and pitch controls in Simulink R® convenient block diagram form. The open loop FAST simulink model is provided in Figure 2. The next sections present the proposed nonlinear dynamic torque and linear pitch controller designs.

9.4.1 TORQUE CONTROLLER

The electrical power-tracking error is defined as

$$e = P_e - P_{\text{ref}} \tag{1}$$

where P_e is the electrical power and P_{ref} is the reference power. We impose a first-order dynamic to this error,

$$\dot{e} = -ae - K_\alpha \mathrm{sgn}(e) \;\; a, K_\alpha > 0 \tag{2}$$

and consider that the electrical power is described as [10,15,17,19]

$$P_e = T_e \omega_g \tag{3}$$

where τ_c is the torque control and ω_g is the generator speed. By substitution of Equations (1) and (3) into (2), and assuming that P_{ref} is a constant function, we obtain

$$\dot{\tau}_c \omega_g + \tau_c \dot{\omega}_g = -a(\tau_c \omega_g - P_{\mathrm{ref}}) - K_\alpha \mathrm{sgn}(P_e - P_{\mathrm{ref}})$$

which, can also be written as

$$\dot{\tau}_c = -\frac{1}{\omega_g}\left[\tau_c(a\omega_g + \dot{\omega}_g) - aP_{\mathrm{ref}} + K_\alpha \mathrm{sgn}(P_e - P_{\mathrm{ref}})\right] \tag{4}$$

Theorem 4.1

The proposed controller 4 ensures finite time stability [20]. Moreover, the settling time can be chosen by properly defining the values of the parameters a and K.

Proof

We now present the Lyapunov function

$$V = \frac{1}{2}e^2 \tag{5}$$

Then, based on Equation (2), the time derivative along the trajectory of the system yields

$$\dot{V} = e\dot{e} = e(-ae - K_\alpha \text{sgn}(e)) = -ae^2 - K_\alpha |e| < 0 \tag{6}$$

Thus, V is globally positive definite and radially unbounded, while the time derivative of the Lyapunov-candidate-function is globally negative definite; so the equilibrium is proven to be globally asymptotically stable. Moreover, finite time stability can be proven. Equation (6) can be written as

$$\dot{V} \leq -K_\alpha |e| = -K_\alpha \sqrt{2}\sqrt{V}$$

Thus, $\dot{V} + K_\alpha \sqrt{2}\sqrt{V}$ is negative semidefinite and Theorem 1 in [20] can be applied to conclude that the origin is a finite time stable equilibrium. Furthermore, from [20], the settling time function t_s is described as

$$t_s \leq \frac{1}{K_\alpha \sqrt{2}} (V)^{1/2}$$

and using Equation (5) leads to

$$t_s \leq \frac{e}{K_\alpha} \tag{7}$$

For $K_\alpha = 0$, an exponentially (but not finite time) stable controller is obtained

$$\dot{e} = -ae \tag{8}$$

Next, we compute an approximate settling time (for practical purposes) for the exponentially stable controller to choose a settling time that is much smaller for the finite time stable approach. For this purpose, we compare the exponentially stable error dynamic, Equation (8), with the simplest resistor-capacitor (RC) circuit. This circuit is composed of one resistor, R, and one capacitor, C, in series. When a circuit only consists of a charged capacitor and a resistor, the capacitor will discharge its stored energy through the resistor. The voltage, v, across the capacitor, which is time dependent, can be obtained with Kirchhoff's current law. This results in the linear differential equation described as

$$C\dot{v} + \frac{v}{R} = 0 \tag{9}$$

It is well known that the solution of this first order differential equation is an exponential decay function,

$$v(t) = v_0 e^{\frac{-t}{RC}}$$

where v_0 is the capacitor voltage at time t = 0. The time required for the voltage to decrease to v_0/e is the time constant, $\tau = RC$. The capacitor is considered to be fully discharged (0.7%) after approximately 5τ s, as described in [21].

Comparison of the RC circuit ODE, Equation (9), with the exponentially stable error dynamic, Equation (8), leads to the equality a = 1/RC, where τ = 1/a. An exponentially stable error dynamic will require 5τ to achieve (0.7% error) the desired value. Because our proposed controller is finite time stable, from Equation (7) we can choose parameter values to obtain the desired value in 0:2(5τ) s. Thus, assuming values close to t = 0, the error is bounded by $|e| < 1{:}5 \times 10^6$ (which is the rated power of the wind turbine)

$$t_s \leq \frac{1.5\times10^6}{K_\alpha} < 0.2(5\tau) = 0.2\left(5\frac{1}{\alpha}\right)$$

For a = 1, the estimated settling time is less than one second,

$$t_s \leq \frac{1.5\times10^6}{K_\alpha} < 1 \tag{10}$$

and, by rearranging terms, the value of K_α should be,

$$K_\alpha > 1.5\times10^6$$

Note that Equation (4) depends on ω_g. One way to compute this derivative is to use the one-mass model of a wind turbine that is presented in Section 2, in which all of the following WT parameters are required: turbine total inertia, turbine total external damping, aerodynamic torque, generator torque in rotor side, and gearbox ratio. Another way to compute this derivative is to use the estimator proposed in [22] (transfer function in the Laplace domain),

$$\frac{s}{0.1s + 1} \tag{11}$$

Input to Equation (11) is ω_g and the output is an estimation of $\dot{\omega}_g$. The proposed simple nonlinear torque control Equation (4) does not require information from the turbine total external damping or the turbine total inertia. This control only requires the generator speed and electrical power of the WT. Thus, our proposed controller used with Equation (11), to approximate requires few WT parameters. By contrast, most of the torque controllers in the literature [10,15–17] require many WT parameters, which restricts controller applicability when not all of the required parameters are available.

9.4.2 PITCH CONTROLLER

To assist the torque controller with regulating the wind turbine electric power output, while avoiding significant loads and maintaining the rotor speed within acceptable limits, a pitch proportional integral (PI) controller is added to the rotor speed tracking error:

$$\beta = K_p(\omega_r - \omega_n) + K_1 \int_0^t (\omega_r - \omega_n)dt, \quad K_p > 0, K_i > 0$$

where ω_r is the rotor speed and ω_n is the nominal rotor speed, at which the rated electrical power of the wind turbine is obtained. To disable the proportional term when $\omega_r < \omega_n$, the final proposed controller is described with the following expression

$$\beta = \frac{1}{2} K_p(\omega_r - \omega_n)[1 + \mathrm{sgn}(\omega_r - \omega_n)] + K_1 \int_0^t (\omega_r - \omega_n)dt, \quad K_p > 0, K_i > 0$$

9.5 SIMULATION RESULTS

Numerical validations with FAST on Matlab-Simulink were performed with the NREL WP 1.5-MW wind turbine. The wind turbine characteristics are summarized in Table 1.

TABLE 1: Wind Turbine Characteristics.

Number of blades	3
Height of tower	82:39 m
Rotor diameter	70 m
Rated power	1:5 MW
Gearbox ratio	87:965
Nominal rotor speed (ω_n)	20 rpm

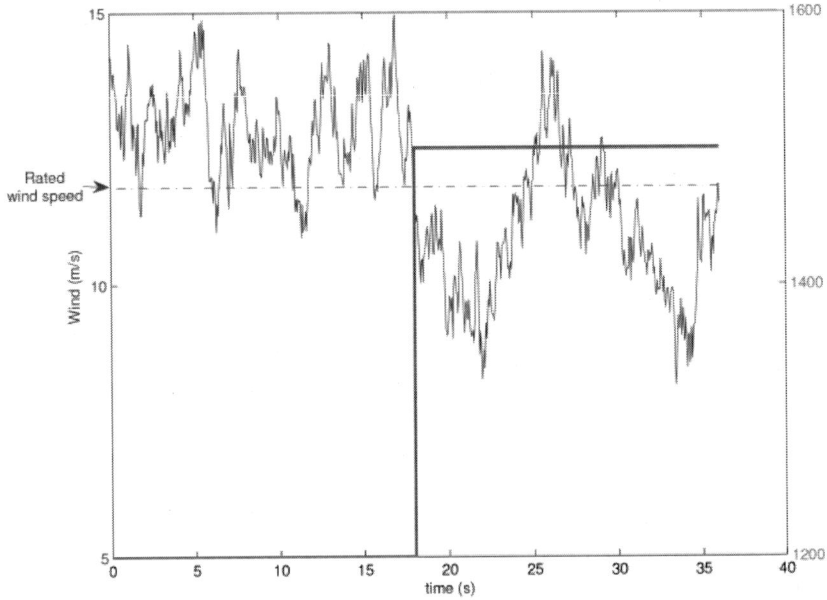

FIGURE 3: Wind speed profile with a mean of 11:8 m/s that corresponds to the rated wind speed of the WT (left y-axes). Reference power (right y-axes).

The wind inflow for the simulations is shown in Figure 3. A variable reference set point is imposed on the WT electrical power. When the wind park manager requires a given electrical power, he/she must dispatch this reference over different wind turbines and impose a variable reference for each turbine to meet a specific request for the grid. This wind inflow, for the simulated NREL WP 1.5-MW wind turbine, reaches wind speeds that are above the rated power operating conditions. From Figure 3, the rated wind speed for the wind turbine is 11:8 m/s, which coincides with the mean wind speed profile. Figure 3 also shows the reference power (right y-axes).

9.5.1 TORQUE AND PITCH CONTROL

The FAST simulator outputs with torque and pitch control are computed with a = 1, $K_p = 1$, $K_i = 1$ and two values for K_α (different settling times),

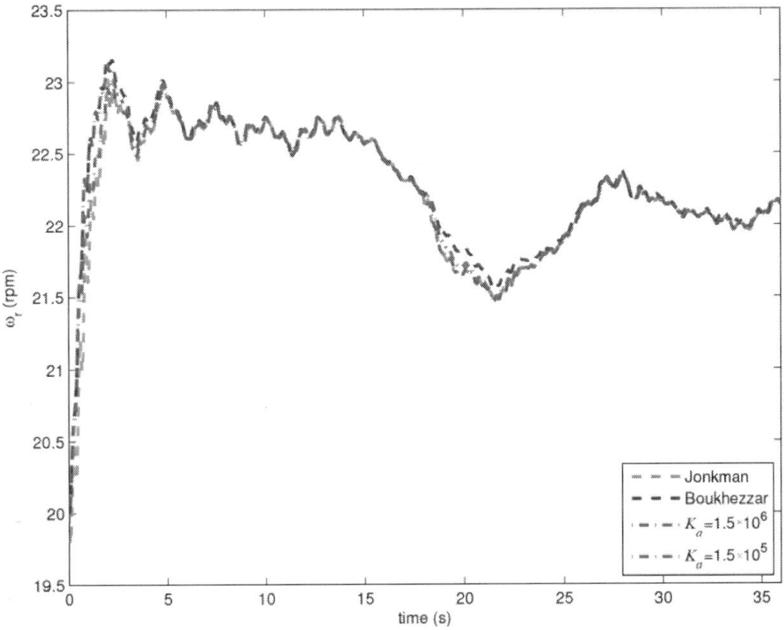

FIGURE 4: Rotor speed.

which are K = 1:5 × 10^6 and K = 1:5 × 10^5. These results are compared to those obtained with the controllers that were proposed by [10] (Bukhezzar's controller) and [11] (Jonkman's controller).

For all the tested controllers, the rotor speed, as shown in Figure 4, is near its nominal value of (20 rpm) due to the pitch control action. From Figure 5, with the Boukhezzar controller, an exponential convergence is observed and the desired value is reached in approximately 5 s when the reference electrical power is changed. By contrast, with the Jonkman controller, an almost perfect power regulation is obtained; however, this torque controller generates high loads that can exceed the design load, which will be shown later. Our proposed controller has an intermediate behavior between Jonkman's and Boukhezzar's controllers. The electrical power follows the reference, independently of the wind fluctuations, with a settling time of one second, as can be expected [see Equation (10)] when using parameter K_α = 1:5×10^6. When parameter K_α = 1:5 × 10^5 is used, similar results are obtained but the settling time is increased. Our controller allows for selection of the settling time to obtain a controller that is closer to Jonkman's or Boukhezzar's controllers. However, for any given settling time, our controller more precisely reaches the reference power compared to the Boukhezzar's controller because it has finite convergence. This trend can be seen in the magnified image of Figure 5.

Typical maximum pitch rates range from 18°/s for 600 kW research turbines to 8°/s for 5 MW turbines [23]. From Figure 6, for all the tested controllers, the blade pitch angle is always within the authorized variation domain without exceeding a variation of 10°/s.

From Figure 7, the torque action of the proposed controller is smooth and achieves reasonable values, similar to those obtained by the Jonkman and Boukhezzar controllers. The generator may not be able to supply the desired electro-mechanic torque depending on the operating conditions. To avoid this excessive overloading, the torque control should be saturated

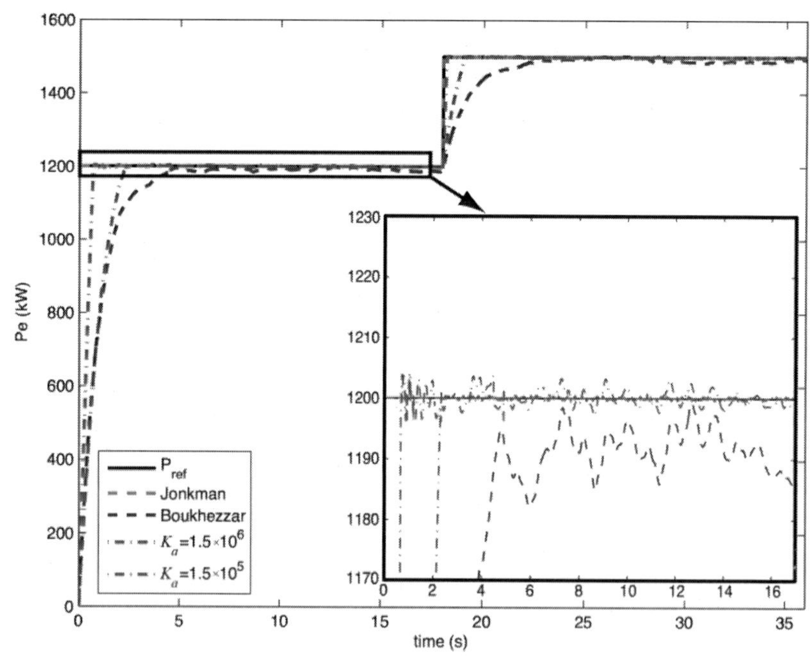

FIGURE 5: Power output.

to a maximum of 10% above the rated value, or 7:7 kN·m, see [11]. This value is represented in Figure 7; none of the tested controllers reach this extreme value.

The effect of loads on the control behavior is also important. The relevant loads to consider are the tower bottom side-to-side moment (shown in Figure 8), the drive shaft torsion (shown in Figure 9), the tower top/yaw bearing roll moment (shown in Figure 10), and the tower top/yaw bearing side-to-side shear force (shown in Figure 11). The Jonkman controller achieves high loads that almost exceed the design load in all cases, although it achieves nearly perfect power regulation. By contrast, Boukhezzar's controller uses intermediate loads but shows a poor performance for power regulation. Finally, our controller achieves the desired compromise between loads and the ability to track changes in the desired power.

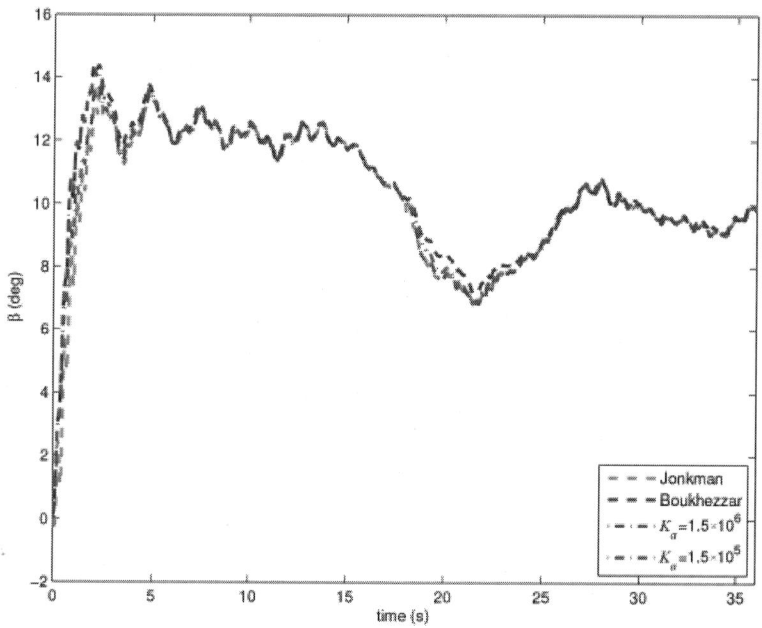

FIGURE 6: Pitch control.

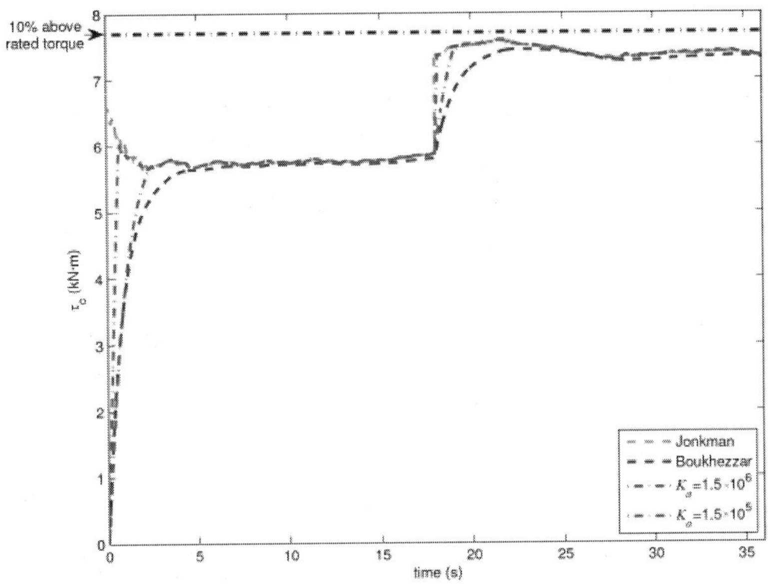

FIGURE 7: Torque control.

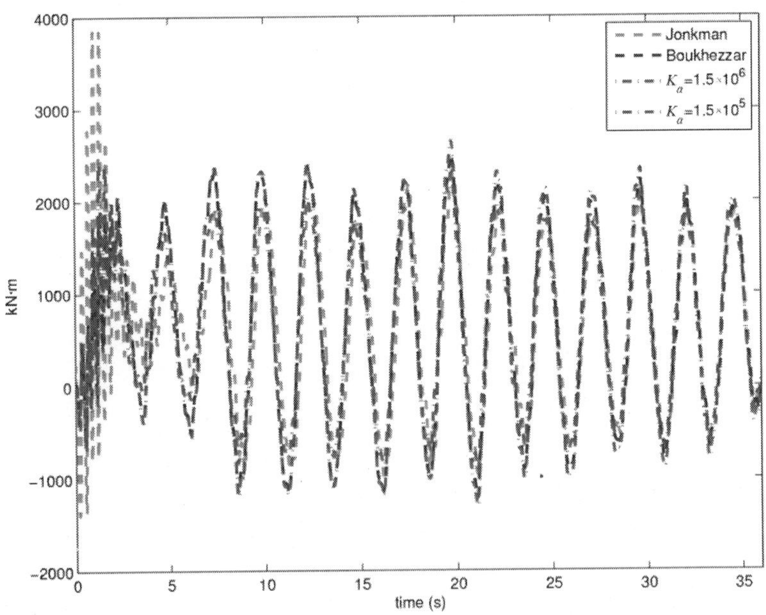

FIGURE 8: Tower bottom side-to-side moment.

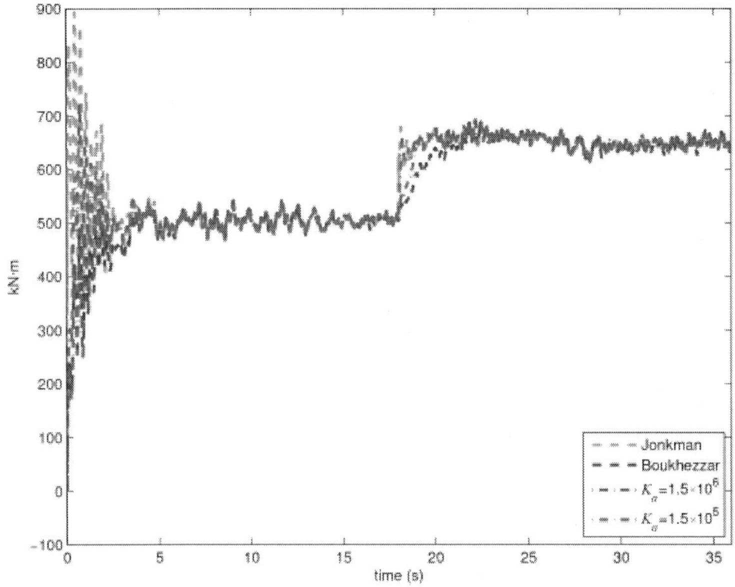

FIGURE 9: Drive shaft torsion.

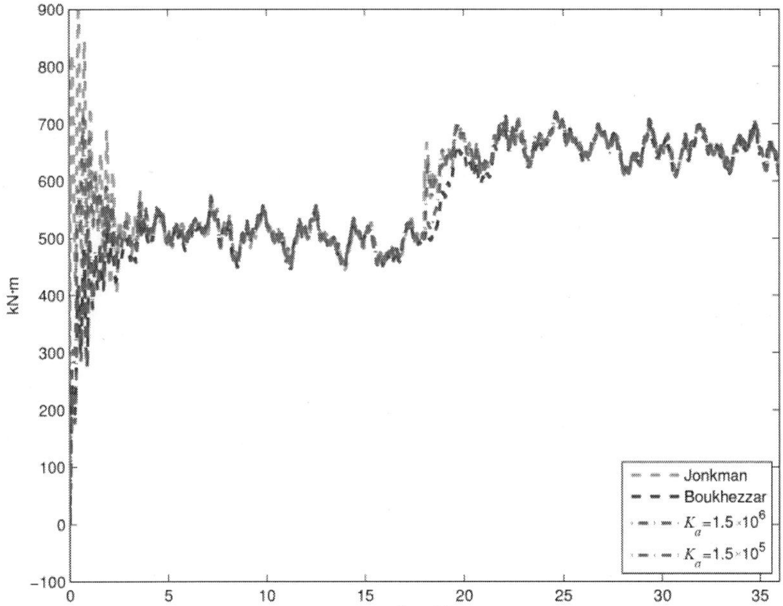

FIGURE 10: Tower top/yaw bearing roll moment.

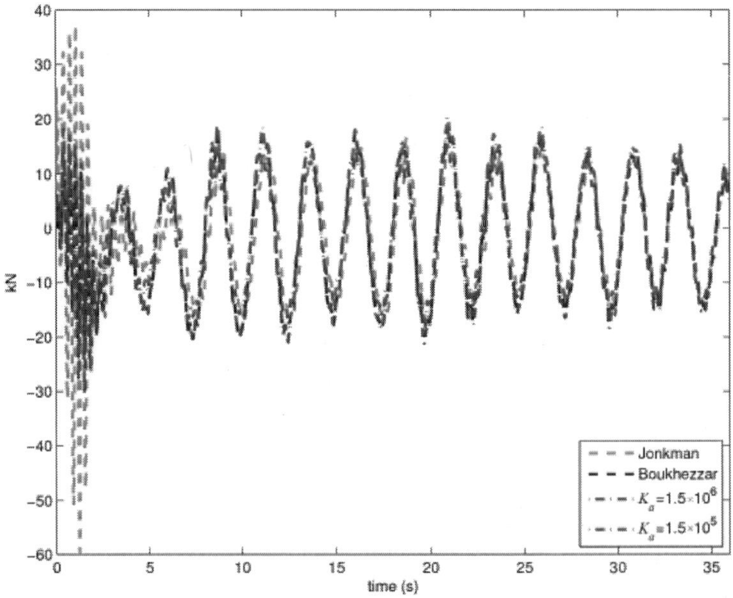

FIGURE 11: Tower top/yaw bearing side-to-side shear force.

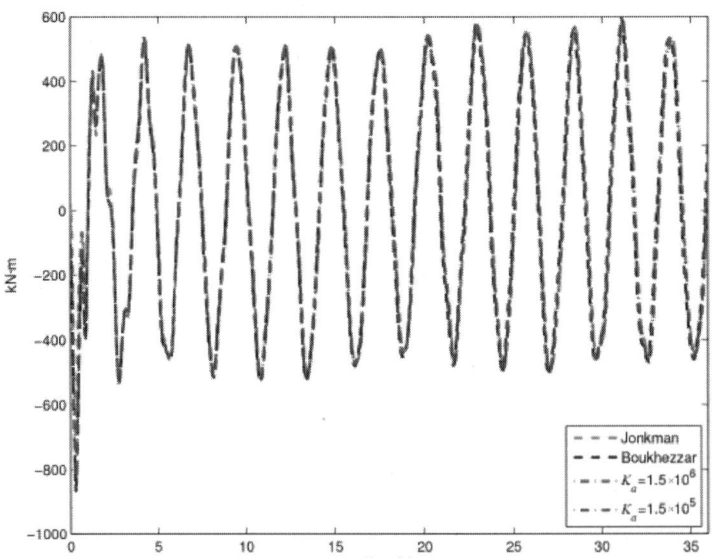

FIGURE 12: Blade edge-wise bending moment.

The blade edge-wise bending moment shown in Figure 12 is another relevant load, that, in this case, achieves similar results for all the tested controllers.

Finally the MatLab-based postprocessor MCrunch [24] for wind turbine data analysis has been used to perform a fatigue analysis. Table 2 shows the damage equivalent loads and Figure 13 shows the cumulative rainflow cycles of relevant loads from simulations up to 600 s and the reference power changing every 18 s between the values 1200 and 1500 kW. The fatigue design SN slopes are extracted from the publication that documents the WindPACT turbines [25]. It is appreciated that the Jonkman's controller presents a marked fatigue variation for the first cumulative cycles per seconds for relevant loads as drive shaft torsion and tower top/yaw bearing roll moment. This agrees with the results observed in the previous section where this controller achieves high loads that almost exceed the design load.

TABLE 2: Table of damage-equivalent loads.

	Units	SN Slope	$K_\alpha = 1.5 \times 10^5$	$K_\alpha = 1.5 \times 10^6$	Boukhezzar	Jonkman
Tower bottom side-to-side	(kN·m)	3	1.255×10^3	1.195×10^3	1.174×10^3	1.418×10^3
Drive shaft	(kN·m)	6.5	1.386×10^2	1.450×10^2	1.295×10^2	3.080×10^2
Tower top/yaw bearing roll	(kN·m)	3	7.699×10^1	8.144×10^1	7.338×10^1	1.083×10^2
Tower top/yaw side-to-side	(kN)	3	1.555×10^1	1.501×10^1	1.473×10^1	1.443×10^1
Blade edge-wise bending	(kN·m)	8	1.237×10^3	9.599×10^2	9.562×10^2	9.595×10^2

9.5.2 TORQUE AND PITCH CONTROL WITH NOISY SIGNALS

As is typical for the utility-scale multi-megawatt wind turbines, the proposed generator torque and blade pitch controllers use the generator speed measurement as the sole feedback input. To consider signals noise (which is present in real applications), the generator speed measurement is modified

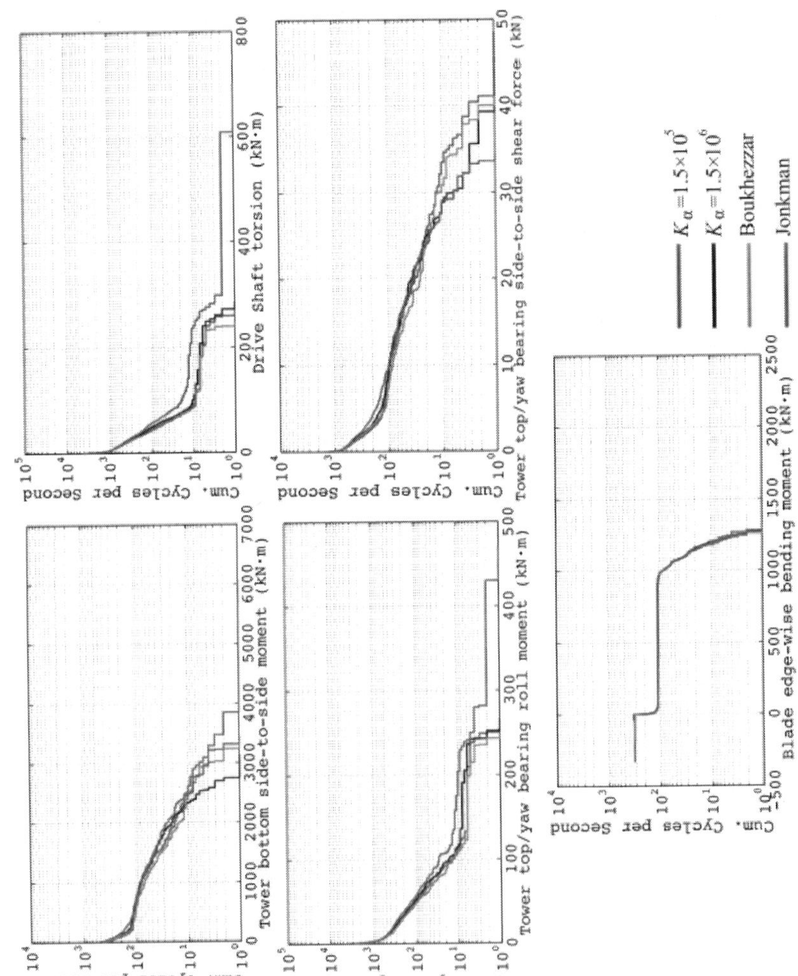

FIGURE 13: Cumulative rainflow cycles.

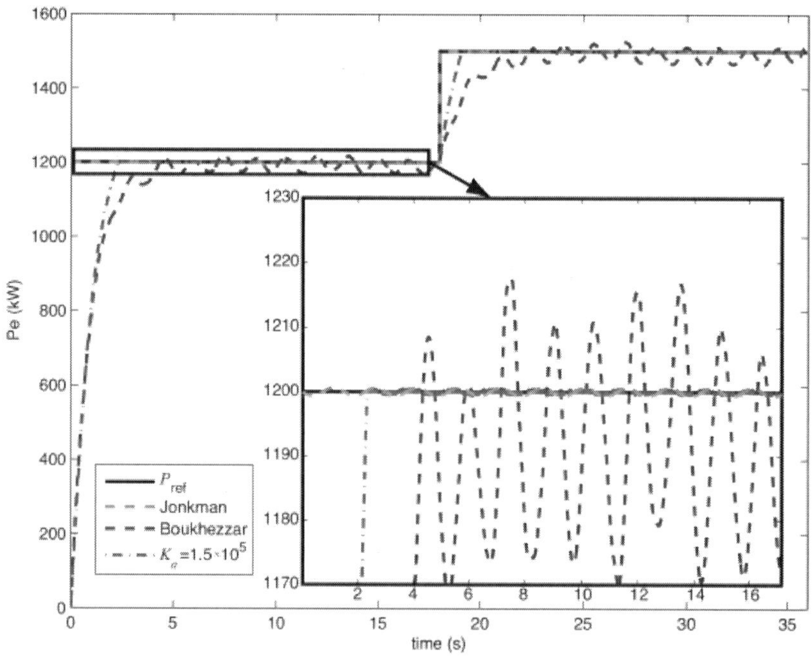

FIGURE 14: Power output with a periodic noise signal.

by adding a sine wave with an amplitude of 0:1 and a frequency of 0:^6 Hz which is proportional (two times) to the nominal rotor speed. A periodic noise signal is first tested as periodic disturbances appear in rotating mechanical systems and it is important to reject them (see [26,27]). From the magnified image in Figure 14, our proposed controller is more robust to periodic noise signals than the other tested controllers. When comparing these results with Figure 5, Boukhezzar's controller is much more affected by the noise. Jonkman's controller is an almost perfect power regulation control; however, when noisy signals are used, the results are also affected. Jonkman's controller has a low-pass filter, as described in [11], but, in this case, the noisy signal is not filtered because it has a frequency of 0:25 Hz, which is the corner frequency of the low-pass filter. A more suited filter can be used for Jonkman's controller and also certain filter types can be used with Boukhezzar's controller. However, our controller shows good performance without filters. Finally, a white noise signal is tested.

From the magnified image in Figure 15, Boukhezzar's controller is again much more affected by the noise. Our proposed controller and Jonkman's controller have a similar performance in this case.

9.6 CONCLUSIONS

A WT controller for turbulent wind conditions is presented in this paper. The proposed controller achieves strong performances in rotor speed and electrical power regulation with acceptable control activity. These results show that the proposed controller allows the WT generated power to transit between different desired set values. This achievement implies that it is possible to increase or decrease the WT power production in response to the power consumption of the network and to participate in the primary grid frequency control, which allows for a higher level of wind penetration

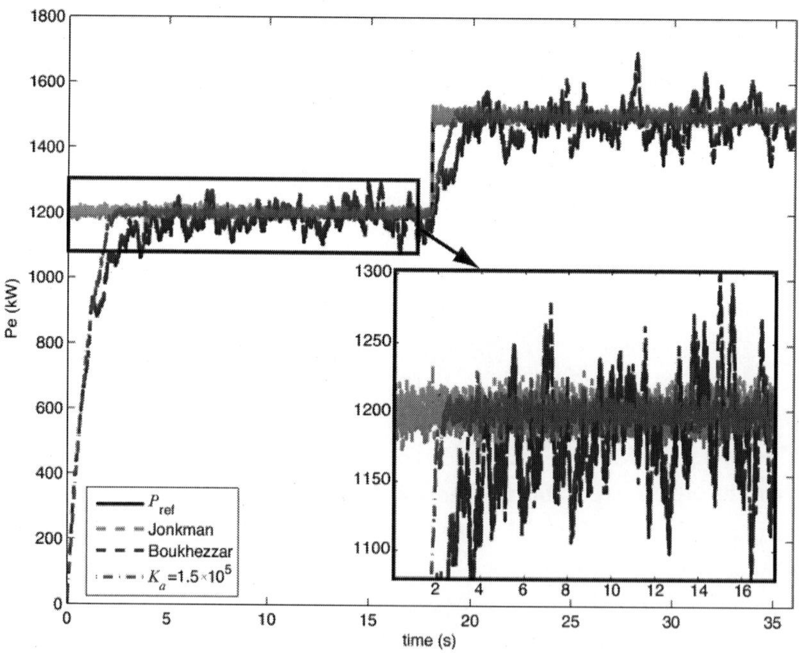

FIGURE 15: Power output with a white noise signal.

in electric networks without affecting the quality of the generated electric power. Finally, the improvements of the proposed controller versus the other tested strategies are described as follows:

- The proposed controller ensures finite time stability. Thus, the proposed controller more precisely reaches the desired power reference than exponentially stable controllers, such as [10].
- The proposed controller allows for selection of the settling time by properly defining the values of the parameters a and K_α in Equation (4). Thus, our controller can be adjusted to obtain intermediate controllers with settling times that are closer to the Jonkman or Boukhezzar controller.
- The proposed simple nonlinear torque controller does not require information regarding the turbine total external damping or the turbine total inertia; it only requires the generator speed and electrical power of the WT. Thus, the proposed controller is easily applicable to other WTs. Using a simpler model than in [10], better results can be obtained.
- The proposed controller achieves the desired compromise between loads and the ability to track changes in the desired power.
- The proposed controller is more robust to periodic noise signals and does not require filters in this case.

REFERENCES

1. Burton, T.; Sharpe, D.; Jenkins, N.; Bossanyi, E. Wind Energy Handbook; Wiley: Chichester, UK, 2001.
2. Zinger, D.; Muljadi, E. Annualized wind energy improvement using variable speeds. IEEE Trans. Ind. Appl. 1997, 33, 1444–1447.
3. Kusiak, A.; Zhang, Z. Control of wind turbine power and vibration with a data-driven approach. Renew. Energy 2012, 43, 73–82.
4. Hassan, H.M.; Eishafei, A.L.; Farag, W.A.; Saad, M.S. A robust LMI-based pitch controller for large wind turbines. Renew. Energy 2012, 44, 63–71.
5. Sandquist, F.; Moe, G.; Anaya-Lara, O. Individual pitch control of horizontal axis wind turbines. J. Offshore Mech. Arctic Eng.-Trans. ASME 2012, 134, doi:10.1115/1.4005376.
6. Joo, Y.; Back, J. Power regulation of variable speed wind turbines using pitch control based on disturbance observer. J. Electr. Eng. Technol. 2012, 7, 273–280.
7. Diaz de Corcuera, A.; Pujana-Arrese, A.; Ezquerra, J.M.; Segurola, E.; Landaluze, J. H-infinity based control for load mitigation in wind turbines. Energies 2012, 5, 938–967.
8. Soliman, M.; Malik, O.P.; Westwick, D.T. Multiple Model MIMO Predictive Control for Variable Speed Variable Pitch Wind Turbines. In Proceedings of the American Control Conference, Baltimore, MD, USA, 30 June–2 July 2010.

9. Jonkman, J. NWTC Design Codes (FAST). Available online: http://wind.nrel.gov/designcodes/ simulators/fast/ (accessed on 8 March 2012).
10. Boukhezzar, B.; Lupu, L.; Siguerdidjane, H.; Hand, M. Multivariable control strategy for variable speed, variable pitch wind turbines. Renew. Energy 2007, 32, 1273–1287.
11. Jonkman, J.M.; Butterfield, S.; Musial,W.; Scott, G. Definition of a 5-MW Reference Wind Turbine for Offshore System Development; Technical Report NREL/TP-500-38060; National Renewable Energy Laboratory: Golden, CO, USA, 2009.
12. Slootweg, J., Polinder, H.; Kling, W. Dynamic Modelling of a Wind Turbine with Doubly Fed Induction Generator. In Proceedings of the Power Engineering Society Summer Meeting, 15–19 July 2001; Volume 1, pp. 644–649.
13. Song, Y.; Dhinakaran, B.; Bao, X. Variable speed control of wind turbines using nonlinear and adaptive algorithms. J. Wind Eng. Ind. Aerodyn. 2000, 85, 293–308.
14. De Battista, H.; Puleston, P.; Mantz, R.; Christiansen, C. Sliding mode control of wind energy systems with DOIG-power efficiency and torsional dynamics optimization. IEEE Trans. Power Syst. 2000, 15, 728–734.
15. Khezami, N.; Braiek, N.B.; Guillaud, X. Wind turbine power tracking using an improved multimodel quadratic approach. Int.Soc. Autom. Trans. 2010, 49, 326–334.
16. Acho, L.; Vidal, Y.; Pozo, F. Robust variable speed control of a wind turbine. Int. J. Innov. Comput. Inf. Control 2010, 6, 1925–1933.
17. Beltran, B.; Ahmed-Ali, T.; Benbouzid, M. High-order sliding-mode control of variable-speed wind turbines. IEEE Trans. Ind. Electr. 2009, 56, 3314–3321.
18. Manjock, A. Design Codes FAST and ADAMS for Load Calculations of Onshore Wind Turbines, 2005; National Renewable Energy Laboratory (NREL): Golden, CO, USA, 2005.
19. Beltran, B.; Ahmed-Ali, T.; El Hachemi Benbouzid, M. Sliding mode power control of variable-speed wind energy conversion systems. IEEE Trans. Energy Convers. 2008, 23, 551–558.
20. Bhat, S.; Bernstein, D. Finite-Time Stability of Homogeneous Systems. In Proceedings of the American Control Conference, Albuquerque, NM, USA, 4–6 June 1997; Volume 4, pp. 2513–2514.
21. Beaty, H.W. Handbook of Electric Power Calculations, 3rd ed.; McGraw-Hill: New York, NY, USA, 2001; Volume 1.
22. Spong, M.W.; Vidyasagar, M. Robot Dynamics and Control; John Wiley and Sons: Hoboken, NJ, USA, 1989.
23. Pao, L.; Johnson, K. A Tutorial on the Dynamics and Control of Wind Turbines and Wind Farms. In Proceedings of the American Control Conference, Boulder, CO, USA, 10–12 June 2009; pp. 2076–2089.
24. Hayman, G. NWTC Design Codes (MCrunch). Available online: http://wind.nrel.gov/designcodes/postprocessors/mcrunch/ (accessed on 6 June 2012).
25. Malcolm, D.J.; Hansen, A.C. WindPACT Turbine Rotor Design Study; Technical Report NREL/SR 500-32495; National Renewable Energy Laboratory: Golden, CO, USA, 2002.
26. Brown, L.J.; Zhang, Q. Periodic disturbance cancellation with uncertain frequency. Automatica 2004, 40, 631–637.
27. Wu, B.; Bodson, M. Direct adaptive cancellation of periodic disturbances for multivariable plants. IEEE Trans. Speech Audio Process. 2003, 11, 538–548.

CHAPTER 10

H_∞ BASED CONTROL FOR LOAD MITIGATION IN WIND TURBINES

ASIER DIAZ DE CORCUERA, ARON PUJANA-ARRESE, JOSE M. EZQUERRA, EDURNE SEGUROLA, AND JOSEBA LANDALUZE

10.1 INTRODUCTION

The continuous increase of the size of wind turbines, due to the demand of higher power production installations, has led to new challenges in the design of the turbines. Moreover, new control strategies are being developed. Today's strategies trend towards being multivariable and multi-objective in order to fulfill the numerous control design specifications. To be more precise, one important specification is to mitigate loads in the turbine components to increase their life time. This can be done through the components mechanical design, the introduction of new materials or by improving the control itself. In addition to this, the behaviour of a wind turbine is non-linear, which implies that the designed control performance has to be robust.

Over the last few years, several modern control techniques used to replace the classical PI controllers (see Section 3) have been developed. These techniques are fuzzy controllers [1], adaptive control strategies [2], linear quadratic controllers [3] like the Disturbance Accommodating Control (DAC) [4] developed by NREL and tested in the CART real wind turbine [5], QFT controllers [6], Linear Parameter Varying (LPV) controllers

This chapter was originally published under the Creative Commons Attribution License. Diaz de Corcuera A, Pujana-Arrese A, Ezquerra JM, Segurola E, and Landaluze J. H_∞ Based Control for Load Mitigation in Wind Turbines. Energies ***2012**,5 (2012). doi:10.3390/en5040938.*

[7] and controllers based on the H_∞ norm reduction. H_∞ controllers have the capacity for robustness and these controllers are multivariable and multi-objective, so their applications in wind turbine control offer a lot of advantages and they achieve interesting results. One article dealing with this topic [8] shows the design of two controllers based on the H_∞ norm reduction applied to a simple and analytical model of a wind turbine. The first one reduces the loads on the tower with the tower fore-aft acceleration displacement measurement and controls the generator speed reference with a pitch collective control in the above rated zone. The second controller also reduces the loads on the blades with a cyclic pitch controller based on the H_∞ norm reduction. Control strategies using SISO and MISO state-space controllers based on the H_∞ norm are tested and compared in the CART3 experimental wind turbine [9]. In this article, torque controllers are used to damp the drive train mode and the tower side-to-side bending mode.

This article presents the design of two H_∞ MISO (Multi-Input Single-Output) controllers in the above rated zone (see Section 5). These controllers not only control the generator speed and reduce the fore-aft displacements on the tower using a collective pitch controller, but they also reduce the side-to-side displacements on the tower and the loads on the drive train if a generator torque H_∞ controller is used. Furthermore, in terms of the controller design, instead of using a simple analytical model of a wind turbine, complex linear plants extracted from GH Bladed 4.0 are used, although the design methodology could be applied by using linear models obtained from any modeling package. Regarding the H_∞ controller design, some notch filters are included in the controller dynamics by means of the correct definition of the weight functions in the augmented plant of the mixed sensitivity problem. In the design process of this control strategy based on H_∞ controllers, two software packages are used: GH Bladed 4.0 and MATLAB. GH Bladed is a software package commercialized by Garrad Hassan Company, commonly used by major wind turbine manufacturers to model and simulate wind turbines. The controller synthesis and discretization is carried out in MATLAB and, finally, simulations of the closed loop system are carried out using GH Bladed with different perturbed production winds. Results using H_∞ controllers are compared to the baseline controller results, based on classical control strategies, in order to

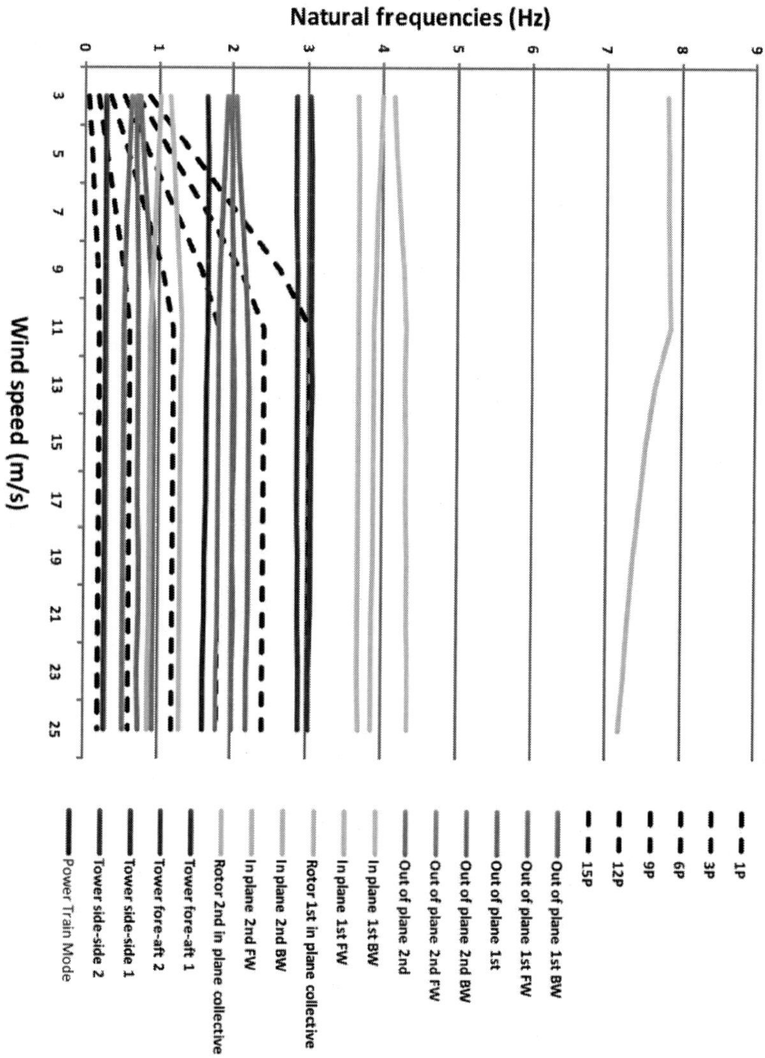

FIGURE 1: Campbell diagram for the Upwind model.

do a load mitigation analysis to test the load mitigation capacity of the new designed control strategy. In the load analysis, both fatigue damage cases (DLC1.2 in IEC61400-1 Second Edition) and some extreme load cases (DLC1.6 in IEC61400-1 Second Edition) are taken into account.

10.2 WIND TURBINE MODEL

10.2.1 NON-LINEAR MODEL

The Upwind wind turbine defined in the Upwind European project was developed in GH Bladed 4.0 and it is the non-linear model used in this research project. The Upwind model consists of a 5 MW offshore wind turbine [10,11] with a monopile structure in the foundation. It has three blades and each blade has an individual pitch actuator. The rotor diameter is 126 m, the hub height is 90 m, it has a gear box ratio of 97, the rated wind speed is 11.3 m/s, the cut-out wind speed is 25 m/s and the rated rotor rotational speed is 12.1 rpm.

10.2.2 LINEAR MODELS

The wind turbine linear models are obtained in different operational points from the GH Bladed (version 4.0) non-linear model using the linearization tool of this software. Twelve operational points are defined from 3 m/s to 25 m/s. The Campbell diagram shows the frequencies of the structural modes of linear model family with respect to the operational points (see Figure 1).

In Table 1, the frequencies of these modes are more accurately shown for the operational point of 11 m/s wind speed and some abbreviations are defined as well as referring to the modes used throughout this article. Linear models (1) are expressed by the state-space matrices and have different inputs and outputs. Inputs are the collective pitch angle and generator torque control signals u(t) and the disturbance output w(t) caused by the wind speed. The outputs y(t) are the sensorized measurements used to design the controller. In this case, these outputs are the generator speed wg, the tower top fore-aft acceleration a_{Tfa} and the tower top side-to-side acceleration a_{Tss}. Due to the non-linear model complexity, and the number of modes taken into account, the order of the linear models is 55. The linear models are not reduced because, after carrying out an analysis, the best quality of the controller syntheses are obtained using high order linear plants and reducing the higher order obtained controllers:

$$\begin{aligned} \dot{X}(t) &= A \cdot X(t) + B_{11} \cdot u(t) + B_{12} \cdot w(t) \\ y(t) &= C \cdot X(t) + D_{11} \cdot u(t) + D_{12} \cdot w(t) \end{aligned} \quad (1)$$

TABLE 1. Modal analysis of the Upwind model (BW: backward whirl; FW: forward whirl).

Elem.	Mode	Freq. (Hz)	Abbrev.
Rotor	In plane 1st	3.68	M_{R1ip}
	In plane 1st FW	1.31	M_{R1ipfw}
	In plane 1st BW	0.89	M_{R1ipbw}
	In plane 2st	7.85	M_{R2ip}
	In plane 2nd FW	4.30	M_{R2ipfw}
	In plane 2nd BW	3.88	M_{R2ipbw}
	Out of Plane 1st FW	0.93	M_{R1opfw}
	Out of Plane 1st	0.73	M_{R1op}
	Out of Plane 1st BW	0.52	M_{R1opbw}
	Out of Plane 2nd FW	2.20	M_{R2opfw}
	Out of Plane 2nd	2.00	M_{R2op}
	Out of Plane 2st BW	1.80	M_{R2opbw}
Drive Train	Drive Train	1.66	M_{DT}
Tower	1st tower side-to-side	0.28	M_{T1ss}
	1st tower fore-aft	0.28	M_{T1fa}
	2nd tower side-to-side	2.85	M_{T2ss}
	2nd tower fore-aft	3.05	M_{T2fa}
Non-str.	1P	0.2	$1P$
	3P	0.6	$3P$

10.3 BASELINE CLASSICAL CONTROL STRATEGY (C1)

The wind turbine control strategy is defined by a curve (see Figure 2) which relates the generator torque and the generator speed [12]. Three control zones are distinguished in this curve: below rated zone, transition zone and above rated zone. In the below rated zone the control objective is to maintain the power coefficient (C_p) in the optimum value. In the Upwind baseline controller, this is done by means of a generator torque control depending on the generator speed measurement (2). The generator torque T_{br} is proportional to the square of the generator speed by a constant K_{opt}.

$$T_{br} = K_{opt} \cdot w_g^2$$

$$K_{opt} = 2.14\left[\frac{\text{Nm}}{(\text{rad/s})^2}\right] \tag{2}$$

The aim in the transition zone is the control of generator speed by varying the generator torque. In the Upwind model, this can be done with a torque proportional-integral PI (3) controller [13] or with an open loop torque control which produces a ramp [14] to relate the generator torque and the generator speed. In the C1 control strategy, the PI values in the transition zone (wind speed of 11 m/s) used in the Upwind baseline controller are K_{pt} and K_{it} (3), where u(s) is the generator torque control signal and e(s) is the generator speed error:

$$\frac{3^k}{2}\log_2\frac{m}{3^k} + \frac{2k}{2}\log_2 m \tag{3}$$

In the above rated zone, the goal is the generator speed control at the nominal value of 1173 rpm varying the collective pitch angle in the blades to maintain the electric power at the value of 5 MW. To do this, a gain-scheduled (GS) PI controller [15] is used. In this case, the controller input

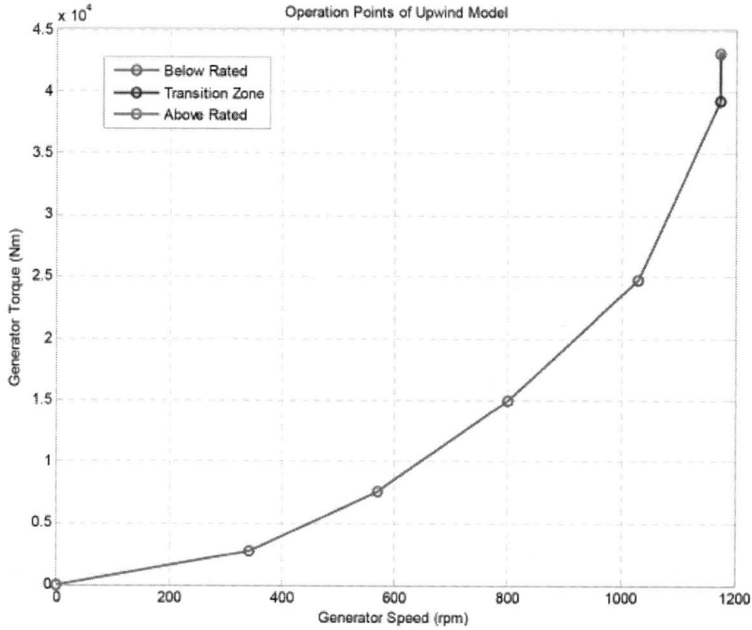

FIGURE 2: Curve of power production control zones for the Upwind wind turbine.

u(s) is the generator speed error, and the controller output $\beta_{col}(s)$ is the collective pitch angle control signal. The linear plants used to tune the gain-scheduled PI controller are the plants which relate pitch angle and generator speed. These plants have different gains, so gain-scheduling is used to guarantee the stability of the closed loop system in spite of the gain differences. To develop the gain-scheduling, two PI controllers (4) in two operational points, winds of 13 m/s and 21 m/s, are tuned:

$$K_{pt_{13}} = 0.009;\ K_{it_{13}} = 0.003$$
$$K_{pt\_21} = 0.0039;\ K_{it\_21} = 0.0013 \quad (4)$$

In the other operational points, the PI parameters are extrapolated by a first order approximation. A similar gain-scheduling strategy is proposed in [14]. Instead of using the wind speed signal from the anemometer, this

PI is scheduled by the collective pitch angle in the blades. The corresponding steady-state collective pitch angle is 6.42° for the operational point with a wind speed of 13 m/s, and the corresponding steady-state collective pitch angle value is 18.53° for the operational point with a wind speed of 21 m/s. Finally, some series notch filters are useful to improve the PI controller response [16]. Some design criteria are established to tune these controllers in these operational points:

1. Output sensitivity peak: 6 dB approximately.
2. Open loop phase margin between 30 and 60 degrees.
3. Open loop gain margin between 6 and 12 dB.
4. To maintain constant the PI zero frequency.

The drive train damping filter (DTD) is included. The aim of the DTD is to reduce the wind effect on the drive train mode [15,17]. The DTD for the Upwind model (5) consists of one gain, with one differentiator, one real zero and a pair of complex poles:

$$T_{DTD}(s) = \left[K_1 \cdot \frac{s\left(1 + \frac{1}{w_1} s\right)}{\left(\left(\frac{1}{w_2}\right)^2 s^2 + 2\xi_2 \frac{1}{w_2} s + 1\right)} \right] \cdot w_g(s) \tag{5}$$

Where $K_1 = 641.45$ Nms/rad; $w_1 = 193$ rad/s; $w_2 = 10.4$ rad/s; $\xi_2 = 0.984$.

The input of the filter is the generator speed wg and the output is a contribution TDTD to the generator torque set-point signal. Finally, the tower fore-aft damping filter (TD) is designed to reduce the wind effect on the tower first fore-aft mode in the above rated power production zone [15,17]. For the Upwind baseline controller, the filter (6) consists of a gain with one integrator, a pair of complex poles and a pair of complex zeros:

$$B_{fa}(s) = K_{TD} \cdot \frac{1}{s} \cdot \left[\frac{1 + (2 \cdot \zeta_{T1} \cdot s / w_{T1}) + (s^2 / w_{T1}^2)}{1 + (2 \cdot \zeta_{T2} \cdot s / w_{T2}) + (s^2 / w_{T2}^2)} \right] \cdot a_{Tfa}(s) \tag{6}$$

Where $K_{TD} = 0.035$; $w_{T1} = 1.25$ rad/s; $\zeta_{T1} = 0.69$; $w_{T2} = 3.13$ rad/s; $\zeta_{T2} = 1$.

The input of the filter is the fore-aft acceleration measured in the tower top a_{Tfa} and the output is a pitch contribution β_{fa} to the collective pitch angle. In conclusion, the baseline control strategy is defined in Figure 3. Other strategies to reduce the loads on the wind turbine can be developed, but they are not included in the considered baseline controller.

10.4 OBJECTIVES FOR DESIGNING THE NEW PROPOSED CONTROL STRATEGY

The control objectives for the developed wind turbine control strategy working in the above rated power production zone are as follows:

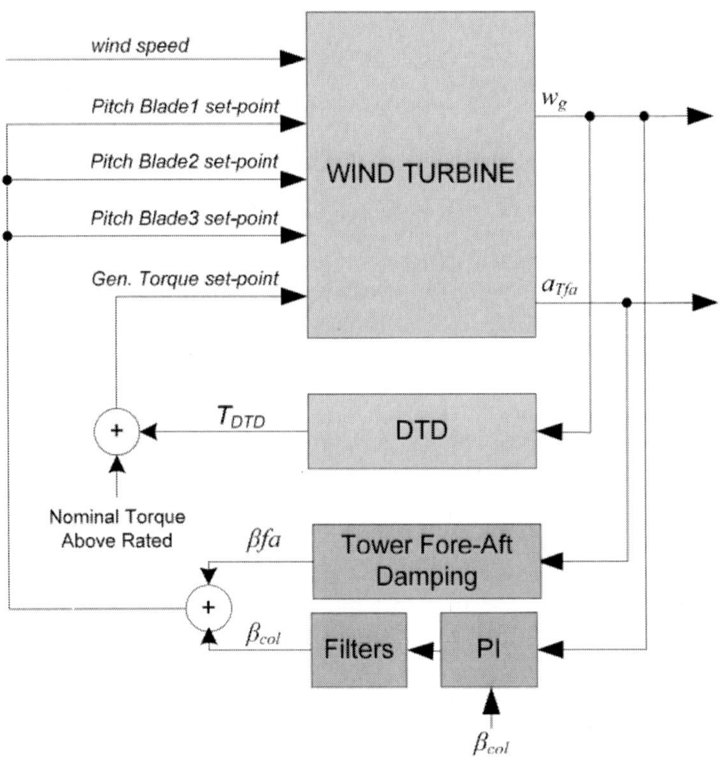

FIGURE 3: Baseline C1 control strategy.

1. Generator speed control (increase of the output sensitivity bandwidth and reduction of the peak in comparison with the baseline controller).
2. To mitigate the load on the drive train reducing the wind effect on the drive train mode.
3. To mitigate the load on the tower reducing the wind effect on the tower first modes (side-to-side and fore-aft).
4. To improve the load mitigation in comparison to a baseline controller based on the classical baseline control strategy.

To achieve these control objectives, a generator speed sensor and an accelerometer on the tower top are used [18].

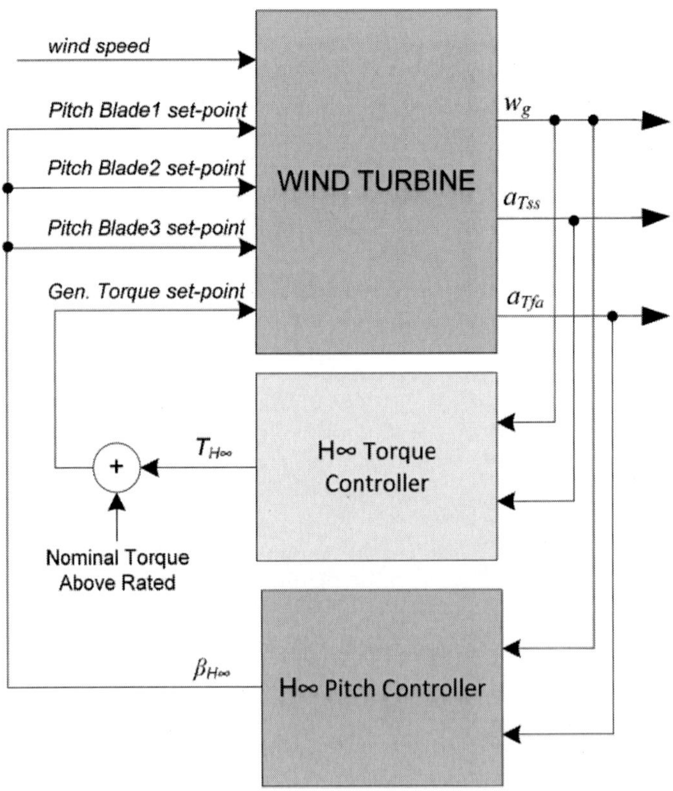

FIGURE 4: C2 control strategy based on the H_∞ norm reduction.

10.5 NEW PROPOSED CONTROL STRATEGY BASED ON H_∞ NORM REDUCTION (C2)

10.5.1 DESIGN OF CONTROL STRATEGY BASED ON H_∞ NORM REDUCTION

This strategy consists of two robust, multivariable and multi-objective controllers based on the H_∞ norm reduction (see Figure 4). The generator torque controller and the pitch controller are designed separately [19]. The torque controller has two inputs (generator speed wg and tower top side-to-side acceleration a_{Tss}) and one output (generator torque control signal TH_∞). On the other hand, the pitch controller has two inputs (generator speed wg and tower top fore-aft acceleration a_{Tfa}) and one output (collective pith control signal $\beta_{H\infty}$). The collective pitch angle set-point value is the pitch control signal $\beta_{H\infty}$. However, the generator torque set-point value is the addition of the generator torque control signal $T_{H\infty}$ and the generator torque nominal value in the above rated zone.

The control design method can be divided into the following steps:

1. To extract the wind turbine linear models from the GH Bladed non-linear model. The wind turbine used for this design is the 5 MW Upwind model.
2. To analyze the linear models in Simulink extracting the Campbell Diagram.
3. To design the torque H_∞ controller in MATLAB.
4. To design the pitch H_∞ controller in MATLAB taking into account the previous designed H_∞ torque controller.
5. To analyze the controller robustness in MATLAB.
6. To test the controllers in Simulink.
7. To include the controllers in the GH Bladed External Controller.
8. To simulate the GH Bladed non-linear model using the designed two MISO H_∞ controllers.
9. To compare the time domain and frequency domain results to the baseline classical controller.

10. To analyze the fatigue loads and extreme loads reduction of the proposed control strategy compared to the baseline control strategy.

10.5.2 GENERATOR TORQUE CONTROLLER (H_∞ TORQUE CONTROLLER)

The designed generator torque controller based on the H_∞ norm reduction solves two of the control objectives proposed in Section 4:

1. To reduce the wind effect on the drive train mode M_{DT}.
2. To reduce the wind effect on the tower side-to-side mode M_{T1ss}.

To design the controller, a mixed sensitivity problem (7) will be solved. The nominal plant G(s) is selected at the operational point of 19 m/s wind speed and has one input T (generator torque), two outputs w_g and a_{Tss} and 55 states (see Figure 5). $G_{11}(s)$ is the plant with a generator torque input and a generator speed output, while $G_{12}(s)$ is the plant with a generator torque input and a tower top side-to-side acceleration output. p_1 and p_2 are the disturbance outputs of the plant, u is the control signal, y_1 and y_2 are the controller inputs, and Z_{p11}, Z_{p12}, Z_{p2}, Z_{p31} and Z_{p32} are the performance outputs. The augmented plant (see Figure 6) of this mixed sensitivity problem is scaled using the constants Du, De_1, De_2, Dp_1 and Dp_2 (8).

$$\begin{pmatrix} Zp_{11} \\ Zp_{12} \\ Zp_2 \\ Zp_{31} \\ y_1 \\ y_2 \end{pmatrix} = \begin{pmatrix} -\frac{Dp_1}{De_1}\cdot W_{11} & 0 & \frac{Du}{De_1}\cdot G_{11}(s)\cdot W_{11} \\ 0 & -\frac{Dp_2}{De_2}\cdot W_{12} & \frac{Du}{De_2}\cdot G_{12}(s)\cdot W_{12} \\ 0 & 0 & W_2 \\ 0 & 0 & \frac{Du}{De_2}\cdot G_{11}(s)\cdot W_{31} \\ 0 & 0 & \frac{Du}{De_1}\cdot G_{12}(s)\cdot W_{32} \\ -\frac{Dp_1}{De_1} & 0 & \frac{Du}{De_2}\cdot G_{11}(s) \\ 0 & -\frac{Dp_2}{De_2} & \frac{Du}{De_2}\cdot G_{12}(s) \end{pmatrix} \cdot \begin{pmatrix} p_1 \\ p_2 \\ u \end{pmatrix} \tag{7}$$

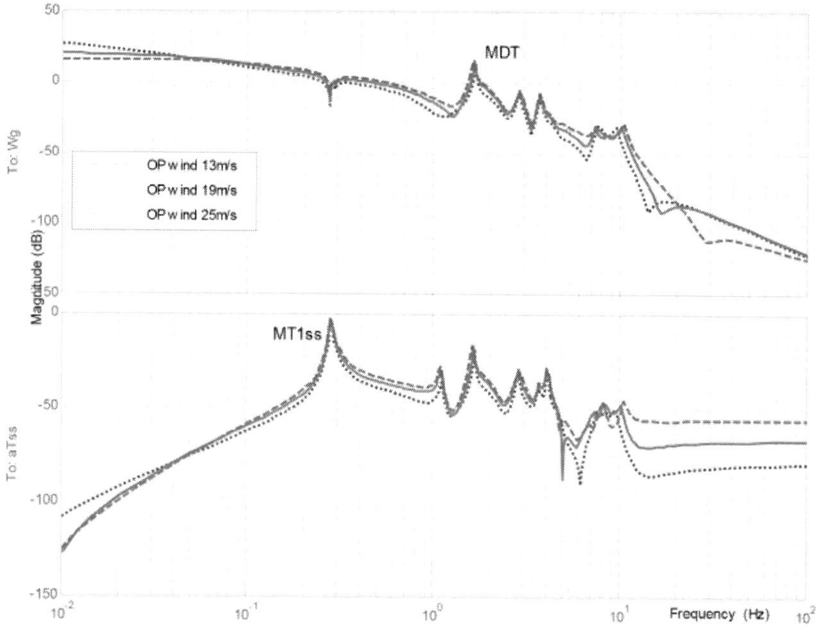

FIGURE 5: Family of plants for the H_∞ torque controller design.

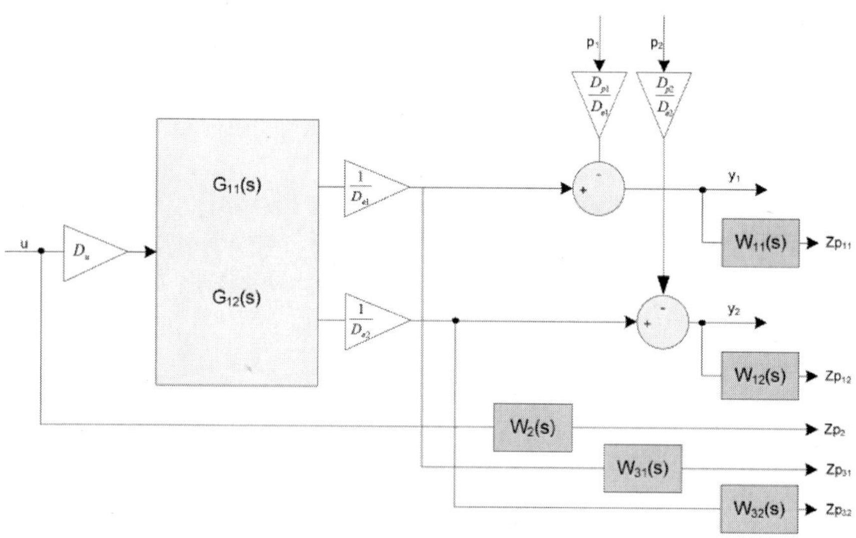

FIGURE 6. Augmented plant for the MISO Mixed-Sensitivity Problem.

The uncertainties of the family of plants are not considered in this mixed sensitivity problem due to the fact that the drive train and tower modes frequencies do not considerably vary in the above rated zone. The weight functions (9) W_{31} and W_{32} are not used, so their values are 1 in order not to consider them in the MATLAB Robust Toolbox [20]. W_{11} is an inverted notch filter centred on the M_{DT} frequency and W_{12} is another inverted notch filter centred on the M_{T1ss} frequency. W_2 is an inverted low-pass filter used to reduce the controller activity in high frequencies (see Figure 7):

$$Du = 90;\ De_1 = 0.1;\ De_2 = 1;\ Dp_1 = 0.1;\ Dp_2 = 1 \tag{8}$$

$$W_{11}(s) = \frac{(s^2 + 6.435s + 104.9)}{(s^2 + 0.1416s + 104.9)}$$

$$W_{12}(s) = \frac{(s^2 + 9.984s + 3.117)}{(s^2 + 0.04437s + 3.117)}$$

$$W_2(s) = \frac{3000(s + 5.027)}{(s + 6.823e5)} \tag{9}$$

After doing the controller synthesis, the obtained controller (see Figure 8) has to be re-scaled to adapt the inputs and the outputs to the real non-scaled plant. The obtained controller order is 39 but, finally, the controller order is reduced to order 25 and discretized using a sample time of 0.01 s. The discretized controller is represented by the state space matrices ATD, BTD, CTD and DTD (10):

$$X_{TD}(k+1) = A_{TD} \cdot X_{TD}(k) + B_{TD} \cdot \begin{pmatrix} e_{wg}(k) \\ a_{Tss}(k) \end{pmatrix}$$

$$T_{H\infty}(k) = C_{TD} \cdot X_{TD}(k) + D_{TD} \cdot \begin{pmatrix} e_{wg}(k) \\ a_{Tss}(k) \end{pmatrix} \tag{10}$$

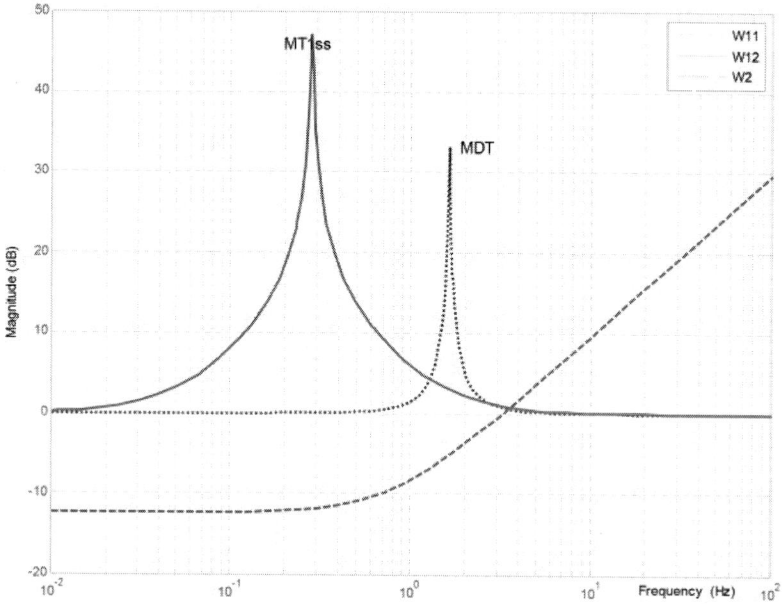

FIGURE 7: Weight functions for H_∞ torque controller design.

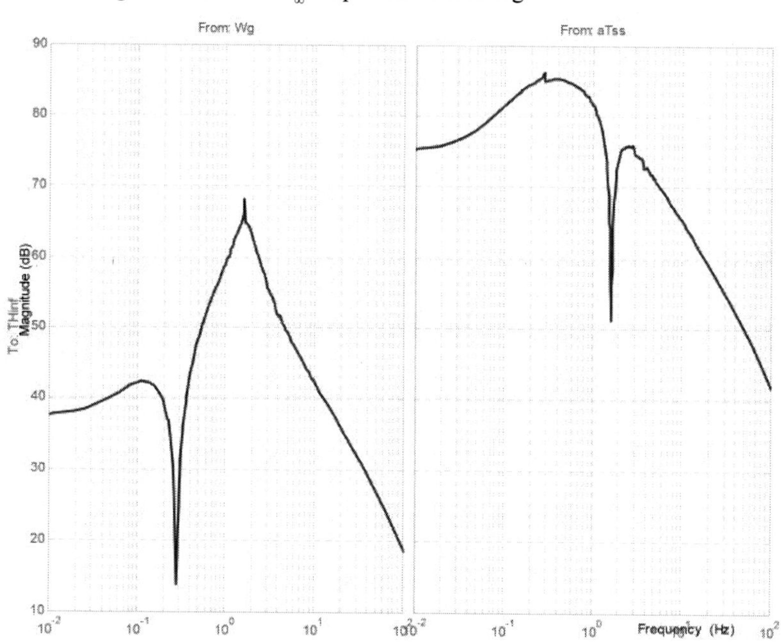

FIGURE 8: H_∞ Torque Controller.

10.5.3 COLLECTIVE PITCH ANGLE CONTROLLER (H_∞ PITCH CONTROLLER)

The collective pitch H_∞ MISO controller solves the other control objectives:

1. Generator speed control increasing the closed loop disturbance attenuation bandwidth.
2. Reduction of the wind effect on the tower fore-aft mode.
3. Inclusion of notch filters at particular frequencies in the controller dynamics to mitigate other excited frequencies (see Table 2) in the nominal plant.

TABLE 2: Frequency of notch filters in the H_∞ Pitch Controller.

Mode	Freq. (Hz)
$1P$	0.20
$3P$	0.60
M_{T2ss}	2.86
M_{R1ip}	3.69
M_{R2ip}	7.36

Another mixed sensitivity problem is proposed to develop this controller. In this case, the nominal plant GI(s) is selected for the operational point of 19 m/s wind speed (see Figure 9), it has one input β (collective pitch angle), two outputs wg and aTfa and considers the coupling caused by the inclusion of the H_∞ MISO torque controller designed in the previous section. G11(s) is the plant with a collective pitch input and a generator speed output and G12(s) is the plant with a collective pitch input and the tower top fore-aft acceleration output. This control scenario has new scaled constants (11) and the family of plants is considered as an additive uncertainty model due to the variations of the linear plants according to the operational point in the above rated zone:

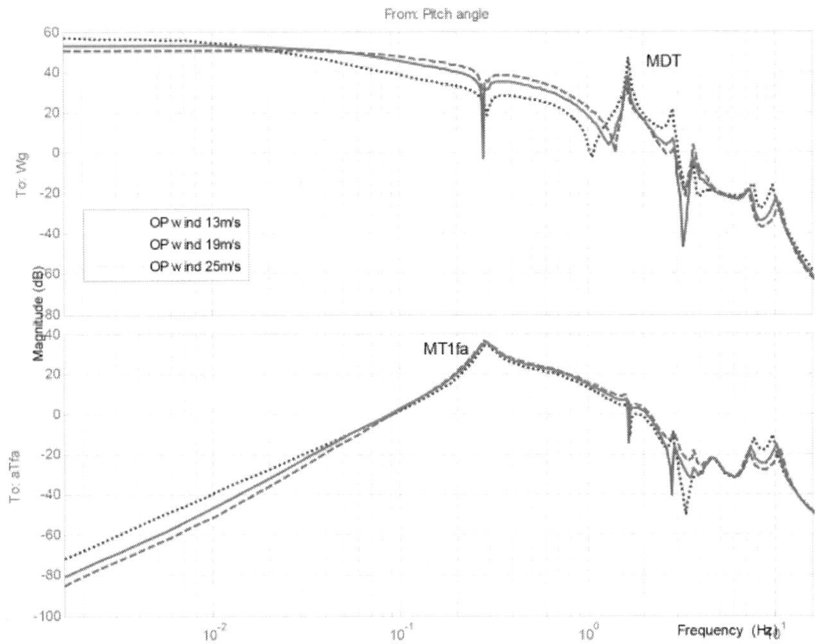

FIGURE 9: Family of plants for the H_∞ pitch controller design.

$$Du = 1; De_1 = 10; De_2 = 0.1;\ Dp_1 = 10; Dp_2 = 0.1 \tag{11}$$

Regarding the weight functions (12) in this mixed sensitivity problem, the W11 is an inverted highpass filter which determines the desired profile of the output sensitivity function. W12 is an inverted notch filter centred on the MT1fa and W2 is an inverted low-pass filter used to reduce the controller activity in high frequencies, including some inverted notch filters centred on excited frequencies (see Table 2) to include notch filters in the pitch controller dynamics (see Figure 10).

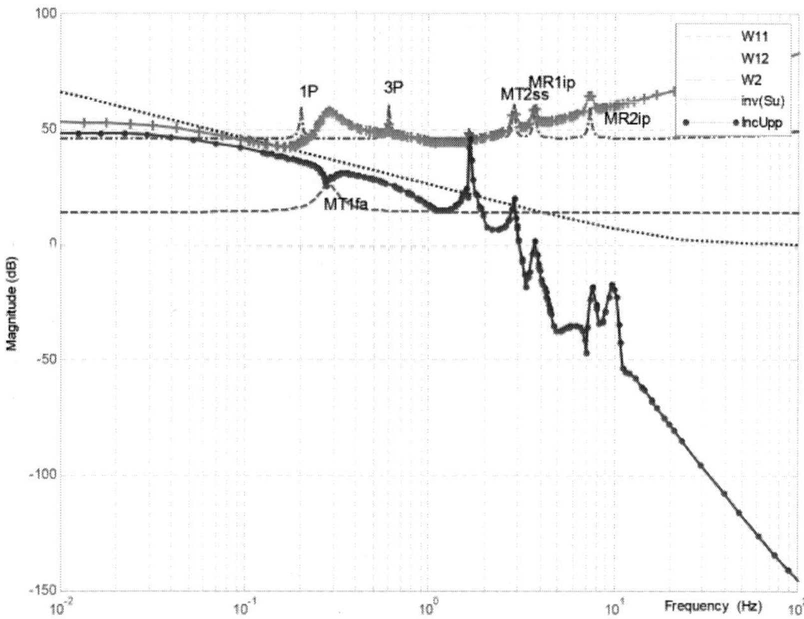

FIGURE 10: Weight functions for the H_∞ pitch controller design.

$$W_{11}(s) = \frac{(s + 125.7)}{(s + 6.283e - 5)}$$

$$W_{12}(s) = \frac{(5s^4 + 5.733s^3 + 31.58s^2 + 18s + 49.28)}{(s^4 + 0.3117s^3 + 6.288s^2 + 0.9786s + 9.856)}$$

$$W_2(s) = \frac{200000(s + 628.3)(s^2 + 0.1005s + 1.579)(s^2 + 0.3016s + 14.21)}{(s + 6.283e5)(s^2 + 0.02011s + 1.579)(s^2 + 0.06032s + 14.21)}$$

$$\cdot \frac{(s^2 + 1.438s + 322.9)(s^2 + 1.885s + 537.5)(s^2 + 3.7s + 2139)}{(s^2 + 0.2875s + 322.9)(s^2 + 0.371s + 537.5)(s^2 + 0.7399s + 2139)} \qquad (12)$$

The gains of the upper uncertainty model IncUpp are bounded by W_2 weight functions (see Figure 8) to guarantee the robust controller design. After re-scaling the obtained controller (see Figure 11), whose order is 45, it is reduced to order of 24 and discretized using a sample time of 0.01 s. The discretized controller is represented by the state space matrices A_{BD}, B_{BD}, C_{BD} and D_{BD} (13):

$$X_{BD}(k+1) = A_{BD} \cdot X_{BD}(k) \cdot B_{BD} \cdot \begin{pmatrix} e_{wg}(k) \\ a_{Tfa})k) \end{pmatrix}$$

$$\beta_{H\infty}(k) = C_{BD} \cdot X_{BD}(k) \cdot D_{BD} \cdot \begin{pmatrix} e_{wg}(k) \\ a_{Tfa})k) \end{pmatrix} \tag{13}$$

10.5.4 ANALYSIS OF THE H_∞ CONTROL STRATEGY

Gain variations in the generator speed control are only considered in the controller robust analysis due to the fact that the tower and drive train modes for the Upwind model have constant frequencies in the above rated zone. The controller robustness is guaranteed because the gains of the upper uncertainty model IncUpp are bounded by the inverse of the control sensitivity function Su [21] (see Figure 10). To compare the response of the designed controllers to the baseline controller, the two control strategies in the above rated zone are considered:

- C1: Baseline control strategy with drive train damping filter and tower fore-aft damping filter activated (see Figure 3).
- C2: Proposed control strategy with two H_∞ MISO controllers.

Using the C2 control strategy, the generator speed output disturbance attenuation bandwidth DABW in the different operational points is higher than using the baseline control strategy (see Table 3) and the generator speed output disturbance attenuation peak DAP is lower near the designed wind speed nominal operational point of 19 m/s. For the nominal plant, for which the controller is designed, the generator speed output sensitivity function (see Figure 13) shows the peak and the bandwidth to control the generator speed output for a generator speed output disturbance. This sensitivity function clearly shows the increase in the bandwidth achieved with the H_∞ C2 control strategy. These improvements are of interest in order to reduce extreme loads, as will be shown in section 6.The reduction of the wind effect on the MDT drive train mode is critical for the control strategy design, so it has been designed first. This mode reduction appears in the wind effect on different parts of the wind turbine due to the hard coupling of this mode in the system. For example, Figure 12 shows the MDT mitigation in the plant which relates the generator speed frequency response for a pitch angle input. Figure 14 shows the frequency response of the tower side-side acceleration for a wind input where the drive train mode is mitigated clearly with the C1 and C2 control strategies compared to the plant without the control system.

TABLE 3: Comparison of generator speed disturbance attenuation.

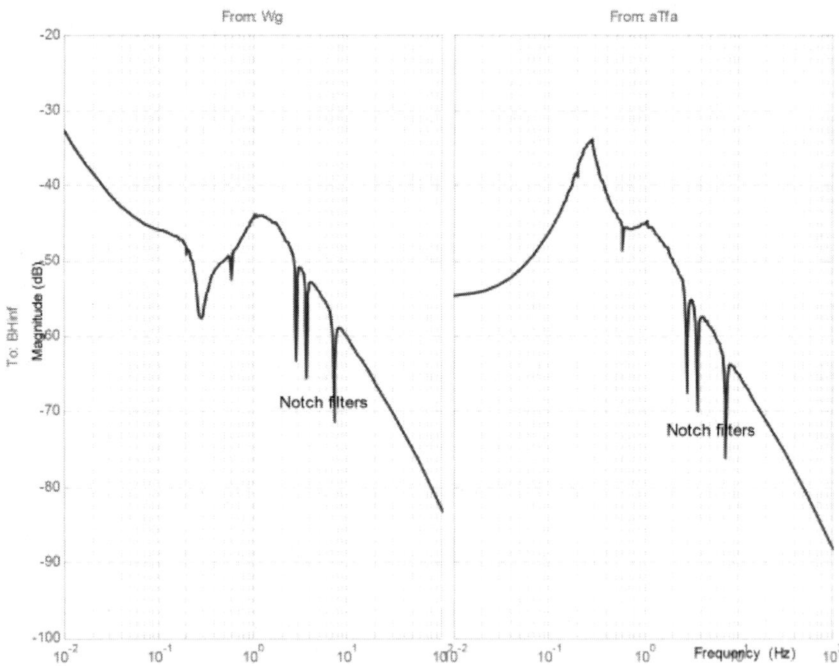

FIGURE 11: H_∞ Pitch Controller.

OP (m/s)	C1		C2	
	DABW (Hz)	DAP (dB)	DABW (Hz)	DAP (dB)
13	0.037	6.06	0.035	3.35
15	0.045	6.06	0.044	3.59
17	0.052	6.09	0.057	4.31
19	0.058	6.31	0.070	5.29
21	0.061	6.00	0.078	5.78
23	0.065	6.05	0.089	6.70
25	0.069	6.04	0.10 7.	84

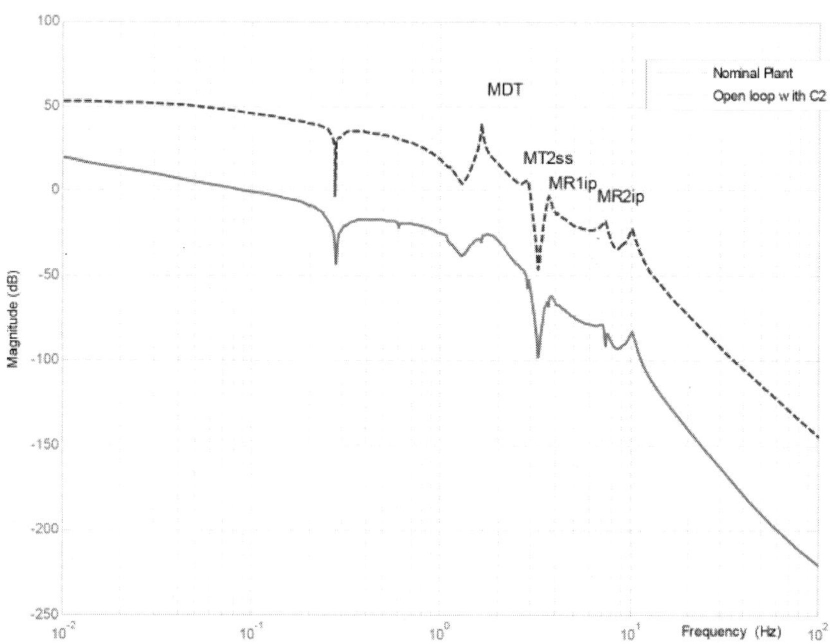

FIGURE 12: Effect of the pitch controller notch filter in open loop.

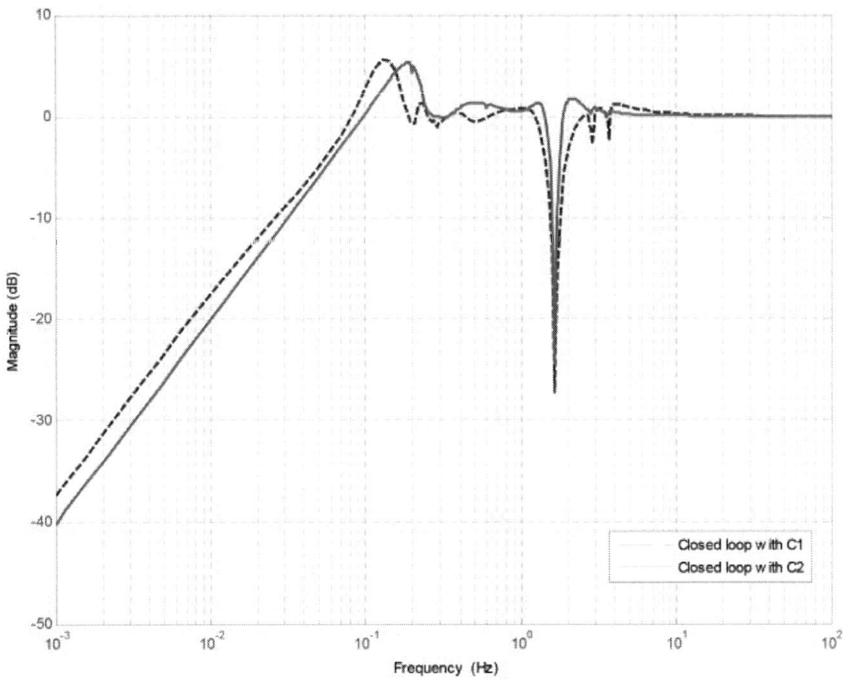

FIGURE 13: Generator speed output sensitivity function.

To analyze the reduction of the fore-aft and side-to-side tower accelerations due to the mitigation of the wind effect on these modes using the H_∞ control strategy, the closed loop response has to be analyzed in time and frequency domains for the two control strategies. The frequency response of the tower top side-to-side acceleration for a wind input (see Figure 14) is mitigated at the M_{T1ss} frequency using the C2 control strategy, but this mode is not reduced when the C1 strategy is used because it was not designed for that. This gain reduction at this frequency involves an amplitude reduction of the tower side-to-side acceleration in time domain (see Figure 14). The frequency response of the tower top fore-aft acceleration for a wind input (see Figure 15) is mitigated at the M_{T1fa} frequency using the C1 and C2 control strategies. This mode is not very excited in the Upwind model, but this mitigation could be more useful in other wind turbine models. This gain reduction at the peak of the M_{T1fa} mode involves an

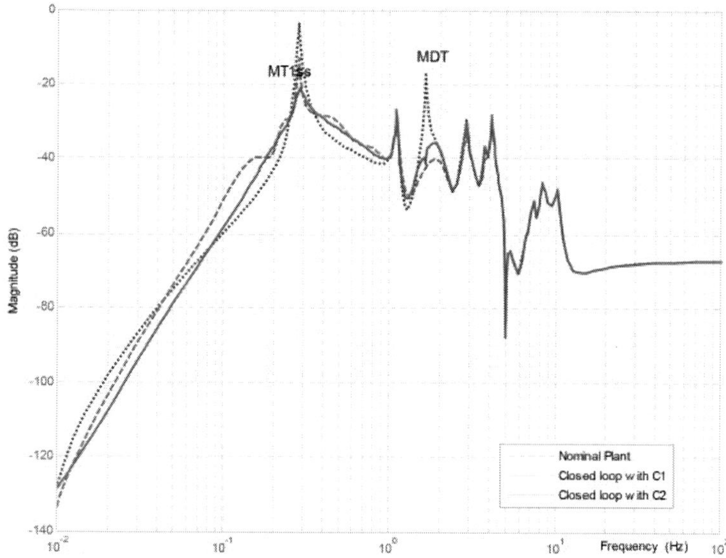

(a)

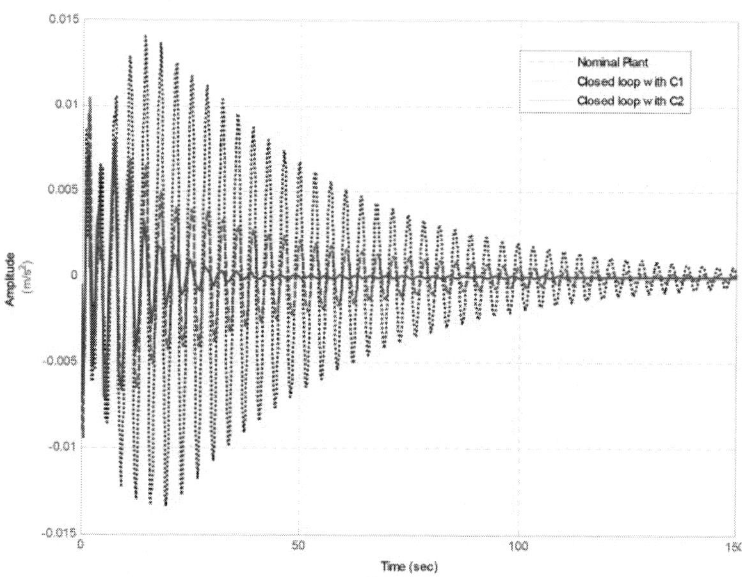

(b)

FIGURE 14: Tower top side-to-side acceleration response for a wind input (a) Frequency response; (b) Time domain wind step response.

amplitude reduction of the tower fore-aft acceleration in time domain. The gain mitigation on the M_{T1fa} and M_{T1ss} frequencies is important to reduce the momentums in the tower y and x axis respectively, and the momentum reductions mean load mitigations on the tower.

Finally, the notch filters included in the pitch controller dynamics are used to mitigate other excited frequencies which appear in the plant which relates the pitch angle with the generator speed. In this plant (see Figure 12), for the operational point of wind 19 m/s, the structural modes $M_{T2ss,}$ M_{R1ip}, M_{R2ip} are excited and they are mitigated using the H_∞ C2 control strategy. The effect of the notch filters at the frequencies 1P and 3P (blade passing frequencies) are only observed in the frequency analysis of the time domain simulations, because the excitations in these frequencies are not expressed in the linear plants extracted from GH Bladed.

10.6 RESULTS IN GH BLADED

10.6.1 EXTERNAL CONTROLLER IN GH BLADED

The two H_∞ MISO controllers are included in the External Controller in GH Bladed to do time domain simulations using the Upwind wind turbine non-linear model. The External Controller [22] is the name of the programmed code to control the wind turbine non-linear model in GH Bladed. GH Bladed calls to the External dynamic library .dll with the frequency determined by the sample time of the control strategy. The C1 and C2 control strategies are included in the External Controller to carry out the control strategies in the above rated power production zone. However, the control strategy in the below rated and transition zones is the same as the baseline control strategy and it is described in section 3. For a more realistic comparison between the results using the C1 control strategy and the results using the C2 control strategy in the above rated zone, the C2 strategy is divided into two cases:

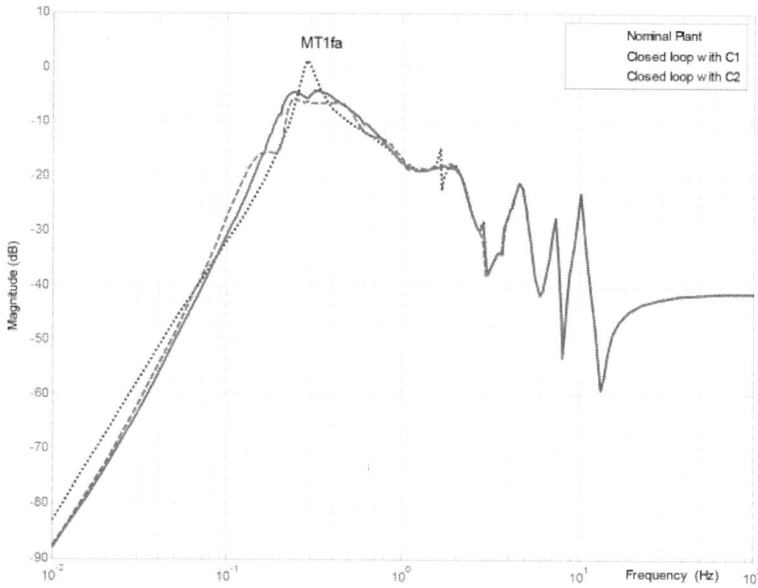

(a)

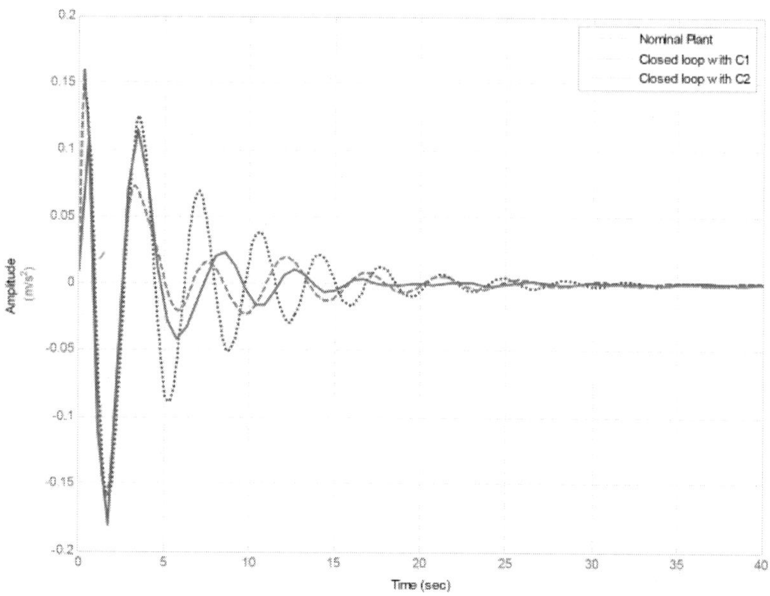

(b)

FIGURE 15: Tower top fore-aft acceleration response for a wind input (a) Frequency response; (b) Time domain wind step response.

- C2.1: The accelerometer to measure the tower top side-to-side acceleration is disabled. This is done to compare C1 and C2 control strategies without tower side-to-side damping.
- C2.2: The tower top side-to-side accelerometer is activated and C2 control strategy works without sensor signals restrictions (see Figure 4).

In the control strategy based on the H_∞ MISO discretized controllers, the control signals are calculated for each sample time (0.01 s) using the present vector of states expressed in the state-representation of the controller dynamics. The sample time has been selected after consulting wind turbine manufacturer references. The strategy to calculate the controller output is divided into four steps:

1. To initialize the controller state-space matrices A, B, C, and D from a static library and initialize the actual state vector X(k).
2. To update the present vector of controller inputs e(k) reading the wind turbine measurements from the sensors.
3. To calculate the vector of present controller outputs u(k) using matrices C, D and the current vectors of controller inputs e(k) and states X(k).
4. To calculate the vector of the next sample time controller states X(k) using matrices A and B and the actual vectors of controller inputs e(k)and states X(k). In the next sample time this vector of controller states will be the current vector of controller states.

10.6.2 FATIGUE ANALYSIS (DLC1.2 IN IEC61400-1 SECOND EDITION)

The rain flow counting algorithm [23,24] is used to analyze the load reduction capacity of the designed controllers. A fatigue analysis is carried out using this algorithm to determine the fatigue damage on the wind turbine components. The fatigue damage analysis, called load equivalent analysis, follows these steps:

1. To carry out time domain simulations using the non-linear wind turbine model and the designed controller. Twelve simulations of

600 s have been carried out using odd production winds from mean speeds from 3 m/s to 25 m/s.

2. To subject some signals of loads in time simulations (stationary hub Mx, stationary hub My, tower base Mx, tower base My, blade MFlap and blade MEdge) to the rain flow counting algorithm (one for each measured variable) using the toolbox in MATLAB [25] to carry out this analysis.
3. To obtain the load equivalent L_{eq} (14) for each kind of material and for each simulated wind. The material is defined by the m value. m is the slope of the SN curve of the material, where S is the fatigue strength and N the number of cycles to failure. N_i, the number of cycles, and L_i, the cycles amplitudes, are extracted from the rain-flow counting and N_{rd} is the number of points of the time domain simulation. For glass fibre m = 10, for cast modular iron m = 7 and for welded steel m = 3:

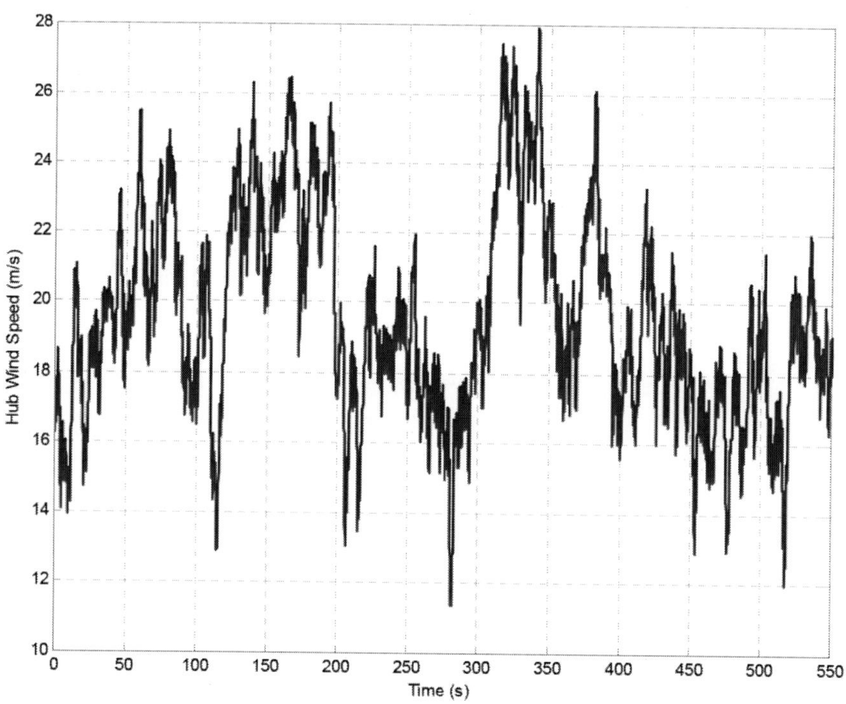

FIGURE 16: Hub wind speed for a turbulent production wind of 19 m/s.

$$L_{eq} = \left(\frac{\sum(n_i \cdot L_i)}{N_{rd}}\right)^{\frac{1}{m}} \tag{14}$$

4. The twelve simulations must be taken into account to calculate the total load equivalent for each material. The load equivalent referring to the Weibull distribution w_{eqm} (15) is calculated for each wind and each material. The total load equivalent for one material L_{eqw} (16) referring to the Weibull distribution is calculated with the summation of the w_{eqm}. w_c is a parameter of the Weibull distribution, slife is the standard life of wind turbines (20 years) and tsim is the simulated time of the considered variable in this load equivalent analysis:

$$w_{eqm} = L_{eq}^{m} \cdot w_c \cdot slife/tsim \tag{15}$$

$$L_{eq} = \left(\sum w_{eqm}\right)^{1/m} \tag{16}$$

5. To compare the wind turbine life variations $comp_{life}$ (17) between two compared load equivalent analysis. L_{eqw1} is the total load equivalent value for twelve simulations and L_{eqw2} is the other total load equivalent value for the other twelve simulations:

$$comp_{life} = \frac{slife}{\left(\frac{L_{eqw1} - L_{eqw2}}{100}\right)^{m}} \tag{17}$$

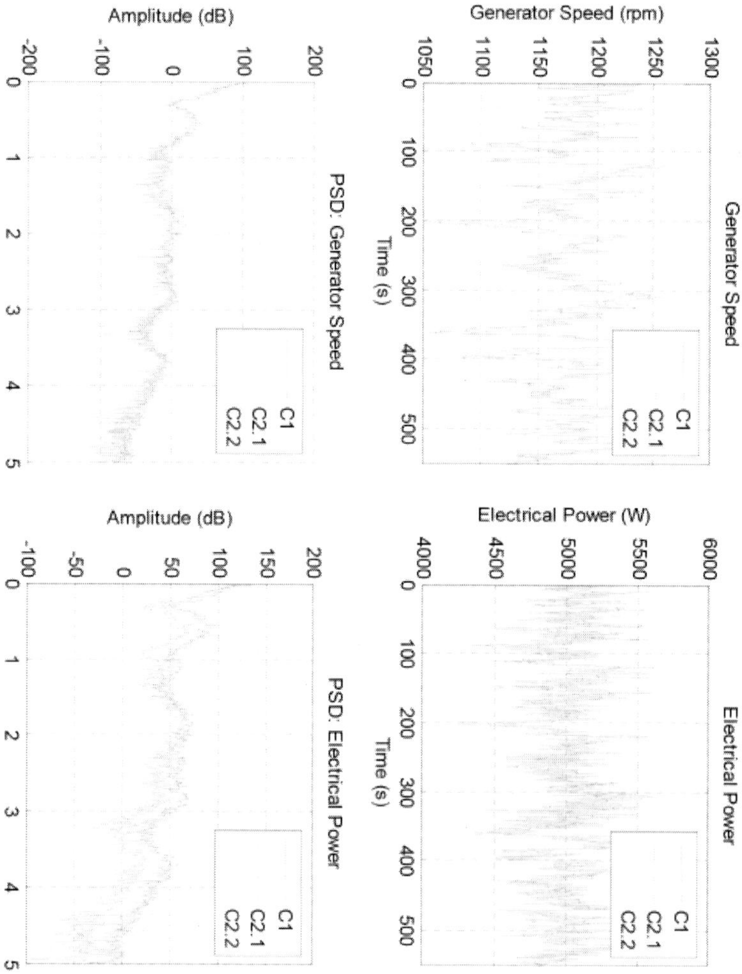

FIGURE 17. Generator speed and electrical power with a turbulent production wind of 19 m/s.

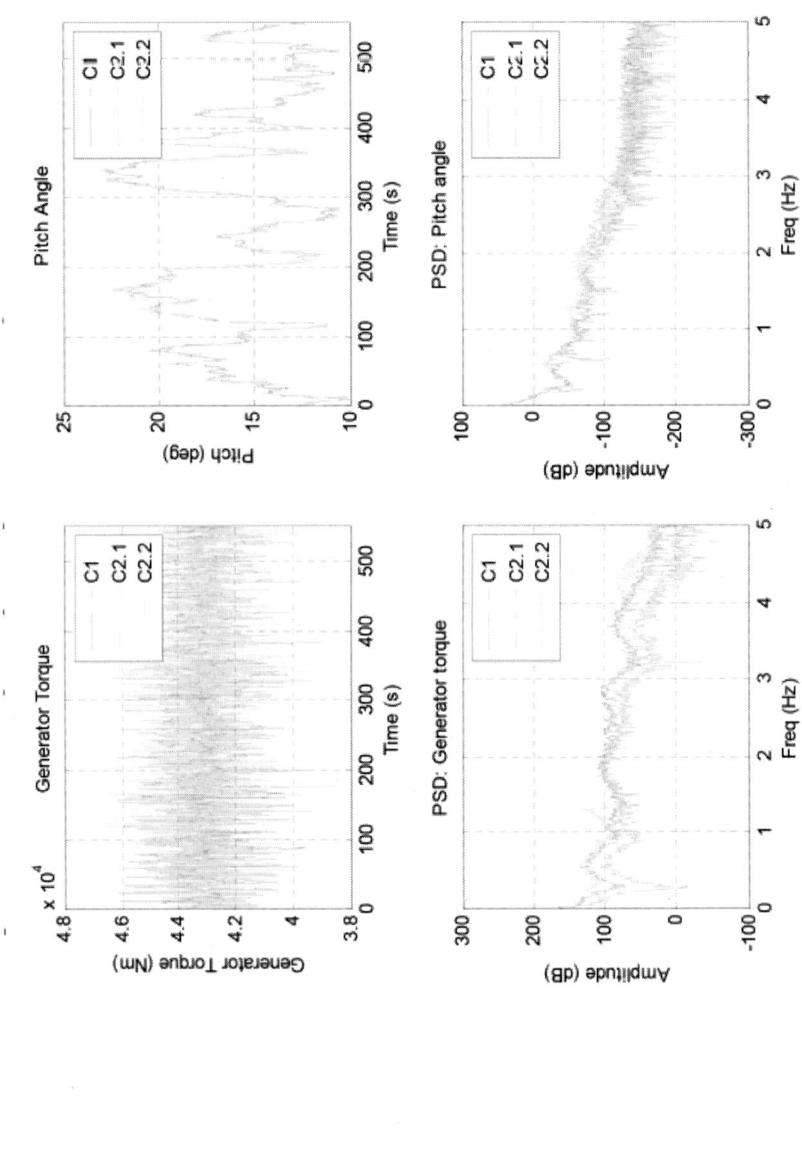

FIGURE 18: Generator torque and pitch angle with a turbulent production wind of 19 m/s.

In Figure 17 the controlled signals (generator speed and electric power) are compared for a turbulent production wind of 19 m/s (see Figure 16) using the C1, C2.1 and C2.2 control strategies. The generator speed is controlled for the nominal value 1173 rpm and the electrical power around 5 MW. The power spectral density (PSD) performs a frequency analysis of time domain simulations. In Figure 18 the control signals (collective pitch angle and generator torque) are compared. The time domain simulation shows the quick response of the pitch angle using the C2.1 and C2.2 strategies and the torque contribution signal of the C2.2 control strategy to mitigate the side-to-side displacement on the tower. Figure 19 shows the reduction of the wind effect on the tower fore-aft mode in the tower base momentum My and the reduction of the wind effect on the tower side-to-side mode and drive train mode in tower base momentum Mx.

Finally, the fatigue damage analysis of the components of the wind turbine is carried out as a result of the load equivalent analysis. Table 4 shows the load reduction percentage of the control strategies on the different components of the Upwind model. C1 is the reference strategy to compare the load reduction achieved with C2.1 and C2.2 control strategies. Results are calculated for three material constants, m, which are commonly used by the commercial companies of wind turbines. If m = 3 using the two H_∞ MISO controllers, the load reduction is 0.4% on the Stationary Hub Mx momentum using the C2.2 control strategy and 4.8% using the C2.1 strategy, 13.4% on the Tower Base Mx momentum with the C2.2 and 2.6% using the C2.1, and 4.7% on the Tower Base My momentum respect to the C1 baseline controller using the C2.2 and 5.2% with the C2.1. If m = 9, the load reduction is 3.1% on the Stationary Hub Mx momentum, 19.6% on the Tower Base Mx momentum and 8.8% on the Tower Base My momentum using the C2.2 control strategy. On the other hand, if m = 9 using the C2.1 control strategy, the load reduction is 4.2% on the Stationary Hub Mx momentum, −0.1% on the Tower Base Mx momentum and 10.9% on the Tower Base My momentum. If m = 12 using the C2.2 strategy, the load reduction is 2.9% on the Stationary Hub Mx momentum, 19.2% on the Tower Base Mx momentum and 10.6% on the Tower Base My momentum. For this m value using the C2.1 control strategy, the load reduction is 4.0% on the Stationary Hub Mx momentum, −0.2% on the Tower Base Mx momentum and 13.6% on the Tower Base My momentum. Load

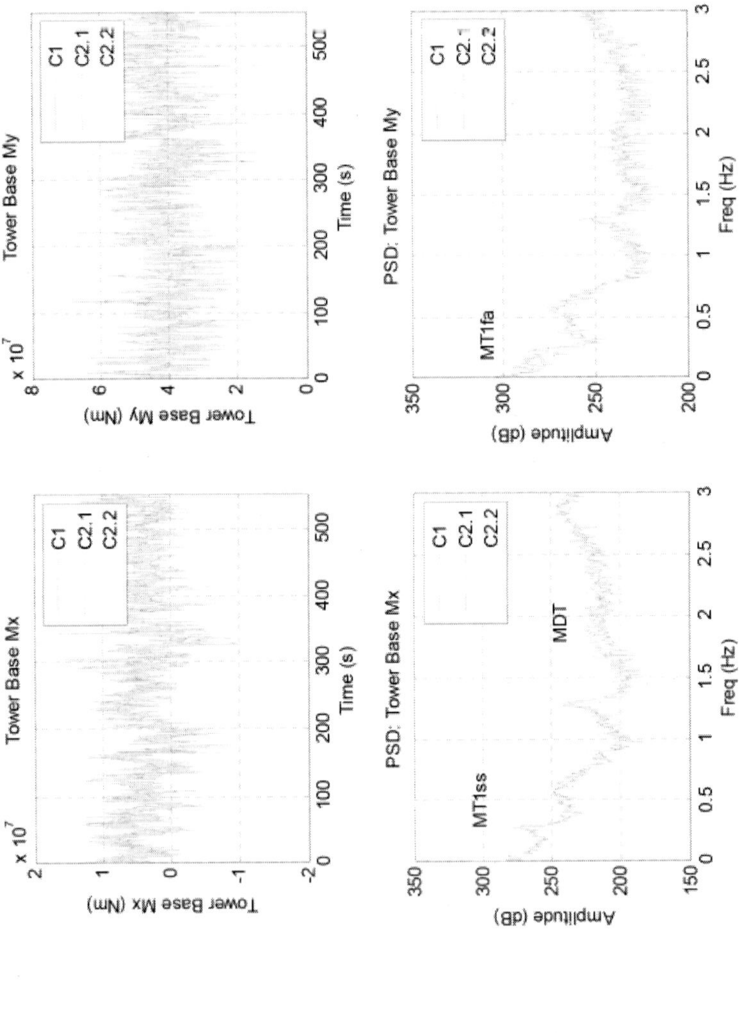

FIGURE 19: Loads on tower base with a turbulent production wind of 19 m/s.

reduction figures less than 0.4% should not be considered because they can be caused by mathematical calculation precision in the load equivalent algorithm (in blue colour in Table 4).

TABLE 4: Comparison of the load equivalent analysis.

	m	C1-C2.1 (%)	C1-C2.2 (%)
Stationary Hub Mx	3	4.8	0.4
	9	4.2	3.1
	12	4.0	2.9
	3	0.2	0.2
Stationary Hub My	9	0.9	1
	12	1.2	1.5
	3	4.8	0.4
Gearbox Torque	9	4.2	3.1
	12	4.0	2.9
	3	2.6	13.4
Tower Base Mx	9	−0.1	19.6
	12	−0.2	19.2
	3	5.2	4.7
Tower Base My	9	10.9	8.8
	12	13.6	10.6
	3	0.1	−0.2
Blade1 MFlap	9	0.1	−0.1
	12	0.1	−0.2
	3	0	0.1
Blade1 MEdge	9	0	0
	12	0	0

In these simulations there is an excitation of the rotor in-plane 1st FW mode M_{R1ipfw} (1.2 Hz). This excitation is not critical from the point of view of the load reduction in a wind turbine system as is proven in this load equivalent analysis. The cause of this excitation is the bandwidth of the torque controller. The torque controller reduces the wind effect on the drive train mode M_{DT} (1.6 Hz) and tower 1st side-to-side mode M_{T1ss} (0.28 Hz). The torque H_∞ MISO controller (see Figure 8) dynamics from tower top side-to-side acceleration to torque set point value introduces a high gain in frequencies between 0.2 Hz and 1.6 Hz which produces the In plane 1st FW mode excitation. To reduce this excitation, a notch filter in the rotor in-plane 1st FW frequency must be included in the weight functions W_2 used to design the torque controller.

10.6.3 EXTREME LOAD ANALYSIS (DLC1.6 IN IEC61400-1 SECOND EDITION)

The extreme load DLC1.6 analysis studies the system response for different kinds of extreme gusts. This analysis is divided into three different steps:

1. To carry out time domain simulations using the non-linear wind turbine model and the C1 and C2 different control strategies. Six simulations of different kinds of gusts have been carried out. The gusts are called Vr-0, Vr-p, Vr-n, Vout-0, Vout-p, Vout-n.
2. To analyze the six simulations and extract the maximum value of the generator speed signal and some momentums (tower base Mx, tower base My, tower base Mxy, hub total bending Myz, blade MFlap and blade MEdge).
3. To compare these maximum values using the C2 control strategy with regard to the baseline C1 control strategy.

Other extreme load cases (as for instance DLC1.5 in IEC61400-1 Second Edition cases) are not taken into account because results depend especially on the stop strategy, which has not been implemented. Moreover, a safety control strategy is not developed in the supervisory control to stop the wind turbine in generator over-speed cases. This article only shows the response of the developed C1 and C2 control strategies in the above rated zone without taking into account any safety control strategy.

The results of the extreme load DLC1.6 analysis are summarized in Table 5. The C2.1 and C2.2 control strategies, based on the H_∞ norm reduction, give better results than the baseline control strategy C1. Using C2.2, the reduction of the generator speed maximum value, compared to the C1

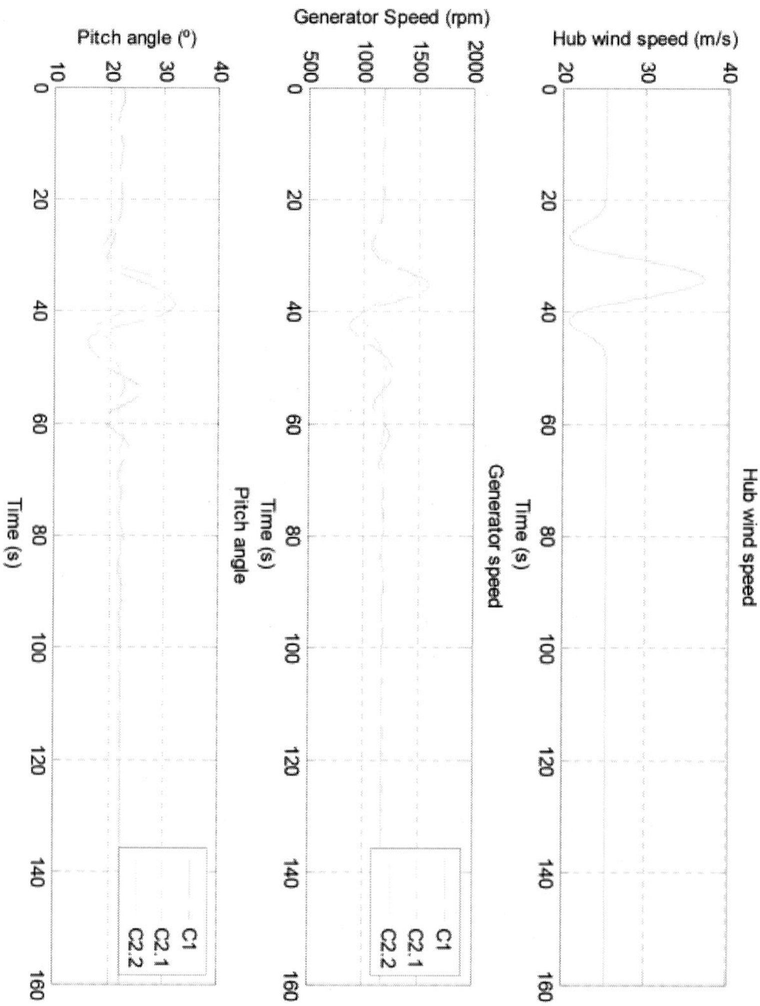

FIGURE 20. Vout-p extreme gust simulation.

strategy, is 7.8%, the tower base Mx momentum is reduced by 7.8% and the blade MEdge momentum is reduced by 26.3%. The tower base My momentum, tower base Mxy momentum and hub total bending Myz momentum are reduced by around 1.5% when using the C2.2 control strategy. Using C2.1, the reduction of the generator speed maximum value is 7.8%, the tower base Mx momentum is not reduced and the blade MEdge momentum is reduced by 25.9%. However, the tower base My momentum, tower base Mxy momentum and hub total bending Myz momentum are not considerably reduced using the C2.1 control strategy. The blade MEdge momentum is considerably reduced due to the increase in the generator speed output disturbance bandwidth and the reduction in the peak of this sensitivity function. In Figure 20, the results of the simulation in GH Bladed using an input of wind of a Vout-p gust and using the C1 control strategy are compared to the same wind input using the C2 control strategy without including any safety system to avoid generator overspeeds. The higher bandwidth of the generator speed output sensitivity function obtained with the C2 control strategy means a quick response of the collective pitch angle signal and the consistent reduction of the generator speed maximum value. Furthermore, the mitigation of the variations of the generator speed using the H_∞ controllers is the main reason for the mitigation of the extreme load on the blade MEdge momentum. The most useful advantage of this reduction of extreme loads using the H_∞ control strategy is to avoid the activation of special safety strategies to stop the wind turbine. Usually, these special safety strategies are activated when the generator speed is higher than a critical value and involves losses of the electric power and critical momentary increases of loads in the wind turbine.

10.7 CONCLUSIONS

The work carried out and presented in this article can be summarized as follows:

1. The offshore Upwind 5 MW wind turbine model is developed using the GH Bladed 4.0 software package.
2. A classical control strategy for wind turbines is defined and it is considered the baseline controller for comparing with the new developed control strategies.

3. New design process of a control strategy based on H_∞ controllers is defined and validated in GH Bladed. The new strategies are applied in above rated power production zone in wind turbines. The results obtained in the closed loop simulations using GH Bladed 4.0 software package show the fatigue load reduction on the desired components (tower and drive train) compared to the classical baseline control strategy (see Figure 21). Using the designed H_∞ controllers, the extreme load reduction in case DLC1.6 does not appear only in the tower, but also in the three blades. Results obtained using H_∞ controllers have these outstanding benefits from the load reduction point of view due to some interesting properties:

TABLE 5: Comparison of the extreme load analysis.

	C1	C2.1	C1-C2.1 (%)	C2.2	C1-C2.2 (%)
Generator Speed	1589 rpm	1464 rpm	7.86	1465 rpm	7.8
Tower Base Mx	29278 KNm	29285 KNm	0.02	26983 KNm	7.8
Tower Base My	158258 KNm	155500 KNm	1.74	155473 KNm	1.7
Tower Base Mxy	158311 KNm	155500 KNm	1.77	155555 KNm	1.7
Hub total bending Myz	12991 KNm	12780 KNm	1.62	12817 KNm	1.3
Blade MFlap	18341 KNm	18400 KNm	−0.32	18355 KNm	−0.07
Blade MEdge	9946 KNm	7366 KNm	25.94	7327 KNm	26.3

- The attenuation of the generator speed output disturbance bandwidth is higher than that obtained using the classical control strategy.
- The attenuation of the generator speed output disturbance peak is higher than that obtained using the classical control strategy.
- The proposed control strategy based on the H_∞ norm reduction takes into account the coupling between variables in the wind turbine system. The designed controller is multivariable and multi-objective.
- The controller robustness is guaranteed due to the small gain theorem properties applied to the H_∞ controller synthesis.
- Some notch filters can be included in the controller dynamics using a correct definition of the mixed sensitivity problem. This is very useful for reducing excited modes on non-desired frequencies.

REFERENCES

1. Caselitz, P.; Geyler, M.; Giebhardt, J.; Panahandeh, B. Hardware-in-the-Loop development and testing of new pitch control algorithms. In Proceeding of European Wind Energy Conference and Exhibition (EWEC), Brussels, Belgium, March 2011; pp. 14–17.
2. Johnson, K.E.; Pao, L.Y.; Balas, M.J.; Kulkarni, V.; Fingersh, L.J. Stability analysis of an adaptive torque controller for variable speed wind turbines. In Proceeding of IEEE Conference on Decision and Control, Atlantis, Bahamas, December 2004; pp. 14–17.
3. Nourdine, S.; Díaz de Corcuera A.; Camblong, H.; Landaluze, J.; Vechiu, I.; Tapia, G. Control of wind turbines for frequency regulation and fatigue loads reduction. In Proceeding of 6th Dubrovnik Conference on Sustainable Development of Energy, Water and Environment Systems, Dubrovnik, Croatia, September 2011; pp. 25–29.
4. Wright, A.D. Modern Control Design for Flexible Wind Turbines; NREL/TP-500-35816; Technical Report for NREL: Colorado, CO, USA, July 2004.
5. Wright, A.D.; Fingersh, L.J.; Balas, M.J. Testing state-space controls for the controls advanced research turbine. In Proceeding of 44th AIAA Aerospace Sciences Meeting and Exhibit, Reno, NV, USA, January 2006; pp. 9–12.
6. Sanz, M.G.; Torres, M. Aerogenerador síncrono multipolar de velocidad variable y 1.5 MW de potencia: TWT1500. Rev. Iberoamer. Autom. Informát. 2004, 1, 53–64.
7. Bianchi, F.D.; Battista, H.D.; Mantz, R.J. Wind turbine control systems. In Principles, Modelling and Gain Scheduling Design; Springer-Verlag: London, UK, 2007.
8. Geyler, M.; Caselitz, P. Robust multivariable pitch control design for load reduction on large wind turbines. J. Sol. Energy Eng. 2008, 130, 12.
9. Fleming, P.A.; van Wingerden, J.W.; Wright, A.D. Comparing state-space multivariable controls to multi-siso controls for load reduction of drivetrain-coupled modes on wind turbines through field-testing. NREL/CP-5000-53500; NREL: Colorado, CO, USA, 2011.
10. Jonkman, J.; Butterfield, S.; Musial, W.; Scott, G. Definition of a 5 MW Reference Wind Turbine for Offshore System Development; NREL/TP-500-38060; Technical Report for NREL: Colorado, CO, USA, February 2009.
11. Upwind Home page. Available online: http://www.upwind.eu (accessed on 12 December 2011).
12. Bossanyi, E.A. The design of closed loop controllers for wind turbines. Wind Energy 2000, 3, 149–163.
13. Bossanyi, E.A. Controller for 5 MW reference turbine. In European Upwind Project Report; Garrad Hassan & Partners Ltd.: Bristol, UK, 2009. Available online: http: // www.upwind.eu (accessed on 12 December 2011).
14. Wright, A.D.; Fingersh, L.J. Advanced Control Design for Wind Turbines Part I: Control Design, Implementation, and Initial Tests; NREL/TP-500-42437; NREL: Colorado, CO, USA, 2008.
15. Bossanyi, E.A. Wind turbine control for load reduction. Wind Energy 2003, 6, 229–244.

16. Van der Hooft, E.L.; Schaak, P.; van Engelen, T.G. Wind Turbine Control Algorithms; DOWEC-F1W1-EH-03094/0; Technical Report for ECN: Petten, The Netherlands, 2003.
17. Wright, A.D.; Balas, M.J. Design of controls to attenuate loads in the controls advanced research turbine. J. Sol. Energy Eng. 2004, 126, 1083.
18. Hau, M. Promising Load Estimation Methodologies for Wind Turbine Components; Technical Report for European Upwind Project; ISET, Kassel, Germany, 2009. Available online: http: //www.upwind.eu (accessed on 12 December 2012).
19. Bossanyi, E.A.; Ramtharan, G.; Savini, B. The importance of control in wind turbines design and loading. In Proceedings of the 17th Mediterranean Conference on Control & Automation, Thessaloniki, Greece, June 2009; pp. 24–26.
20. Balas, G.; Chiang, R.; Packard, A.; Safonov, M. MATLAB robust control toolbox. In Getting Started Guide; The MathWorks, Inc.: Natick, MA, USA, 2009.
21. Doyle, J.C.; Francis, B.A.; Tannenbaum, A.R. Feedback Control Theory; MacMillan: Toronto, Canada, 1992.
22. Bossanyi, E.A. Bladed User Manual; Garrad Hassan & Partners Ltd.: Bristol, UK, 2009.
23. Frandsen, S.T. Turbulence and Turbulence Generated Structural Loading in Wind Turbine Clusters. Ph.D. Thesis, Technical University of Denmark, Roskilde, Denmark, 2007.
24. Söker, H.; Kaufeld, N. Introducing low cycle fatigue in IEC standard range pair spectra. In Proceeding of 7th German Wind Energy Conference, Wilhelmshaven, Germany, October 2004; pp. 20–21.
25. MATLAB Rainflow Counting Algorithm Toolbox. Available online: http://www.mathworks.com/ MATLABcentral/fileexchange/3026 (accessed on 12 December 2011).

PART V

ENVIRONMENTAL ISSUES

CHAPTER 11

ELECTROMAGNETIC INTERFERENCE ON LARGE WIND TURBINES

FLORIAN KRUG AND BASTIAN LEWKE

11.1 INTRODUCTION

Wind turbines (WT) cause electromagnetic interference (EMI) via three principal mechanisms, namely near field effects, diffraction and reflection/scattering [1-4]. Near field effects refer to the potential of a wind turbine to cause interference to radio signals due to electromagnetic fields emitted by the generator and switching components in the turbine nacelle or hub. Diffraction occurs when an object modifies an advancing wavefront by obstructing the wave's path of travel. Diffraction effects can occur when the object not only reflects part of the signal, but also absorbs the signal. Reflection/scattering interference occurs when turbines either reflect or obstruct signals between a transmitter and a receiver. This occurs when the rotating blades of a turbine receive a primary transmitted signal and they act to produce and transmit a scattered signal. In this situation the receiver may pick up two signals simultaneously, with the scattered signal causing EMI because it is delayed in time (out of phase) or distorted compared to the primary signal.

This chapter was originally published under the Creative Commons Attribution License. Krug F and Lewke B. Electromagnetic Interference on Large Wind Turbines. Energies **2009**,2 (2009).doi:10.3390/en20401118.

Other important events for the electromagnetic field distribution of a wind turbine are lightning impacts [5]. These lightning events have strong impact on the electronic systems in a wind turbine. Because of the increasing availability requirements for wind turbines there is a trend of more complex electronic monitoring equipment for large wind turbines [6,7]. State of the art WT control communication is realized via low-bandwidth slip-rings and main-shaft between hub and nacelle. The trend to increase the amount of electronic equipment used leads to a requirement for higher communication bandwidth. Wireless communication links present one solution to this problem. Avoidance of communication loss between operators and control system raises the question of backup communication systems. A GSM transceiver backup system installed to the hub would allow operators to access the control systems, even in case of a communication loss via the nacelle. To optimize such electronic systems in wind turbines an EMI analysis is necessary. On the other hand to prove such complex models efficient measurement methods like the time-domain measurement principle give a deeper understanding of the EMI effects on the electrical energy systems [8].

This paper presents general aspects of EMI with respect to wind turbines. Protection means and measurement techniques are presented. As an example of turbine emitted EMI, the electromagnetic fields caused by a GSM 900 MHz transmitter mounted on a hub of the wind turbine are analyzed by method-of-moments. The transmitter acts as communication backup system for the control systems of the hub.

11.2 CLASSIFICATION OF INTERFERENCES

The EMI originating from the equipment under test (EUT) depends on the frequency, time and geometry of the test setup (position, distance and direction). The interferences may be classified on the basis of the receiver and interference bandwidth [9,10], as shown in Table 1.

Furthermore, EMI signals may be classified on the basis of their statistical behavior as random or deterministic signals. Random signals can be further subdivided into stationary and nonstationary signals [11]. The statistical properties of nonstationary random signals may change considerably over the observation period. Deterministic signals may be periodic, quasi-periodic, nonperiodic, or a combination of these signal types. Periodic and quasi-periodic signals exhibit line spectra. Transients are nonperiodic signals. Nonperiodic signals exhibit continuous spectra. Finally, signals can also be combinations of two or more of the above classes.

TABLE 1: Character of the disturbance.

Class	Description	Condition
A	Continuous narrowband	$\Delta f_{interference} < \Delta f_{receiver}$
B	Continuous broadband	$\Delta f_{interference} < \Delta f_{receiver}$
C	Pulse modulated narrowband	Pulse-duration and -repetion
D	Pulsed broadband	Pulse-duration and -repetion

11.3 EMI AND SHIELDING FOR WIND TURBINE CONTROL SYSTEMS

The critical elements of a wind turbine affected by electromagnetic fields are the control systems inside the hub and nacelle. One of the most important is the pitch control system providing the necessary control over the wind turbine rotor.

Especially for lightning as source of EMI, a redirection of the lightning current to bypass the hub, and its electronics in particular, is not yet feasible. An analysis of possible work around this problem is presented in [12].

The best way to protect the control systems and electronic circuits against electric and magnetic fields is by electromagnetic shielding. It is one of the most important tools in the area of electromagnetic compatibility (EMC) [13]. In addition to shielding devices, filter applications are often installed. Because electronic devices, and electric circuits in particular, need to share data or power with their environment and the operator, conductors have to pass through the shielding device. Therefore, apertures, e.g., due to cable connectors or ventilation slots, represent weaknesses in the shielding devices. Electric and magnetic fields are able to penetrate into the shielded space. Over-voltages and—currents are induced into the electric circuits and may lead to the destruction of circuit elements. In order to be able to specify the need for the shielding effectiveness it is calculated for electric fields according to:

$$a_s = 20\log\left|\frac{E_0}{E_i}\right| \tag{1}$$

where the indices i and o representing the electric field strength at the same spatial position with and without the shielding device, respectively. For magnetic fields, the magnetic field strength H replaces the electric field strength E in Equation 3.1. Depending on the value of shielding effectiveness, an explanation for the shielding classifications is given in Table 2 [13,14].

TABLE 2: Description of damping strength and shielding effectiveness according to [13,14].

Damping	Description
0–10 dB	Very low damping; no real shielding against electromagnetic interference.
10–30 dB	Minimal shielding; slight interferences might by suppressed.
30–60 dB	Average shielding for small problems in high frequency range; high shielding in the low frequency range.
60–90 dB	Very good shielding of problems in hihg frequency domain.
90–120 dB	Maximum shielding effectiveness that can be achieved with excellent shielding.

11.4. EMI MEASUREMENTS ON WIND TURBINES

11.4.1 GENERAL ASPECTS OF EMI MEASUREMENT

Due to the rapid development of new electronic products and due to emerging new technologies the ability to achieve and to improve electromagnetic compatibility is a major challenge in the development of electronic products. EMC and EMI measurement equipment which allows extraction of extensive and accurate information within short measurement times will allow the reduction of the costs and to improve the quality in circuit and system development. In the past and currently, radio noise and electromagnetic interference (EMI) are measured and characterized using superheterodyne radio receivers. The disadvantage of this method is the relatively long measurement time, typically 30 min, for a frequency band from 30 MHz to 1 GHz [15]. Since such a long measurement time results in high test costs, it is important to investigate options for reducing the measurement time without loss of quality. Since conventional measurement systems do not evaluate the phase information of the measured EMI signal, important information is lost.

Novel EMI measurement methods based on a time-domain approach have several advantages. The digital processing of time-domain EMI (TDEMI) measurements using Fourier transform allows the decomposition of the measured signal into its spectral components [15]. The use of Fourier techniques has grown rapidly in recent years because of the economy of programs using the fast Fourier transform (FFT). In general, the digital processing of EMI measurements allows emulation in real-time of the various modes of conventional analogous equipment, e.g., peak, average, rms and quasi-peak detector and also introduces new concepts of analysis, e.g., phase spectra, short-time spectra, statistical evaluation and FFT-based time-frequency analysis methods.

Beyond this, time-domain techniques exhibit additional advantages. Since time-domain techniques allow processing all the amplitude and phase information over the whole signal spectrum in parallel, the measurement time may be reduced by at least one order of magnitude and the information obtained goes far beyond the information obtained with conventional analogue measurement systems.

11.4.2 MEASUREMENT OF LIGHTNING ORIGINATED EMI ON WIND TURBINES

As current peak values of lightning strikes range from values of several tens of Amperes to more than 250 kA [16], with a frequency spectrum ranging from near DC to tens of megahertz [17], the respective lightning detection systems have to be sensitive within these parameter ranges. The most often used detection systems are based on Rogowski coils, shunt resistors or current transformers [18]. Rogowski coils are used to measure alternating currents. They consist of a helical wire coil with both terminals on one side of the coil. In wind turbines, they are wrapped around the down conductor of each blade in order to measure the lightning current flowing in the down conductors. The induced voltage in the coil is proportional to the current change rate in the conductor. Therefore the output of the Rogowski coil is connected to an integrator circuit to provide an output signal proportional to the lightning current.

Shunts consist of precision resistors used to measure DC or AC currents. At the shunt resistor, a voltage signal, proportional to the current, can be measured. Because of its frequency response, a shunt is well suited for lightning current measurements and the estimation of the related lightning parameters. To measure the lightning parameters for a wind turbine blade LPS, the shunt has to be placed in series to the down conductor. By means of an optical signal converter, it is possible to protect the shunt signal against any kind of lightning originated EMI.

The frequency range and accuracy of current transformers also depends on EMI as well as on the rating factor, temperature and physical configuration. A current transformer is designed to provide a current signal in its secondary winding. The signal is proportional to the current conducting in the primary winding. As they are able to safely insulate the measurement circuit from any primary signal, they are commonly used for metering and measuring electric signals.

For research purposes, different lightning current measurement systems have been installed in wind turbines on the Nikon-Kogen wind farm in Japan since 2003 [19]. All sensor types are installed within one turbine for comparison purposes.

Besides these lightning current measurement systems, two further commercial systems designed for lightning detection are on the market. The first one consists of magnetic cards that are to be placed in the blade or at any structure to measure the existence of lightning current [20]. After a lightning strike, these cards can be read out manually using a card reader unit in order to get information on the current peak. Originally, the system was been invented for lightning monitoring in buildings. The cards are not able to detect numerous lightning strikes between two card reading periods.

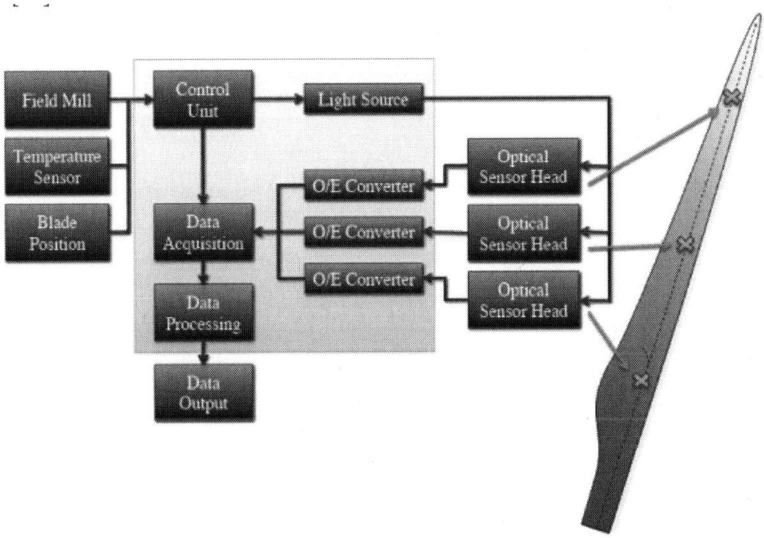

FIGURE 1: Fiber optic sensor network for monitoring lightning impacts on wind turbine blades [18].

A second state-of-the-art lightning detection system has been developed especially for wind turbines by the Association of Danish Energy Companies (DEFU) [21]. The system uses antennas on the wind turbine tower to detect lightning strikes. The antenna signal is transformed into an optical signal and transmitted to the control box via an optical fiber link. After a lightning strike and its detection by the system, it has to be reset by an acknowledgement signal. Lightning parameters like peak current and charge are not recorded.

A new lightning detection system for wind turbine blades merges the advantages of the state-of-the-art lightning current measurement systems with the one of the lightning detection system [22]. It is based on fiber optics and combines online monitoring of lightning current parameters with local lightning detection [18]. Beside the lightning parameters, the point of the lightning impact can be determined. The single sensor heads use the principle of Faraday rotation in ferromagnetic crystals, e.g., Yittrium-Iron Garnets (YIG), to measure magnetic field strengths. For a down conductor based LPS, a magnetic field is induced by the lightning current around the down conductor and the lightning channel. This field can be assessed by the law of Biot-Savart [23]. The general setup of the system is depicted in Figure 1. For a precise localization, a sampling rate of 2 MHz is necessary.

11.5 EXAMPLE TO DEFINE EMI ORIGINATING OF A WIND TURBINE USING METHOD-OF-MOMENTS

11.5.1 WIND TURBINE COMMUNICATION SYSTEM

Modern multi-megawatt wind turbines are equipped with a pitch control system for adjusting the blades' pitch angle. Rotation speed of the turbine is controlled by this system. Communication between the pitch control system in the rotating hub and wind turbine operator is realized over slip-rings at the turbine's main shaft. In case of a communication loss between turbine operators and the pitch control system a backup system is necessary. Such a backup communication system can be established with a GSM transmitter with an operating frequency of 900 MHz that is installed on the wind turbine hub.

11.5.2 FEKO MODEL

Using the commercial method-of-moments (MoM) simulation tool FEKO, a general simulation model of a multi megawatt wind turbine hub was generated [5]. A Hertzian dipole according to the approximation:

$$\Pi(\underline{x}) = \frac{e^{-jkr}}{4\pi\varepsilon_0 r} \int_V \underline{P_0}(\underline{x}') dV' \tag{2}$$

was used to excite the hub model with a GSM based frequency of 900 MHz, with polarization P_0 and the resulting radiated power P:

$$P = \Re\left\{2\pi \int_{0}^{\pi} T_r(r,\vartheta) r^2 \sin\vartheta d\vartheta\right\} \quad (3)$$

and the Poynting vector T_r [24]:

$$T_r = \frac{1}{2}\left(E_\vartheta H_\varphi^* - E_\varphi H_\vartheta^*\right) \quad (4)$$

with the electric and magnetic field components E_φ, E_ϑ, H_φ and H_ϑ.

The electromagnetic model is depicted in Figure 2. According to the wavelength of the GSM signal, the model has 67,744 elements. Model dimensions are 2.09 m × 2.60 m × 2.50 m. Material is cast iron with a relative permeability of μ_r = 1,500 and a conductivity of $\sigma_i = 1.03 \times 10^7$ S/m. Control boxes are simulated as stainless steel with a conductivity of $\sigma_s = 1.1 \times 10^6$ S/m. The man entrance to the hub is sealed by an aluminium plate with conductivity $\sigma_m = 3.816 \times 10^7$ S/m.

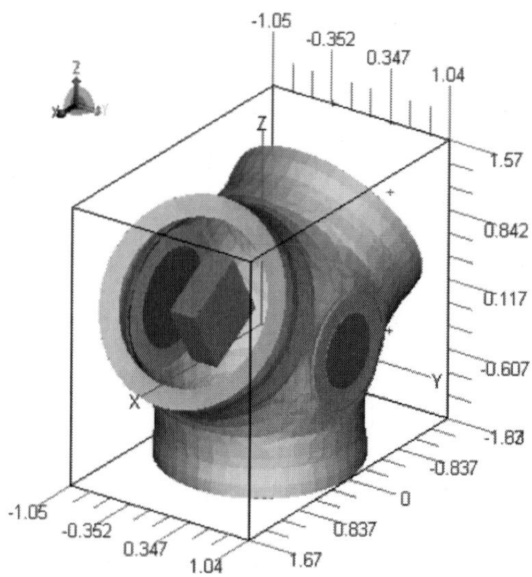

FIGURE 2: Electromagnetic model of wind turbine hub. Figures on the grid show the dimensions of the hub in meters.

For the calculation, the fast multipole method (FMM) was used in combination with the incomplete LU-matrix decomposition. The maximum number of iterations was set to be 10,000.

11.5.3 CAST IRON MATERIAL UNDER ELECTRO-MAGNETIC LOAD

For each of the three materials, the skin effect has been taken into account for the simulation according to [25]:

$$Z_{s,k} = \frac{1-j}{2\sigma_k \delta_k} \frac{1}{\tan\left((1-j)d_k/2\delta_k\right)} \quad (5)$$

with thickness d_k, σ_k as conductivity and skin depth δ_k for k representing either cast iron, stainless steel or aluminum.

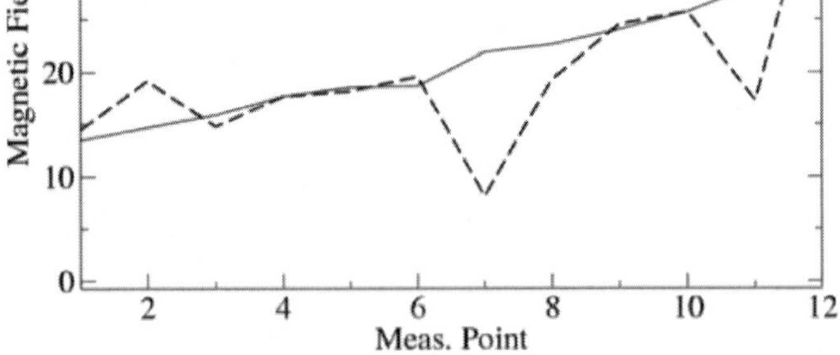

FIGURE 3: Comparison between measurements and simulations of magnetic fields inside a wind turbine hub due to injected current [5]. The solid line represents simulation results with FEKO while the dashed line connects the measured field values at discrete measurement points inside the hub

Magnetic field measurements inside the hub for injected currents of up to 1.3 kA were used to verify the simulation model, see Figure 3. Nonlinear material parameters have to be taken into account only for injected currents higher than 40 kA [5]. Therefore, nonlinear effects may be neglected for the GSM 900 MHz analysis of the cast iron hub.

Field measurements were performed according to Figure 4. An impulse current was injected into the cast iron hub in order to derive the field distribution inside. Field measurements inside the hub were made with a field probe based on the principle of induction. The measurement points 1–12 (see Figure 3) covered the maximum space possible due to probe requirements [5]. Injected currents were generated using a 1 MV impulse generator and were measured using a 4.2 mΩ shunt. The higher deviation between measurement and simulation at positions 7 and 11 in Figure 3 is due to EMI from the impulse generator and the connection lines which could only partly be implemented into the simulation model.

11.6 SIMULATION RESULTS

Wind turbines may cause EMI via three principal mechanisms, namely near field effects, diffraction and reflection/scattering. Near field effects refer to the potential of a wind turbine to cause interference due to electromagnetic fields emitted by the generator and switching components in the nacelle. Diffraction occurs when an object modifies an advancing wavefront by obstructing the wave path of travel. Diffraction effects can

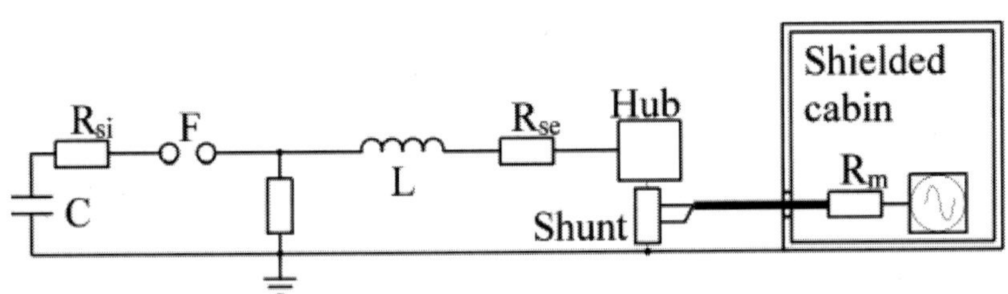

FIGURE 4: Laboratory setup for field measurements inside the wind turbine hub. A 1.2/50 μs impulse current with 1.3 kA amplitude was injected into the hub by an impulse generator.

occur when the object not only reflects part of the signal but also absorbs the signal.

Reflection/scattering interference occurs when turbines either reflect or obstruct signals between a transmitter and a receiver. This occurs because when the rotating blades of a wind turbine receive a primary transmitted signal they act to produce and transmit a scattered signal. In this situation a receiver may pick up two signals simultaneously, with the scattered signal causing EMI because it is delayed in time (out of phase) or distorted compared to the original signal.

The nature and amount of electromagnetic interference from each of these mechanism depends on:

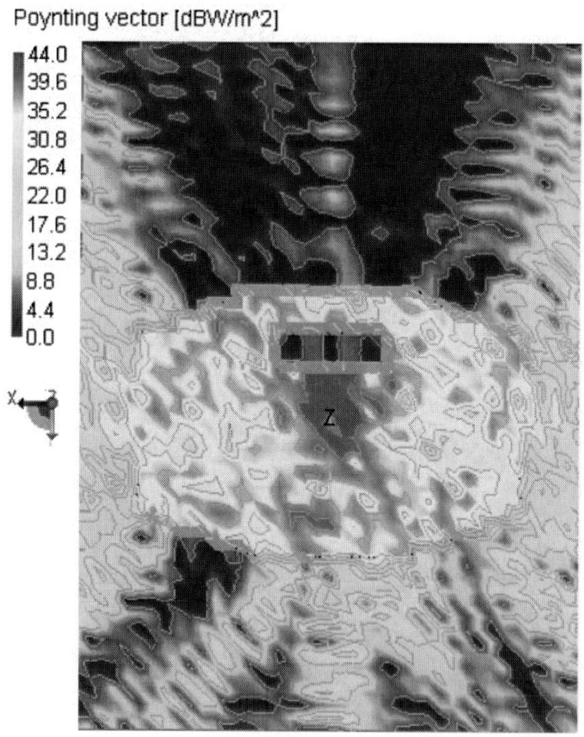

FIGURE 5: Poynting vector radiation pattern due to sinusoidal excitation of the Hertzian dipole with f = 900 MHz and I dl = 1. View is in negative z-direction according to Figure 2.

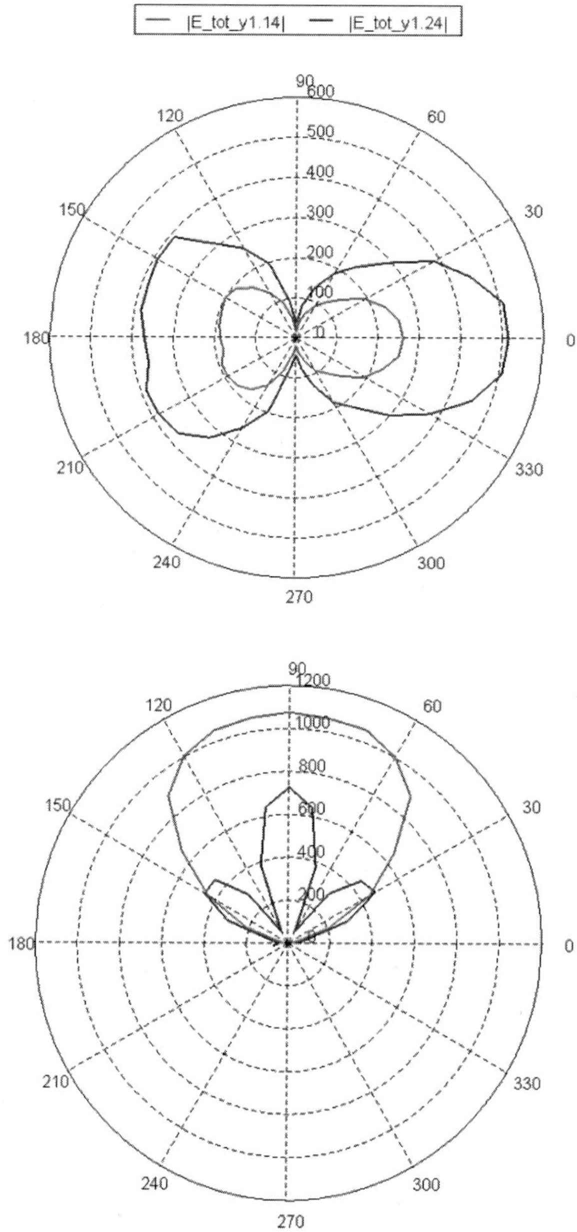

FIGURE 6: Comparison of the 2D radiation pattern of the electric Hertzian dipole at the positions $y_1 = 1.14$ m and $y_2 = 1.24$ m. Radiation frequency is 900 MHz with an amplitude of Idl = 1. Top: Radiation pattern for $\varphi = 0°$ and $\vartheta = 0°–360°$. Bottom: Radiation pattern for $\varphi = 0°–180°$ and $\vartheta = 90°$.

- Location of the mega-watt wind turbine relative to the transmitter and receiver
- Characteristics (design and used material) of the rotor blade
- Signal frequency
- Receiver characteristics
- Radio wave propagation characteristics in the local atmosphere

11.6.1 ANTENNA INSIDE HUB

For the first analysis, the electric Hertzian dipole used as GSM 900 MHz transmitter was placed in the center of the hub. This position would allow for the highest protection of the transmitter against all kinds of EMI, especially against lightning. Excitation is a sinusoidal wave with a magnitude of $Idl = 1$. The resulting Poynting vector inside the hub is depicted in Figure 5. According to Equation 5.2, the Poynting vector holds responsible for the radiated power of the electric Hertzian dipole.

As can be seen in Figure 5, the signal damping of the metallic structure is in the range of 20–40 dB. A good communication link between the transmitter inside the hub and an external receiver and vice versa cannot be established. Therefore the placement of communication transmitters and receivers inside the hub is not practicable.

11.6.2 ANTENNA OUTSIDE HUB

In contrast to the former model, the transmitting Hertzian dipole will now be installed outside the hub.

Because of the described scattering and diffraction effects that occur at wind turbines due to their rotation, the best possible installation point for the electric Hertzian dipole antenna is at the man entrance. An installation between the blades of the wind turbine is therefore not recommended.

For the simulation model this means that the communication unit is placed at positions with $y > 1$ m, for $z = 0$ m and $x = 0$ m. Two different positions of the electric Hertzian dipole were analysed: $y_1 = 1.14$ m and $y_2 = 1.24$ m. In Figure 6 the comparison between the two dimensional radiation patterns of the Hertzian dipole at y_1 and y_2 is given.

11.7 CONCLUSIONS

This paper presents a general overview on electromagnetic interference with respect to wind turbine related aspects. A wind turbine can act as both a transmitter and receiver of electromagnetic interference. The best way to protect a turbine against EMI is by shielding of sensitive components like the control systems. As an example of turbine-made EMI, a GSM 900 MHz transceiver used as communication backup-system for wind turbine control systems is analysed. Electro-magnetic fields resulting from this transmitter mounted on a large wind turbine hub are analysed analytically by method-of-moments. Using a commercial simulation tool, an optimized wireless communication link to a base station is determined. Placement of the GSM transmitter inside the cast iron hub would be preferable in order to minimize EMI due to lightning. Due to strong signal damping of 20–40 dB this is not practicable. The radiation diagrams show that the best position of the transmitter is at the man entrance. Simulations of the Hertzian dipole positioned at different locations show a strong directed radiation pattern, allowing for a good communication link between wind turbine hub and base station.

REFERENCES

1. Tennat, A.; Chambers, B. Radar Signature Control of Wind Turbine Generators. In Proceedings of the IEEE Antennas and Propagation Society International Symposium, Washington, DC, USA, July, 2005; pp. 489-492.
2. Sengupta, D.L. Electromagnetic Interference from Wind Turbines. In Proceedings of the IEEE Antennas and Propagation Society International Symposium, Orlando, FL, USA, July, 1999; pp. 1984-1986.
3. Cavecey, K.H.; Lee, L.Y. Television Interference due to Electromagnetic Scattering by the MOD-2 Wind Turbine Generators. In Proceedings of the IEEE Power Engineering Society Summer Meeting, Los Angeles, CA, USA, 1983.
4. Frye, A. The Effects of Wind Energy Turbines on Military Surveillance Radar Systems. In Proceedings of the German Radar Symposium, Berlin, Germany, 2000; pp. 415-422.
5. Lewke, B.; Krug, F.; Teichmann, R.; Loew, W.; Oberauer, A.; Kindersberger, J. The Influence of Lightning-Induced Field Distribution on the Pitch-Control-System of a Large Wind-Turbine Hub. In Proceedings of the European Wind Energy Conference, Athens, Greece, February, 2006.

6. Krug, F.; Rasmussen, J.R.; Bauer, R.F.; Lemieux, D.; Schram, Ch.; Ahmann, U. Wind Turbine/Generator Drivetrain Condition Based Monitoring. In Proceedings of the European Wind Energy Conference, London, UK, November, 2004.
7. Matsuzaki, R.; Todoroki, A. Wireless detection of internal delamination cracks in CFRP laminates using oscillating frequency changes. Composites Sci. Technol. 2005, 66, 407-416.
8. Krug, F.; Russer, P. Quasi-peak detector model for a time-domain measurement system. IEEE Trans. Electromagn. Compat. 2005, 47, 320-326.
9. Kodali, W.P. Principles, Measurements, Technologies, and Computer Models; Wiley: New York, NY, USA, 2001.
10. Middleton, D. Statistical-physical models of electromagnetic interference. IEEE Trans. Electromagn. Compat. 1977, 19, 106-127.
11. Davenport, W.B.; Root, W.L. An Introduction to the Theory of Random Signals and Noise; Wiley: New York, NY, USA, 1987.
12. Yoh, Y. A New lightning protection system for wind turbines using two ring-shaped electrodes. IEEJ Trans. Electr. Electron. Eng. 2006, 1, 314-319.
13. Gonschorek, K.H.; Singer, H. Elektromagnetische Verträglichkeit, 1st ed.; Teubner, B.G., Ed.; VDE-Verl: Stuttgart, Germany, 1992.
14. Smolke, M. Beitrag zur Wirkung aperturbehafteter Schirme bei magnetischen Blitzimpulsfeldern. Ph.D. Thesis, Technical University of Dresden, Dresden, Germany, 1999.
15. Krug, F.; Russer, P. The time-domain electromagnetic interference measurement system. IEEE Trans. Electromagn. Compat. 2003, 45, 330-338.
16. Diendorfer, G.; Mair, M.; Pichler, H. Blitzstrommessung am Sender Gaisberg. Schriftenreihe der Forschung im Verbund 2005, 89, 1-65.
17. Rakov, V.A. Transient response of a tall object to lightning. IEEE Trans. Electromagn. Compat. 2001, 43, 654-661.
18. Krämer, S.; Puente Léon, F.; Lewke, B.; Méndez Hernández, Y. Lightning Impact Classification on Wind Turbine Blades Using Fiber Optic Measurement Systems. In Proceedings of the Windpower Conference, Los Angeles, CA, USA, June, 2007.
19. Wada, A.; Yokoyama, S.; Hachiya, K.; Hirose, T. Observational Results of Lightning Flashes on the Nikaho-Kogen Wind Farm in Winter (2003-2004). In Proceedings of the XIVth International Symposium on High Voltage Engineering, Tsinghua University, Beijing, China, August, 2005; p. B26.
20. OBO Bettermann GmbH & Co. Kg. Vorrichtung zur Erfassung von Stossströmen an Blitzableitern oder dergleichen, utility patent, DE000009400656U1, 1995.
21. Sørensen, T.; Jensen, F.V.; Raben, N.; Lykkegaard, J.; Saxov, J. Lightning Protection for Offshore Wind Turbines. In Proceedings of the 28th International Conference of Lightning Protection, Kanazawa, Japan, 2006; pp. 555-560.
22. Krämer, S.; Puente Léon, F.; Lewke, B. Use of a Fiber-Optic Sensor System to Review Distributed Magnetic Field Simulation of a Wind Turbine. In Proceedings of the Asia-Pacific Symposium on Electromagnetic Compatibility, Singapore, 2008; pp. 192-195.
23. Jackson, J.D. Klassische Elektrodynamik, 3rd ed.; de Gruyter: Berlin, Germany, 2002.

24. Zinke, O.; Brunswig, H. Hochfrequenztechnik 1–Hochfrequenzfilter, Leitungen, Antennen, 6th ed.; Springer Verlag: Berlin, Germany, 2000.
25. EM Software and Systems. FEKO User Manual, Suite 5.2; Stellenbosch, South Africa, 2006.

CHAPTER 12

NOISE POLLUTION PREVENTION IN WIND TURBINES: STATUS AND RECENT ADVANCES

OFELIA JIANU, MARC A. ROSEN, AND GREG NATERER

12.1 INTRODUCTION

Global warming and greenhouse gas emissions are of great concern. To reduce such emissions, there is a global trend towards cleaner energy sources. Promising alternatives for coal and other fossil fuels are nuclear power and renewable energy sources. One of the most promising renewable sources is wind energy. However, concerns exist with wind turbine technology, and one of the main ones is in the noise that occurs during operation. In order to successfully reduce or prevent the noise generated, the sources of noise must be identified. Two major sources of noise are present during operation: mechanical and aerodynamic. Mechanical noise generally originates from the many different components within the wind turbine, such as the generator, the hydraulic systems and the gearbox. Various mechanical noise prevention strategies exist, such as vibration suppression, vibration isolation and fault detection techniques, which will be described in this paper. Prevention strategies for aerodynamic noise are also discussed because it is the dominant source of noise from wind turbines. The largest contribution to aerodynamic noise comes from the trailing edge of wind turbine blades. Strategies for reducing aerodynamic noise include adaptive solutions and wind turbine blade modification methods. Adaptive noise reduction techniques include varying the speed of rotation of the blades and increasing the pitch angle. Although such strategies have been successfully implemented for noise reduction purposes, they can cause significant power loss. Therefore, alternative adaptive solutions are sought. Blade modification methods such as adding serrations have proven to be beneficial in reducing noise without any power loss.

This paper is organized as follows: noise sources are discussed in Section 2, noise reduction strategies are presented in Section 3 and conclusions are given in Section 4. Section 2 is subdivided into mechanical noise and aerodynamic noise. Section 3 is subdivided into mechanical noise reduction strategies, aerodynamic noise reduction strategies and use of exergy methods.

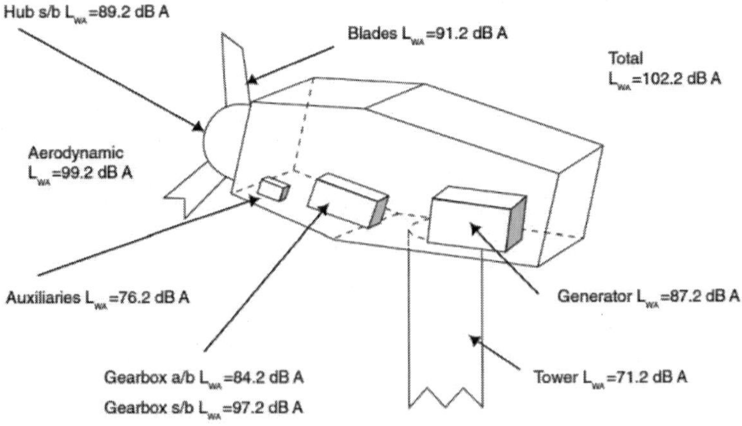

FIGURE 1: Horizontal axis wind turbine noise sources [2].

12.2 NOISE SOURCES

Wind turbines have many components that generate noise. The noise disturbances by wind turbines are related to such factors as distance between the wind turbine and populated areas as well as the background noise where the wind turbine is operating [1]. Operating conditions and maintenance of the wind turbine also affect noise production [1]. In general, there are two main categories of noise sources for wind turbines: mechanical and aerodynamic. In this section, we briefly examine mechanical noise and its causes and solutions but aerodynamic noise is the main focus as it is considered the most significant form of noise and the most difficult to address. Figure 1 shows the different sources of noise and their respective sound power levels; a/b refers to airborne noise and s/b refers to structural noise [2].

12.2.1 MECHANICAL NOISE

Mechanical noise generally originates from the components within the wind turbine, such as the generator, the hydraulic systems and the gearbox. Other elements such as fans, inlets/outlets and ducts also contribute to mechanical noise. The type of noise produced by these mechanical components tends to be more tonal and narrowband in nature, which is more irritating for humans than broadband sound [1]. While the total wind turbine sound pressure level (SPL) only incurs a minor increase due to this noise, the penalty it places on wind turbines is much greater. Many countries have regulations which stipulate distances between wind turbines and the nearest buildings must be increased, or in some cases, outright refusal of installation, due to the negative impact of this noise on humans [1]. There are two ways in which mechanical noise is transmitted: airborne or structural. Airborne noise is straightforward, as the sound is directly emitted to the surroundings. Structural noise is more complex as it can be transmitted along the structure of the turbine and then into the surroundings through different surfaces, such as the casing, the nacelle cover, and the rotor blades [2]. The drive gearbox is a significant source of noise in wind turbines. The structure based noise generated by the tooth mesh propagates through the roller bearings of the gearbox and through the impact noise insulation to the nacelle bedplate and finally to the tower.

12.2.2 AERODYNAMIC NOISE

Aerodynamic noise is more complex and, as can be seen from Figure 1 it is the dominant source of noise from wind turbines, with a sound power level of 99.2 dB A [2].

In general, there are six main regions along the blade (see Figure 2) [1–8]. These regions are considered to create independently their own specific noises, because the noises produced are fundamentally different and, since they occur in different regions along the blade, they do not interfere with each other [5]. The six regions are classified into turbulent boundary layer trailing edge noise, laminar boundary layer vortex shedding noise, separation stall noise, trailing edge bluntness vortex shedding noise, tip vortex formation noise and noise due to turbulent inflow.

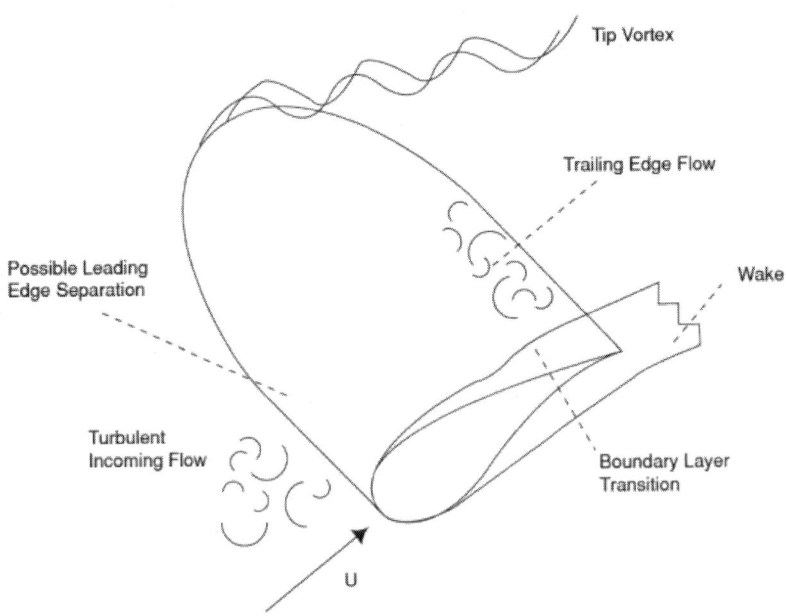

FIGURE 2: Aerodynamic noise sources around a rotor blade due to wind flow with velocity, U [6].

In general, there are six main regions along the blade (see Figure 2) [1–8]. These regions are considered to create independently their own specific noises, because the noises produced are fundamentally different and, since they occur in different regions along the blade, they do not interfere with each other [5]. The six regions are classified into turbulent boundary layer trailing edge noise, laminar boundary layer vortex shedding noise, separation stall noise, trailing edge bluntness vortex shedding noise, tip vortex formation noise and noise due to turbulent inflow.

12.2.2.1 TURBULENT BOUNDARY LAYER TRAILING EDGE NOISE (TBL-TE)

A predominant source of noise, turbulent boundary layer trailing edge noise (TBL-TE), results from the interaction of the boundary layer and the trailing edge of the airfoil, as depicted in Figure 3. Brooks and Hodgson [9] developed a predictor for TBL-TE using measured surface pressures. This predictor can be implemented provided sufficient information about the TBL convective surface pressure field passing the TE is available.

Schlinker and Amiet [10] employed a generalized empirical description of surface pressure to predict measured noise. An approach to model the turbulence within boundary layers as a sum of "hairpin" vortex elements was presented by Langley [6]. Ffowcs and Hall [11] present a simpler approach to the TBL-TE noise problem, based on an edge-scatter formulation. It has been found that the overall sound pressure level depends on velocity to the fifth power, through a number of studies [12]. Also, the Reynolds number and angle of attack have been shown to influence the

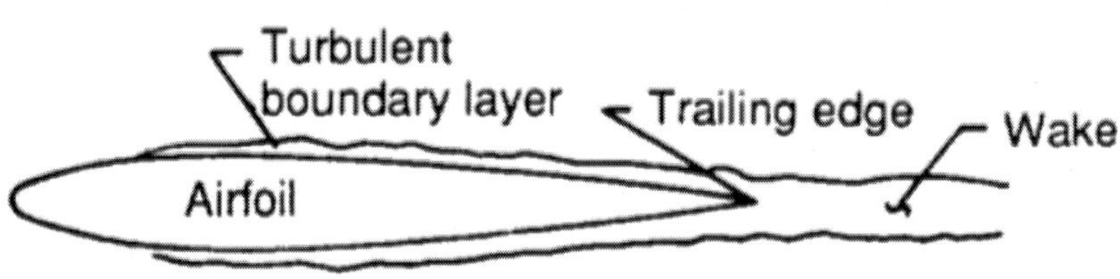

FIGURE 3: Turbulent boundary layer trailing edge noise [6].

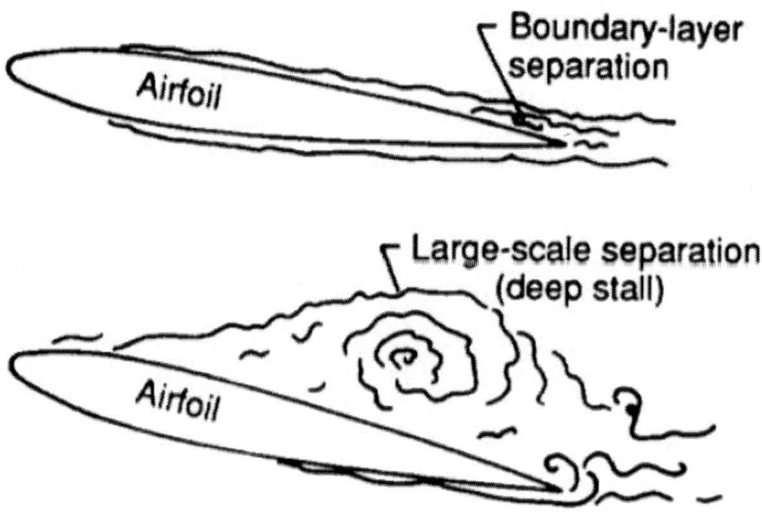

FIGURE 4: Separation-stall noise [6].

turbulent structure [10,13]. Romero-Sanz and Matesanz [2] determined that TBL-TE noise can occur on both the suction and pressure sides of the airfoil and it is affected by the surface finish of the airfoil.

12.2.2.2 SEPARATION-STALL NOISE

Separation-stall noise occurs when the angle of attack increases from moderate to high as depicted in Figure 4. Since wind turbine airfoils operate at high angles of attack for significant portions of time, this source of noise is of significant interest. As the angle of attack increases, the boundary layer on the suction side increases and large-scale unsteady structures begin to form. It has been found that in such cases the noise increases by more than 10 dB relative to TBL-TE noise [4]. It has also been determined through far-field cross correlations that the noise is emitted from the trailing edge for mildly separated flow and from the chord for large-scale separation [13]. Empirical relations for separated-stall noise have been determined, and they are similar to those for TBL-TE noise with different scaling factors [2].

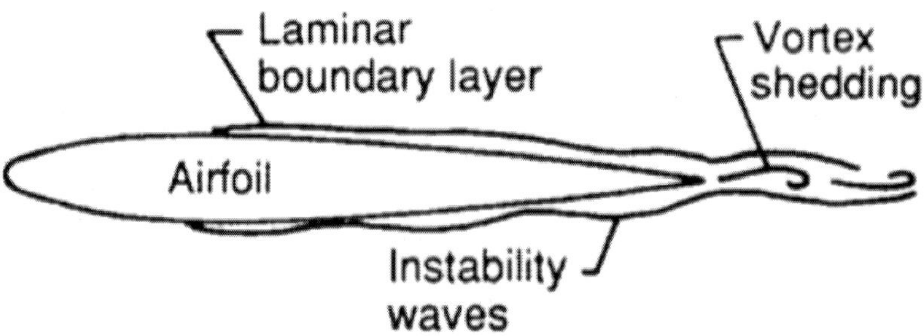

FIGURE 5: Laminar-boundary-layer vortex shedding noise [6].

12.2.2.3 LAMINAR-BOUNDARY-LAYER VORTEX-SHEDDING (LBL VS) NOISE

This type of self-noise occurs when a laminar boundary layer is present over most or one side of the airfoil, as shown in Figure 5. The noise from this source is coupled to acoustically excited feedback loops taken between the trailing edge and instability waves (Tolmien-Schlichting waves) upstream of the trailing edge [6,7,14–19]. Pressure waves due to vortex shedding leaving the trailing edge propagate upstream and instabilities are amplified in the boundary layer. A feedback loop is created when the instabilities reach the trailing edge and vortices with similar frequency content form.

12.2.2.4 TIP VORTEX FORMATION NOISE

Unlike other noise sources due to its three dimensionality, this source of self-noise results from the interaction of the thick viscous turbulent core tip vortex with the trailing edge near the tip (see Figure 6) [6]. Experimental studies have isolated tip noise quantitatively [20]. A prediction model based on spectral data from delta wing studies, mean flow studies of several tip shapes and trailing edge noise analysis was proposed by George and Chou [13]. A relation for an untwisted, constant chord blade was also developed by Brooks, Pope and Marcolini [6,12,20].

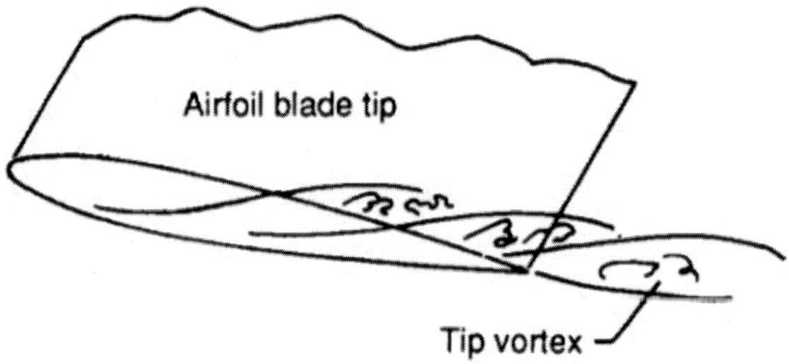

FIGURE 6: Tip vortex formation noise [6].

12.2.2.5 TRAILING-EDGE-BLUNTNESS VORTEX-SHEDDING NOISE

Another important source of noise as determined by Brooks and Hodgson [9] is noise due to vortex shedding from blunt trailing edges, as represented in Figure 7. The frequency and amplitude of this noise source is given by the geometry of the trailing edge [2]. Empirical relations to predict this type of noise have been developed, and they are dependent on the trailing edge thickness and proportional to the sixth power of the velocity [2].

12.2.2.6 TURBULENT INFLOW NOISE

At low frequencies, the interaction of the turbulent inflow with the leading edge of the turbine blades proves to be a significant source of noise. Figure 2 illustrates such sources of noise. Romero-Sanz [2] determined that depending on the size of the length scale relative to the leading edge radius of the airfoil, a dipole noise source (low frequency) or a quadrupole noise source (high frequency) could be created. Furthermore, the dipole noise source is dependent on the Mach number to the sixth power whereas the scattered quadrupole noise source is dependent on the Mach number to the fifth power [2]. Empirical relations have been developed by Lowson

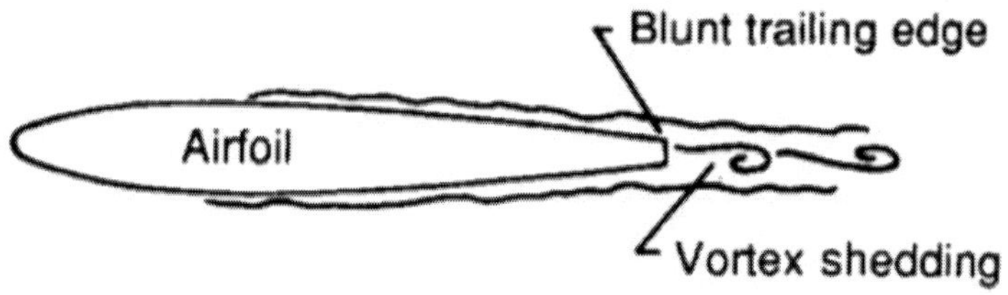

FIGURE 7: Trailing-edge-bluntness vortex-shedding noise [6].

[21] for both low and high frequencies, based on the experimental results of Amiet [22].

12.3 NOISE REDUCTION STRATEGIES

There are many ways in which sound can be reduced. One is to design the wind turbine with acoustic behaviors in mind. Researchers are focused on reducing noise without affecting the power generated by the wind turbine. Strategies for reducing mechanical and aerodynamic noise will be discussed in this section.

12.3.1 MECHANICAL NOISE REDUCTION

One source of mechanical noise is vibrations induced by the rotating components. Vibration control is used to suppress or eliminate unwanted vibrations. Depending on the case, different control laws can be chosen in order to minimize unwanted vibration. Additionally, damping or increasing the effective mass can be realized by the controller [23]. Inferentially, the absorber works as an active system. This includes the use of sound isolating materials, insulation, and closing the holes in the nacelles which would decrease the sound transmitted to the air [6]. Aside from loss of power and increased maintenance costs, faulty gearboxes also increase noise levels in wind turbines. As a result, researchers are developing fault diagnostic systems for gearboxes with applications to wind turbines. A system has been developed to integrate singular value decomposition noise reduction, time-frequency analysis and order analysis methods in order to identify weak faults objectively and effectively [24]. More recently, efforts have been taken to develop intelligent techniques for online condition monitoring in machinery systems such as wind turbines. Several neural fuzzy classification techniques have been proposed for fault detection [25–29].

12.3.2 AERODYNAMIC NOISE REDUCTION

12.3.2.1 ADAPTIVE APPROACHES

There are a number of adaptive noise reduction approaches for aerodynamic noise, including varying the speed of rotation of the blades. Since an increase in rotational speed will also lead to increased noise production, lowering the rotational speed will lead to decreased sound. However the rotational speed decrease reduces power output, and therefore should only be implemented within a certain range of wind velocities, since high winds also have the added benefit of masking the sound of the wind turbine with the sound of the wind itself [2]. The pitch angle of the wind turbine blades also has an important role in noise production. An increase in pitch angle will lead to a reduction in the angle of attack. As the angle of attack increases, the size of the turbulent boundary layer on the suction side of the airfoil grows, thereby increasing noise production in the wind turbine. Therefore, if the pitch angle is increased, a thinner boundary layer results on the suction side, which is considered the strongest source of noise production [2]. This also implies that, on the pressure side, the effect is the opposite; therefore when using this method for noise control, it is important to find the appropriate pitch angle range for optimal noise control. As with the previous method, the major drawback to this adaptive noise control method is the corresponding reduction of power since the angle of attack is decreased. Despite a potential loss in power due to pitch angle changes that reduce noise, more wind turbines can potentially be built within a specified area [2].

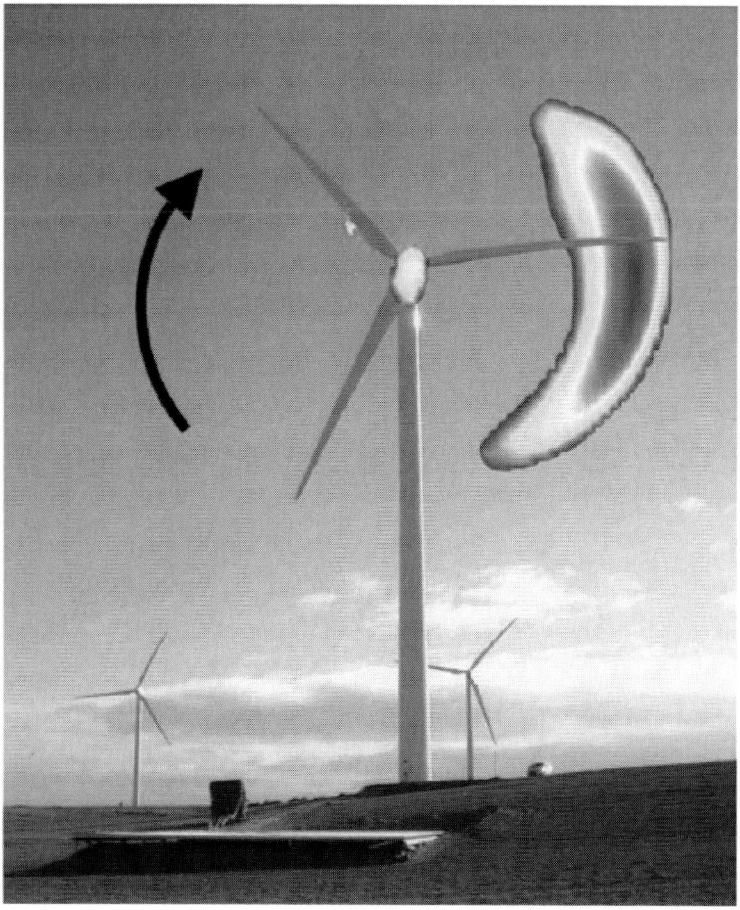

FIGURE 8: Area on a turbine blade with largest sound production [2].

12.3.2.2 WIND TURBINE BLADE MODIFICATION METHODS

The main drawback to adaptive methods (an overall reduction of power) is a hindrance to that method of noise control. By breaking down the noise sources it can be seen that the maximum noise contribution occurs within the trailing edge [30,31]. Different aeroacoustic prediction models such as semi-empirical airfoil self-noise models and simplified theoretical models are available in the literature [32]. Kamruzzaman et al. [32] presented results using a well-known TNO-Blake model with Computational Aeroacoustics (CAA) and validated the predictions against wind tunnel measurements. The predictions are based on Reynolds Averaged Navier-Stokes simulation results. Such predictions are beneficial in determining the region with the highest aeroacoustic levels. Researchers established that the region between about 75–95% span is exposed to the maximum flow velocities and it has the highest aero-acoustic noise levels [30]. Furthermore, experimental tests showed that most of the noise is generated when the blade is moving downwards in a clockwise rotation, as shown in Figure 8. Therefore, the majority of modification procedures are aimed at reducing the noise in this area. Research had been conducted into the

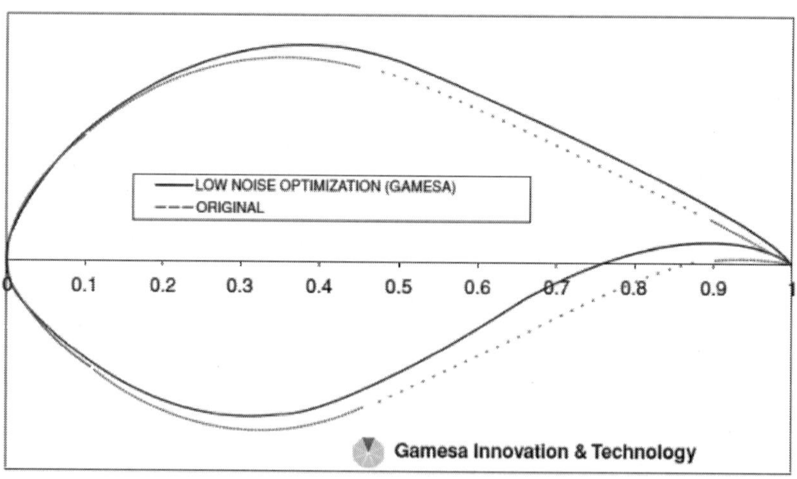

FIGURE 9: Comparison between original and optimized airfoil [2].

use of aero-acoustically optimized airfoils and trailing edge serration [5], while trailing edge brushes have also been considered to control the noise generated from this portion of wind turbine blades [31].

Many studies have focused on reducing noise from the trailing edge. One such method is through acoustically optimized airfoils. The "silent rotors by acoustic optimization" (SIROCCO) project was conducted in 2003–2007 in Europe [5], and involves having silent airfoils replace existing airfoils in the outer part of a baseline blade in the areas exposed to maximum flow velocities and highest aero-acoustic noise levels between 75–95% span. The airfoil design is shown in Figure 9. The SIROCCO project aimed to modify existing blades with a different trailing edge in the outer region of the blade, so designing an airfoil anew would lead to enhanced performance [5]. This project studied two different wind turbines: the Gamesa 850 kW turbine (G58) in Zaragoza, Spain with a rotor diameter of 58 m, and the GE 2.3 MW turbine in Wieringermeer, Netherlands, with a rotor diameter of 94 m. The acoustically optimized airfoils were initially tested in wind tunnels and then mounted on their respective turbines. Both turbines were tested using a hybrid rotor, and two baseline blades with one modified SIROCCO blade, which allowed for direct comparison of noise production with similar conditions (since all blades were on the same rotor).

The noise reduction was found to be about 1–1.5 dB A for the G58 with a chord-based Reynolds number of 1.6×10^6 and 2–3 dB A for the GE94 with a chord-based Reynolds number of 3×10^6. It was difficult to analyze the aerodynamic performance differences since only 1 blade is different in the hybrid rotor. However, the power production of the hybrid rotor on the G54 with an average wind speed of 8 m/s was reduced by 1.4%, which was below the measurement uncertainty, but which the study attributed to an erosion trip used on the SIROCCO blade, and not due to the modification. For the GE94 turbine, the power production was higher than baseline; 2.8% annual energy production at an average wind speed of 8 m/s [1].

In addition to having a SIROCCO blade, one of the blades on the GE turbine incorporated serrations on the baseline blades, as shown in Figure 10. The serrations were 2 mm thick, and mounted on the outer 12.5 m of the blade (on the pressure side). They were smoothed out using an epoxy filler to maintain the aerodynamics of the blade. The lengths of the serra-

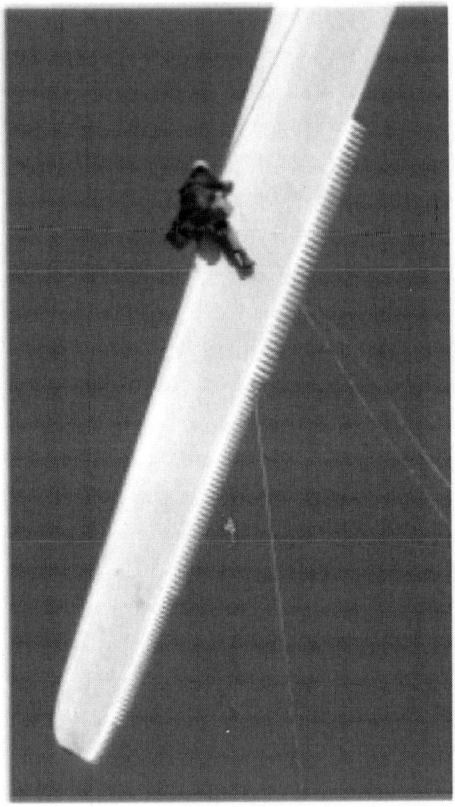

FIGURE 10: Trailing edge serrations [31].

tions occurred from about 20% of the local chord, and varied as a function of radius. For example, they had a 10 cm tooth length at the tip and 30 cm at the most inboard position. The plane of serrations aligned with the flow direction at the blade trailing edge to maintain the aerodynamics of the blade. These serrations were found to reduce the noise by about 3.2 dB A at low frequencies. At higher frequencies, however, the noise production from the serrations is actually higher than the baseline blade [31]. The bluntness of the trailing edge also contributes to the overall noise production. The thickness of the trailing edge causes vortices which in turn generate sound.

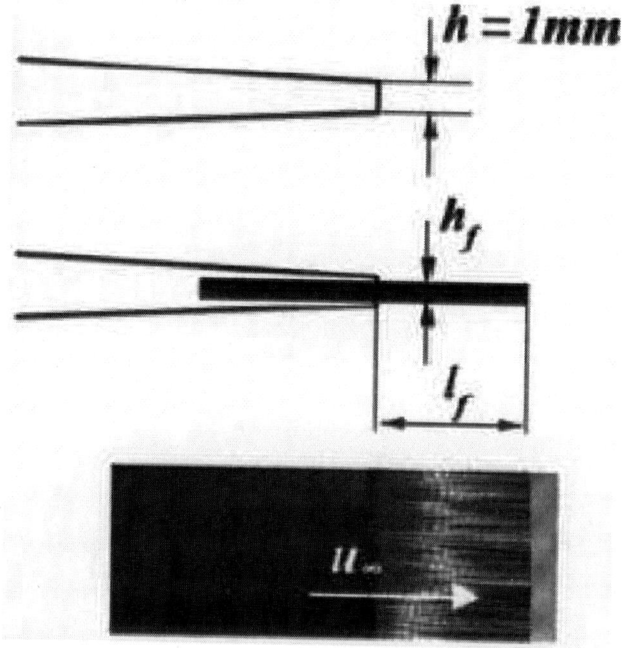

FIGURE 11: Trailing edge brushes [6].

In order to minimize this effect, a single row of polypropylene fibres can be connected to the trailing edge, as shown in Figure 11. These brushes work similar to serrations, except that the tip angles in this case are extremely sharp. These brushes can reduce the sound by an amount depending on the brush design characteristics. Three fibre lengths lf (15, 30 and 60 mm) and fibre diameters hf (0.3, 0.4, 0.5 mm) are considered [33]. These brushes were aligned automatically with trailing edge flow and showed significant noise reduction. Depending on the configuration and frequency, noise reductions from 2 to 10 dB were achieved. A possible problem to research with this modification is how well these brushes will perform in different weather conditions, such as snow and ice.

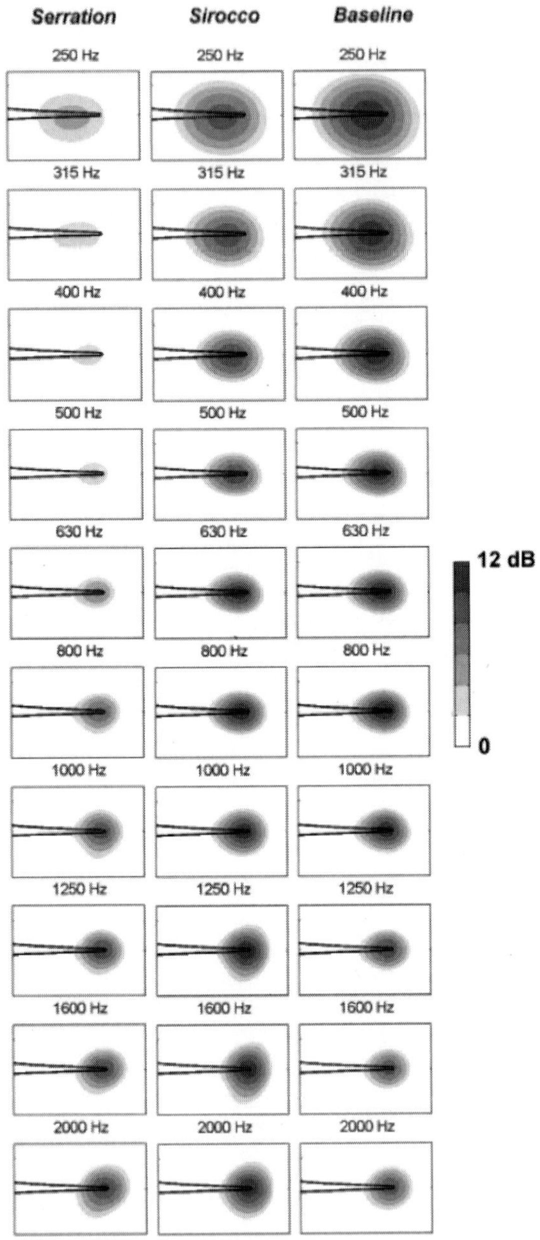

FIGURE 12: Comparison of serrations vs. sirocco and baseline [30].

As shown in Figure 12, the serrations and optimized airfoils work very well at low frequencies, but in fact produce more noise at higher frequencies. At present, wind turbines contain controllers which control the angle of attack to optimize the power generation of the turbine [1]. Similar controllers could be used to change the blade between the different modes, such as using serrations at low frequencies, and then retracting them at higher frequencies to reduce the noise production at high frequencies. Furthermore, trailing edge brushes have been found to work well at high frequencies. In future designs, trailing edge brushes could be incorporated into blade design and, with a controller, could be retracted so they would only function within a specific frequency range.

12.3.3 USE OF EXERGY METHODS

An investigation has been undertaken by the authors to correlate the noise pollution to exergy, a factor not normally used to design wind turbine airfoils. The main objective was to determine a correlation between the sound pressure level resulting from flow over a solid object and the exergy destroyed within the fluid medium. This correlation has the potential to reveal relationships between noise pollution and exergy destruction. Such correlation may be useful in efforts to minimize noise pollution in commercial wind turbines.

12.4 CONCLUSIONS

Noise production in wind turbines and recent advances to prevent it have been critically reviewed and compared. To successfully reduce or prevent the noise generation, the sources of noise must be identified. Two major sources of noise are present during operation: mechanical and aerodynamic. Mechanical noise generally originates from the many different components within the wind turbine, such as the generator, the hydraulic systems and the gearbox. Different mechanical noise prevention strategies such as vibration suppression, vibration isolation and fault detection techniques are utilized for this type of noise. Aerodynamic noise is the dominant source of noise from wind turbines. It occurs at high velocities when turbulent boundary layers develop over the airfoil and they pass over the trailing edge or at lower velocities as a result of laminar boundary layers leading to vortex shedding at the trailing edge. Other factors presented include flow separation and blunt trailing edge flow leading to vortex shedding. Strategies for reducing aerodynamic noise include adaptive approaches and wind turbine blade modification methods.

REFERENCES

1. Klug, H. Noise from Wind Turbines: Standards and Noise Reduction Procedures. Paper presented on the Forum Acusticum, Sevilla, Spain, 16–20 September 2002.
2. Romero-Sanz, I.; Matesanz, A. Noise management on modern wind turbines. Wind Eng. 2008, 32, 27–44.
3. Oerlemans, S.; Sijtsma, P.; Mendez Lopez, B. Location and quantification of noise sources on a wind turbine. J. Sound Vib. 2007, 299, 869–883.
4. Moriarty, P.; Migliore, P. Semi-Empirical Aeroacoustic Noise Prediction Code for Wind Turbines; National Renewable Energy Laboratory: Golden, CO, USA, 2003.
5. Schepers, J.G.; Curvers, A.; Oerlemans, S.; Braun, K.; Lutz, T.; Herrig, A.; Wuerz, W.; Mantesanz, A.; Garcillan, L.; Fischer, M.; et al. SIROCCO: Silent Rotors by Acoustic Optimization. Presented at the Second International Meeting on Wind Turbine Noise, Lyon, France, 20–21 September 2007; ECN-M-07-064.
6. Brooks, T.F.; Pope, D.S.; Marcolini, M.A. Airfoil Self-Noise and Prediction; NASA Reference Publication 1218; National Aeronautics and Space Administration, Washinton, DC, USA, 1989.
7. Leloudas, G.; Zhu, W.J.; Sorensen, J.N.; Shen, W.Z.; Hjort, S. Prediction and reduction of noise from 2.3 MW wind turbine. J. Phys. Conf. Ser. 2007, 75, doi:10.1088/1742-6596/75/1/012083.
8. Oerlemans, S.; Schepers, J.G. Prediction of wind turbine noise and validation against experiment. Int. J. Aeroacoustics 2009, 8, 555–584.
9. Brooks, T.F.; Hodgson, T.H. Trailing edge noise prediction from measured surface pressures. J. Sound Vib. 1981, 78, 69–117.
10. Schlinker, R.H.; Amiet, R.K. Helicopter Rotor Trailing Edge Noise; NASA CR-3470; NASA: Washington, DC, USA, 1981.
11. Ffowcs Williams, J.E.; Hall, L.H. Aerodynamic sound generation by turbulent flow in the vicinity of a scattering half plane. J. Fluid Mech. 1970, 40, 657–670.
12. Brooks, T.F.; Marcolini, M.A. Scaling of airfoil self-noise using measured flow parameters. AIAA J. 1985, 23, 207–213.
13. Chou, S.-T.; George, A.R. Effect of angle of attack on rotor trailing-edge noise. Am. Inst. Aeronautics Astronaut. J. 1984, 22, 1821–1823.
14. Paterson, R.W.; Amiet, R.K.; Munch, C.L. Isolated airfoil-tip vortex interaction noise. J. Aircraft 1975, 12, 34–40.

15. George, A.R.; Najjar, F.E.; Kim, Y.N. Noise Due to Tip Vortex Formation on Lifting Rotors. In Proceedings of the 6th Aeroacoustics Conference on American Institute of Aeronautics and Astronautics, Hartford, CT, USA, 4–6 June 1980.
16. Arakawa, C.; Fleig, O.; Iida, M.; Shimooka, M. Numerical approach for noise reduction of wind turbine blade tip with earth simulator. J. Earth Simul. 2005, 2, 11–33.
17. Tam, C.K.W. Discrete tones of isolated air-foils. J. Acoust. Soc. Am. 1974, 55, 1173–1177.
18. Fink, M.R. Fine structure of airfoil tone frequency. J. Acoust. Soc. Am. 1978, 63, doi:10.1121/1.2016551.
19. Wright, S.E. The acoustic spectrum of axial flow machines. J. Sound Vib. 1976, 45, 165–223.
20. Brooks, T.F.; Marcolini, M.A. Airfoil tip vortex formation noise. Am. Inst. Aeronautics Astronaut. J. 1986, 24, 246–252.
21. Lowson, M. Assessment and Prediction of Wind Turbine Noise; Flow Solutions Report 92/19, ETSU W/13/00284/REP; Energy Technology Support Unit: Harwell, UK, September 1992.
22. Amiet, R. Acoustic radiation from an airfoil in a turbulent stream. J. Sound Vib. 1975, 41, 407–420.
23. Kelly, S.G. Fundamentals of Mechanical Vibrations, 2nd ed.; McGraw Hill: New York, NY, USA, 2000.
24. Wang, F.; Zhang, L.; Zhang, B.; Zhang, Y.; He, L. Development of Wind Turbine Gearbox Data Analysis and Fault Diagnosis System. In Proceedings of the Power and Energy Engineering Conference (APPEEC), Whan, China, 25–28 March 2011.
25. Angelov, P.; Filev, D. An approach to online identification of Takagi-Sugeno fuzzy models. IEEE Trans. Syst. Man Cyber. Part B 2004, 34, 484–498.
26. Song, Q.; Kasabov, N. NFI—Neuro-fuzzy inference method for transductive reasoning and applications for prognostic systems. IEEE Trans. Fuzzy Syst. 2005, 13, 799–808.
27. Kasabov, N.; Song, Q. DENFIS: Dynamic, evolving neural-fuzzy inference systems and its application for time-series prediction. IEEE Trans. Fuzzy Syst. 2002, 10, 144–154.
28. Wang, W.; Ismail, F.; Golnaraghi, F. A neuro-fuzzy approach for gear system monitoring. IEEE Trans. Fuzzy Syst. 2004, 12, 710–723.
29. Jianu, O. An Evolving Neural Fuzzy Classifier for Machinery Diagnostics. M.Sc. Thesis, Lakehead University, Thunder Bay, ON, Canada, 2010.
30. Oerlemans, S.; Schepers, J.G.; Guidati, G.; Wagner, S. Experimental Demonstration of Wind Turbine Noise Reduction Through Optimized Airfoil Shape and Trailing Edge Serrations. In Proceedings of the European Wind Energy Conference and Exhibition, Copenhagen, Denmark, 2–6 July 2001.
31. Oerlemans, S. Reduction of Wind Turbine Noise Using Optimized Airfoils and Trailing-Edge Serrations. In Proceedings of the 14th AIAA/CEAS Aeroacoustics Conference, Vancouver, BC, Canada, 5–7 May 2008.
32. Kamruzzaman, M.; Lutz, T.; Wurtz, W.; Shen, W.Z.; Zhu, W.J.; Hansen, M.O.L.; Bertagnolio, F.; Madsen, H.A. Validations and improvements of airfoil trailing-edge noise prediction models using detailed experimental data. Wind Energy 2012, 15, 45–61.

33. Herr, M. Experimental study on noise reduction through trailing edge brushes. New Results Numer. Exp. Fluid Mech. V 2006, 92, 365–372.

AUTHOR NOTES

CHAPTER 2

Acknowledgments

This work was supported by five organizations including a Grant-in-Aids for Scientific Research, No.14205139, sponsored by the Ministry of Education, Culture, Sports, Science and Technology, Japan, Environment Protection Research sponsored by the Sumitomo Fund, Fluid Machinery Research sponsored by the Harada Memorial Fund, and the Program and Project for Education and Research of Kyushu University. It was also supported by NEDO (New Energy Development Organization) of the Ministry of Economy, Trade and Industry. We gratefully acknowledge our laboratory staff, Messrs. N. Fukamachi and K. Watanabe, Research Institute for Applied Mechanics, Kyushu University, for their great cooperation in the experiments and data analysis.

CHAPTER 5

Acknowledgments

The authors are grateful to Ontario Power Authority (OPA), Ontario Centres of Excellence (OCE), and University of Ottawa for their financial support of this project.

CHAPTER 6

Acknowledgments

The authors wish to acknowledge the support from the Research Council of Norway through the Centre for Ships and Ocean Structures at the Norwegian University of Science and Technology in Trondheim, Norway. The gearbox and wind turbine model was obtained courtesy of the Gearbox Reliability Collaborative (GRC) project at the National Renewable

Energy Laboratory, Golden, CO, USA. The GRC initiative is funded by the Wind and Water Power Program of the United States Department of Energy.

CHAPTER 7

Acknowledgments

This paper was supported by the Fundamental Research Funds for the Chinese Central University under Grant 12MS58 and National Natural Science Foundation of China under Grant 61074094.

CHAPTER 8

Acknowledgments

This work was supported by the National Research Foundation of Korea (NRF) grant funded by the Korea government(MEST) (No. 2011-0012420).

CHAPTER 9

Acknowledgments

We want to express our deepest gratitude to the reviewers. We believe our manuscript was greatly strengthened in responding to their valuable comments and suggestions. This work was supported by the Ministerio de Ciencia e Innovaci´on projects numbers DPI2011- 27567-C02 and DPI2011-28033-C03-01.

CHAPTER 10

Acknowledgments

The work described in this paper has been supported in part by the Basque Country Government (Spain) and the Regional Council of Aquitaine (France), in the frame of Cooperation Commons Funds Euskadi-Aquitaine (Project Bladed).

CHAPTER 12

Acknowledgments

The authors acknowledge the financial support from Natural Sciences and Engineering Council of Canada. The authors also acknowledge Mr. Ali Sherazee for his input.

Conflict of Interest

The authors declare no conflict of interest.

INDEX

A

aerodynamics, xv, xviii, xix, xxi, 1, 4–6, 8, 14–17, 19–21, 23–26, 28, 30–32, 34, 41, 56, 61, 79, 81–82, 85, 87, 89, 93, 105, 119–120, 145, 154, 174, 181, 185, 189–190, 192, 194–195, 199, 202–203, 225, 229–230, 236, 311–314, 319–320, 323–324, 327–328
  aerodynamic lift, 4–5, 15, 24, 30, 32, 185
  aerodynamic load, 23–24, 26, 145, 189, 195, 225
  aerodynamic performance, 15–16, 21, 32, 81, 105, 323
aerofoil, xv, 3, 5–6, 9, 14–18, 21–22, 24, 28–33
  airfoil constraints, 91
algebraic multigrid (AMG), 95
alloys, 21
anemometer, 4–5, 7, 257
angle of twist, 17, 21–22
Artificial Neural Network (ANN), 34, 179
Association of Danish Energy Companies (DEFU), 299
axis of rotation, 79, 81, 86, 101
azimuthal, 81–82, 86, 95–96, 174, 202

B

batteries, 51
Betz limit, 3, 5, 9
blade
  blade angle, xvii, 18, 174–175, 181, 184–186, 188–189, 192–194
  blade element momentum (BEM), 9, 24, 26
  blade root, 30, 64, 71, 201–202
  blade shape, 4–5, 17, 21–22, 32, 40, 87, 101, 109, 113, 119
Boukhezzar's controller, 240–241, 247
brim, xv, 36–37, 39–48, 50, 55–56

C

cantilever beam, 25–26, 28–29
capacitor, 126–129, 130–133, 137–138, 235
carcinogenic, 58
centrifugal force, 24
China, xi, 50, 52, 55, 138, 225, 308, 329, 332
chord
  chord dimensioning, 10
  chord length, 9–11, 22, 84, 90, 109
coefficient of performance (COP), 87, 106–109, 114–115, 117
Coleman
  Coleman frame, 206–207, 211, 213, 222, 224
  Coleman transform, 205, 213, 224
composite manufacturing, 58
computational fluid dynamics (CFD), xvi, 22, 56, 82–83, 86, 89, 91–92, 119
computational modeling, 81

contact fatigue, xvii, 142–143, 149, 154, 159–161, 167, 169
convergence, 99–100, 103–104, 108, 114, 239–240
coupling, 82, 94, 142, 174, 194, 266, 270, 287
cyclic loading, 113, 119

D

Darcy's law, 66–67, 70
Darrieus rotor, 7, 80
differential evolution (DE), xi, xvi, xviii, 77, 79, 81, 83, 85, 87, 89, 91, 93, 95, 97–101, 103, 105, 107–109, 111, 113–115, 117, 119, 121, 169, 249–251, 288, 308, 332
diffraction, 293, 303, 306
diffuser, xv, 36–50, 55–56
diffuser-augmented wind turbine (DAWT), 36
Disturbance Accommodating Control (DAC), 251
downwash, 5
drag, 3–5, 7, 9, 15, 17, 24, 31–32, 80–81, 85–86, 113, 185
  drag factor, 3
drivetrain, 142, 169, 288, 308
  drive train bearing, 173

E

ecomoulding, 57, 59, 61, 63, 65, 67, 69, 71, 73, 75, 77
edgewise bending, 25, 28–30
efficiency, xv–xvi, 2–8, 10–11, 17–18, 22, 28, 31–32, 47, 55, 57, 81–82, 86–87, 89, 101, 106–107, 109, 113, 117, 119, 126, 128, 132, 134, 138, 174, 250, 341
  maximum theoretical efficiency, 5

electromagnetic
  electromagnetic compatibility (EMC), 131, 295–296, 308
  electromagnetic fields, xix, 293–295, 303
  electromagnetic interference (EMI), xix, 293–301, 303–309
energy
  energy capture, 19, 181, 199
  energy consumption, 58
  energy extraction, 1–3
  kinetic energy, 2–3, 8
environmental, xv–xvi, 13, 35, 50, 57–60, 75, 227, 291
excitation, 126–127, 130, 133, 137–139, 283–284, 304, 306

F

FAST, xviii, 21, 98, 121, 145, 148, 155–156, 169, 173, 228, 232, 237–238, 249–250, 297, 302
fast multipole method (FMM), 302
fatigue damage analysis, 276, 281
feathering, 14, 18
feedback, 209, 213, 225–226, 245, 289, 317
FEKO, 300, 302, 309
FLUENT, 94, 96–97, 101, 103, 120
fluid dynamics, xvi, 22, 56, 82, 119, 121
fossil fuels, xix, 35, 227, 311
fouling, 15
Fourier transform (FFT), 173, 297

G

Gauss-Seidel solver, 95

gear, xv, xvii, 123, 141–143, 148–150, 153, 155, 157, 159–162, 167–169, 174, 205, 229, 254, 329
gearbox, xvii, 14, 18, 81, 141–143, 145–149, 151, 153, 155, 157, 159, 161, 163, 165, 167–169, 173–174, 184, 195–196, 236–237, 283, 311, 313–314, 319, 327, 329, 331
gearbox failure, 141, 168, 174
Gearbox Reliability Colloborative (GRC), 143, 169, 331–332
generator, xv–xix, 2, 14, 17–18, 23–24, 33, 56, 79, 81, 123, 125–130, 132–134, 137–139, 143, 145–146, 148–149, 152–155, 157–158, 162, 164, 166–168, 174, 184, 196, 199, 201, 205, 208, 228–230, 232–233, 236, 240, 245, 249–250, 252, 254–258, 260–262, 266, 269–272, 274, 279–281, 284, 286–287, 293, 303, 307–308, 311, 313, 327
generator controller, 157–158, 167
generator controllers, 149, 152, 167–168
geometry, xvi, 3, 21–22, 31, 63, 82–84, 87, 89, 91–94, 101, 104–107, 109–110, 113–114, 116–117, 119–120, 132, 148, 161, 294, 318
baseline geometry, 101, 105–107, 109, 113, 117, 119
global warming, 35, 311
gravitational centrifugal forces, 24
greenhouse gas, 311
grid, 24, 50, 52–53, 91–95, 101–105, 126, 128–129, 137–138, 154, 227, 238, 248, 301
grid code, 128, 138
grid generation, 91–94, 105
hybrid grid, 93–94, 102–105
harmonic suppression, 132
Hertzian dipole, 300, 304–307
horizontal axis wind turbine (HAWT), xv, 1–2, 6–9, 22, 34, 80–81, 312
hysteresis, 128

I

induction, vii, xvi–xvii, 125–139, 250, 303
infrastructure, 50
injection port, 70–71
irrigation, 50–52, 55

J

Japan, xii–xiii, 35, 51, 54–56, 134, 298, 308, 331
Jonkman's controller, 239, 245, 247–248

K

Kalman filter, 201, 209–211, 213, 224
Kirchhoff's current law, 235

L

leakage reactance, 133
lightning, 13, 294–295, 297–300, 306–308
Linear Parameter Varying (LPV), 251
linearization, 10, 21, 95, 224, 254
load
aerodynamic load, 23–24, 26, 145, 189, 195, 225
fatigue load, xix, 287
gyroscopic loads, 23
load current, 137
load equivalent analysis, 276, 278, 281, 283

load magnitude, 23
loading scenario, 23

M

maintenance, 13–14, 126, 129, 227, 313, 319
MATLAB, 232, 237, 245, 252, 261, 264, 277, 289
Maximum Power Point Tracking (MPPT), 181, 187
mean camber line, 90
mean contact forces, 152–153, 155, 162, 164, 167

N

National Advisory Committee for Aeronautics (NACA), 16, 83, 89–90, 98, 105–106, 109–114, 116–119
National Renewable Energy Laboratory (NREL), xvii–xviii, 16, 142–143, 145, 149, 168–169, 225–226, 228, 237–238, 249–251, 288, 328, 331
noise, viii, xix–xx, 6, 8, 16, 31, 33, 41, 209, 211, 245, 247–249, 297, 308, 311–325, 327–330
aerodynamic noise, xix, 41, 311–314, 319–320, 327–328
mechanical noise, 311–313, 319, 327
noise reduction, 312, 319–320, 323, 325, 328–330
separation-stall noise, 316
turbulent boundary layer trailing edge noise (TBL-TE), 314–316
Nonlinear State Estimation Technique (NSET), xvii, 173–176, 178–180, 186–189, 191, 194, 196
nonrenewable energy, 79
notch filter, 208, 264, 267, 271, 284

O

optimization, 9, 33, 79, 81–83, 85, 87–91, 93–95, 97–99, 101, 103–109, 111, 113–115, 117, 119–121, 225, 250, 323, 328
oscillation, 81, 96, 113, 117, 199–200, 208, 218

P

performance, xv–xviii, 6, 15–16, 18–19, 21, 32–33, 40–41, 43–48, 50, 56, 60, 81–84, 86–87, 101, 105–106, 109–111, 116–119, 125–127, 129–131, 133–135, 137–139, 145, 173, 201, 210, 212, 216, 224, 226, 228, 241, 247–248, 251, 262, 323
performance envelope, 106, 109–110, 116–117
permeability, 66–70, 74, 77, 301
pitch, xviii–xix, 2, 13, 18–19, 24, 31, 33–34, 153, 158, 160, 181, 184–185, 189, 194–195, 199–201, 203, 205–226, 228–229, 232, 237–241, 245, 249–250, 252, 254, 256–259, 261, 266–268, 270–271, 274, 280–281, 286, 288, 295, 300, 307, 312, 320
pitch actuator, 201, 254
pitch controller, 200–201, 207–210, 213, 224–225, 232, 237, 249, 252, 261, 266–268, 270–271, 274
pitching, 18–19, 22–23
Pointwise, 94, 102
polystyrene, 62
power factor, xvii, 126, 129–130, 132–138
Principal Components Analysis (PCA), 180

proportional integral (PI), xviii, 208, 217, 228, 237, 251, 256–258
propulsion, xv, 3–4, 7
pulse width modulation (PWM), 14, 127, 138

R

radio, 293, 297, 306
relative wind velocity, 4–6, 30
resin, xvi, 57–58, 65–67, 70–77
  resin transfer moulding (RTM), xvi, 57–58, 65, 71, 74, 76–77
  resin viscosity, 74
resistor-capacitor (RC), 235
ring-type, 39
Rogowski coils, 297–298
rotation, 3, 11, 13, 24, 79, 81, 85–86, 96–97, 101, 103–104, 113, 117, 125, 143, 167, 174, 199, 205, 207, 299–300, 306, 312, 320, 322
  reverse rotation, 167
  rotational axis, 1
  rotation reversal, 143
  rotational speed, 13–14, 17–18, 45, 96, 173–174, 181, 185, 194, 254, 300, 320
rotor, xvii–xviii, 1–3, 5–7, 9–11, 13, 15, 18–19, 21–23, 28, 30, 33–34, 40, 43–44, 46–48, 50, 55, 80–81, 84, 101, 106, 109–7, 219–220, 222–224, 229, 236–237, 239, 247–248, 250, 254–255, 283–284, 295, 306, 313–314, 323, 328
  cup type differential drag rotor, 5
  rotor aerodynamics, 190
  rotor blade velocity, 6
  rotor design, 2, 15, 250
  rotor dynamics, 174, 194
  rotor speed, xviii, 2–3, 5, 19, 181, 199–200, 203, 207–210, 213–217, 219–220, 222–224, 229, 237, 239, 247–248
  Savonius rotor, 5, 7, 80

S

safety, 13, 19, 42, 57, 195, 284, 286
selection, xv, 13, 37, 45, 57, 61, 65, 100–101, 176, 187, 240, 249
self-excited induction generators (SEIG), 125, 127, 132, 138–139
sensor, 45, 173, 175, 225, 260, 276, 298–299, 308
shaft, 1–2, 14, 79, 81, 128, 134, 142, 145–146, 148, 152, 154, 168, 181, 201, 230, 241, 243, 245, 294, 300
shroud, xv, 35–37, 39–42, 45, 56
SIMPACK, 145–149, 162, 169
Simulink, 230, 232, 237, 261
smart blade, 19
soiling, 15, 17
solidity, xvi, 5, 8, 10, 33, 82–84, 94, 98–99, 101, 104, 106–107, 109, 113–114, 117, 119–120
sound pressure level (SPL), 313, 315, 327
speed ratio, xvi, 1, 4, 6, 8–9, 17, 33, 41, 46–47, 82–85, 89, 98–99, 101, 105–107, 109, 113, 117, 119–120, 229
squirrel cage, 125–127
  squirrel cage induction generator (SCIG), 127, 129, 134–135
stall, 13, 15–19, 33, 113, 119, 143, 185, 314–316
static-synchronous compensator, 129
STATCOM, 129, 139
stationary hub, 277, 281, 283
statistical uncertainty, xvii, 143, 154–155, 159
stresses, 25–26

structural integrity, 8, 28, 30
supervisory control and data acquisition system (SCADA), 174, 181, 184, 186–187, 192, 195–196

T

temperature, 66, 74, 174, 180, 196, 298
time domain, xvii, 141–143, 145, 147, 149, 151, 153–155, 157, 159, 161, 163, 165, 167, 169, 210, 212, 224, 261, 272–277, 281, 284
  time domain simulation, 143, 149, 154, 159, 277, 281
tip speed ratio, xvi, 1, 4, 6, 8–9, 17, 33, 41, 46, 82–85, 89, 98–99, 101, 105–107, 109, 113, 117, 119–120
topography, 36
torque, xvi–xix, 5–6, 8, 45, 81–82, 85–87, 93–94, 96–98, 101, 103–104, 106–107, 111, 113, 117–119, 127, 148–149, 152, 155, 161, 168, 184–185, 187, 199, 201, 205, 208, 228–230, 232–233, 236–240, 242, 245, 249, 252, 254, 256, 258, 261–263, 265–266, 280–281, 283–284, 288
  generator torque, xix, 199, 201, 205, 208, 230, 232, 236, 245, 252, 254, 256, 258, 261–262, 280–281
  torque loads, 168
trapezoidal rule, 97
turbine, ix, xv–xx, 1–3, 5–7, 9, 11–13, 15–19, 21–25, 27–37, 39–59, 61, 63, 65, 67, 69, 71, 73, 75–77, 79–89, 91, 93–121, 125–126, 128–130, 132, 134, 136, 138, 141–145, 147–149, 151, 153–170, 173–175, 177, 179–181, 183–187, 189–196, 199–201, 204–205, 207, 213, 216, 220, 222, 224–226, 228–230, 232, 235–238, 245, 249–252, 254, 256–257, 259, 261, 270, 272, 274, 276, 278, 281, 283–284, 286–289, 293–295, 298–304, 306–308, 311–313, 316, 318–323, 327–329, 331
  turbine nacelle, 293
turbulence model, 52, 82, 95, 120

V

variable set, 186
velocity, 3–6, 8–9, 16–19, 24, 30, 36–39, 67–68, 82, 84–85, 94–95, 113, 154, 314–315, 318
vertical axis wind turbine (VAWT), xvi, 1–2, 6–7, 80–85, 88, 91, 93–94, 101, 104–107, 109, 113–114, 119–120
vibration, vii, xvii–xviii, 173–175, 177, 179, 181–195, 228, 249, 311, 319, 327
  drive train vibration (DTV), 181, 184–188, 192
  tower vibration (TV), xvii, 173–175, 177, 179, 181–195
  tower vibration model (TVM), xvii, 186–192, 194
vortex, xv, 3, 33, 37, 55–56, 82, 109, 113–114, 314–315, 317–319, 328–329
  tip vortex, 314–315, 317–318, 328–329

W

wake rotation, 3
Weibull distribution, 278
weight, 11, 13–14, 21, 28, 42–43, 57, 77, 179, 252, 264–265, 267–269, 284
wind-lens, vii, 35–37, 39–55
windage, 128
winding, vii, xvii, 125–139, 298

auxiliary winding, vii, xvii, 125–137, 139

W

windmill, 1, 4–7, 33, 50, 56

X

XFOIL, 15, 33

Y

yaw, 2, 24, 31, 41, 48, 184, 195, 206, 222–223, 232, 241, 243–245

Z

zero flow scenario, 3